Participatory Budgeting in Global Perspective

Participatory Budgeting in Global Perspective

BRIAN WAMPLER,
STEPHANIE MCNULTY,
AND
MICHAEL TOUCHTON

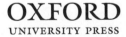
OXFORD
UNIVERSITY PRESS

OXFORD
UNIVERSITY PRESS

Great Clarendon Street, Oxford, OX2 6DP,
United Kingdom

Oxford University Press is a department of the University of Oxford.
It furthers the University's objective of excellence in research, scholarship,
and education by publishing worldwide. Oxford is a registered trade mark of
Oxford University Press in the UK and in certain other countries

First Edition published in 2021

Impression: 1

Published in the United States of America by Oxford University Press
198 Madison Avenue, New York, NY 10016, United States of America

British Library Cataloguing in Publication Data
Data available

Library of Congress Control Number: 2020952844

ISBN 978-0-19-289775-6

DOI: 10.1093/oso/9780192897756.001.0001

Printed and bound by
CPI Group (UK) Ltd, Croydon, CR0 4YY

We dedicate this book to our families.

Acknowledgments

This book was made possible, and greatly improved, with the generous support of countless individuals and institutions. Support from the William and Flora Hewlett Foundation planted the seeds of the book in 2017 when the three authors collaborated with the energetic and dedicated David Sasaki to document and analyze "the state of the art" of Participatory Budgeting. We are grateful to David, Dr. Ruth Levine, and the Global Development and Population team for their support of and feedback on this project.

We were also fortunate to participate in the second phase of Hewlett's work on PB, which was led by Reboot and allowed us to reimagine what a PB community might look like. We are grateful to Panthea Lee, Chelsey LePage, Corey Chao, and Alyssa Kropp for engaging us in conversations about what a more coordinated and impactful PB might look like. Reboot hosted a conference in Barcelona in November 2018; we learned an incredible amount from the thirty plus practitioners and researchers who had come from around the world to participate in the three-day workshop.

We are also very grateful to the Participatory Budgeting Project and the Global PB Research Board for bringing us together for several conferences and workshops, which allowed us to view PB processes and interact with experts from around the world. We are excited to work with Josh Lerner, Clara Bois, and Mariana Gonzalez as the next phase of international PB activism and research kicks off in a more coordinated way. We are also grateful to the Planning and Evaluation office in Jalisco, Mexico, the Open Government Partnership, the Transparency and Accountability Iniative, the World Bank, and the Federal University of Minas Gerais (Brazil), for inviting one or all of us to present our understanding of PB in a variety of formats, including several reports and blogs.

Additionally, we benefited greatly from material we collected through the Making All Voices Count (MAVC) initiative, which was housed at the University of Sussex. MAVC's support allowed us to host a workshop in Nairobi, Kenya, in July 2017 focusing on PB in the Global South, with particular attention on sub-Saharan Africa and Southeast Asia. We had considerable assistance from Rosie McGee and Duncan Edwards at the Institute for Development Studies and support from Osmany Porto de Oliveira for the conference. Fletcher Tembo of Hivos also provided excellent support. We also benefited from helpful contributions that Silvestre Baessa, Andile Cele, Njeri Kagucia, Timothy Kiprono, Patrick Lim, Jacklyn Makaaru, Eliza Meriabe, Ahmad Rifai, and Rohidin Sudamo made to our understanding of PB in sub-Saharan Africa and Southeast Asia. Jason

Lakin of the International Budget Partnership was also able to join us for part of the workshop and provided excellent questions to move our thinking forward.

The World Bank also sponsored a PB learning workshop, focused on Kenya, in 2017. We are grateful to Tiago Peixoto, Annette Omolo, Rose Wanjiru, John Maritim, and Jez Hall for help with this workshop and for valuable knowledge surrounding PB in Kenya, sub-Saharan Africa, and around the world.

The book is possible due to decades of research that we have done individually and together. McNulty's research has been supported by the Fulbright Scholar program, the American Association of University Women, American Political Science Association, and Franklin and Marshall College. Touchton has received support from the World Bank, the Fulbright Scholar program, the Inter-American Development Bank, and regularly benefits from his affiliation with the Institute for Advanced Study of the Americas at the University of Miami. Wampler's research has been supported by the Fulbright Scholar program, the National Science Foundation, the World Bank, and the School of Public Service at Boise State University. At Boise State University, we benefited immensely from the research support provided by Ana Costa and Emily Pape. We also thank Jennifer Morales for her excellent copyediting, which improved the book's flow.

Of course, no book is complete without recognizing the families and friends who supported us as we researched and wrote about democratic innovations. McNulty would like to thank her loving husband, Ramon, and daughters, Maya and Sofia, who patiently support all of her projects. Touchton would like to thank his parents along with his brother, Greg. Wampler would like to thank Paula, Sebastian, and Ginger for their support of his travels, projects, and ramblings.

Our colleagues Benjamin Goldfrank, Wagner Romão, Paolo Spada, Paolo Renzio, Won No, Guillermo Cejudo, Cinthia Michel, Rachel Rumbul, Brian Palmer Rubin, all deserve recognition for giving us valuable information and feedback, which inevitably made this book better.

Finally, we would like to thank our editor at OUP, Dominic Byatt, as well as three anonymous reviewers, all of whom helped us develop a much stronger product.

Contents

List of Tables and Figure   xi
Acronyms   xiii

Introduction   1

1. The Global Adoption of PB   21

2. Theorizing PB's Effects on Individuals and Communities   51

3. Where It All Began: PB in Latin America   81

4. Parallel Paths to Local Democracy in Asia   104

5. Re-engaging Citizens in Europe and North America   133

6. South-to-South and Donor-driven Diffusion in Sub-Saharan Africa   158

Conclusion: The Frontiers of PB   181

References   205
Index   221

List of Tables and Figure

Tables

1.1. Typology of PB global programs   46

3.1. PB in Brazil, Peru, Mexico, and El Salvador   83

4.1. PB in Indonesia, the Philippines, and South Korea   105

4.2. Philippines: Bottom-up Budgeting 2013–16   111

4.3. Percentage of total budget allocated through PB in Indonesian cities   120

5.1. PB programs in Europe and North America   135

6.1. PB programs in sub-Saharan Africa   160

Figure

2.1. PB: Conceptual model of change   53

Acronyms

ANC	African National Congress Party, South Africa
BuB	Bottom-up Budgeting
CCP	Chinese Communist Party
CDD	Community-driven development
CSO	Civil society organization
DFID	Department for International Development, UK
DLGA	Democratic Local Governance Activity, El Salvador
ENDA-ECOPOP	Espaces Co production et d'O res Populaires pour l'Environnement et le Développement en Afrique
FISDL	Social Investment Fund for Local Development, El Salvador
IEED	Institut International pour l'Environnement et le Développement
KDP	Kecamatan Development Project
LPRAT	Local Poverty Reduction Action Team, Philippines
NGO	Non-governmental organization
OIDP	International Observatory of Participatory Democracy
PB	Participatory Budgeting
PBP	Participatory Budgeting Project
PRI	Institutional Revolutionary Party, Mexico
PNPM	*Nasional Pemberdayaan Masyarakat Mandiri* (National Community Empowerment Program)
PT	Worker' Party, Brazil
TCHC	Toronto Community Housing Corporation
URB-AL	European Union-sponsored Urban Program
UCLG	United Cities and Local Governments
UN	United Nations
USAID	United States Agency for International Development

Introduction

In 1999, in a *favela* on the outskirts of Belo Horizonte, Brazil, a group of community leaders led one of this book's authors through their neighborhood, pointing out various public works projects that they had helped select through Participatory Budgeting (PB). During the previous five years, the leaders had participated in PB meetings sponsored by the municipal government; in these meetings, the leaders advocated for a health-care clinic, a sewage system, and the paving of the hilly streets. The *favela*, with thirty-five thousand residents, was surrounded by middle- and upper-class neighborhoods that already had access to these services. During the walking tour, community leaders described how they constructed alliances within and outside their community to secure enough votes to get projects funded. They negotiated with nearby communities by promising to submit no new projects for two years after this round of funding and to support the other communities' projects during the intervening years. In turn, these other communities would support their projects in the third year. These community leaders spoke at length about the solidarity that the process generated, arguing that it had helped to foster inter-neighborhood relationships because they gave and received support from other groups.

During this particular tour, the leaders also talked about their frustrations; government officials dragged their heels on the implementation of four projects that the community had selected in previous years. Their community organization decided to protest these delays by holding a mock funeral procession, in which "PB" would be buried. Teenagers dressed as robed monks carried a coffin through the *favela* to a "burial site"—located alongside a busy avenue; their procession attracted many community residents and also evening commuters on their way home. The procession occurred in the late afternoon and protesters threatened to block rush-hour traffic. While protestors conducted the "funeral," a small group of community leaders went to the city center to meet with the mayor's staff, where the officials eventually agreed to their demands. Construction on all four projects would begin in the near future, and at least one project would begin the next week. Before wrapping up the "funeral," the protestors closed the six-lane avenue for one minute to show the mayor that they had the power to block rush-hour traffic if the government did not fulfill its promise (see Wampler 2007: Chapter 7).

Years later, in Mozambique, the World Bank strongly advocated for the adoption of PB in the capital city of Maputo in 2008 (Nylen 2014). A reform-oriented municipal government accepted the challenge of introducing participatory processes in the country's post-conflict environment. However, the program got off

Participatory Budgeting in Global Perspective. Brian Wampler, Stephanie McNulty, and Michael Touchton,
Oxford University Press. © Brian Wampler, Stephanie McNulty, and Michael Touchton 2021.
DOI: 10.1093/oso/9780192897756.003.0001

to a rocky start, hampered by its institutional placement in the accounting department, limited state capacity, scarce resources, and disorganized civil society. Unfortunately, this start produced few tangible results, leading the World Bank to use external policy experts from Portugal to re-craft and re-institutionalize the program in 2012. Since 2014, PB has been slowly spreading across Mozambique, though it is not clear if it is helping to improve service delivery or deepen local democratic processes.

In Peru, on a June evening in 2018, community leaders attended a public meeting to discuss the budget in Pueblo Libre, a middle-class district in Lima, Peru. This kind of meeting takes place in all districts around the country annually, due to national legislation that mandates citizen participation in budget decisions. The municipal official leading the meeting informed the neighborhood groups in attendance about the new public works projects that would require funding in the coming years, and the final vote to approve the list was about to take place. A middle-aged woman stood up and spoke to the official. "Excuse me, sir. I would like to propose that we cut my neighborhood project's budget so we can give more money to the fire station in our district." Before the vote, two firefighters had told the audience that they needed new equipment. Their proposal to the municipality had been disqualified because it was not considered a "public investment" project. The firefighters explained that they had been awake all night fighting a five-alarm fire in the garment district and told attendees about the need for masks, oxygen, and new hoses. After the community attendee spoke in favor of funding the firefighters, the municipal official asked everyone if they agreed. When they did, the participants voted and unanimously approved making small cuts to the budgets of all approved neighborhood projects to fund the firefighters' new equipment.

These stories—from 1999 Brazil, 2008 Mozambique, and 2018 Peru—illustrate the increased global interest in PB. Recent estimates suggest that there are at least eleven thousand active PB programs around the world (Dias 2018; Dias et al. 2019). These programs generally operate at the subnational level (municipal, town, city, village), but occasionally operate at national and state/provincial levels. For reformers, PB provides a practical, "hands-on" program that allows citizen-participants and government officials to take steps toward achieving lofty democratic and development goals.

The examples above tell us much about the fast-paced adoptions and adaptations of this particular budget-making process. For example, in Belo Horizonte, one of PB's more successful cases in Brazil, political and policy contradictions emerge: notable sighs of improvements paired with conflict among government officials, citizens, and civil society organizations (CSOs). Our incomplete understanding of Mozambique is fairly representative of our knowledge-base in many countries in the Global South: We know PB is being adopted, but we do not have a good handle on how these programs work or the range of impacts that they may generate. And, in some cases, PB can prompt people to make tough decisions that help communities in need, even if that means accepting less funding for their own neighborhood. This book explores the spread, adaptation, and impact of this popular democratic and policy program to improve our understanding of the potential and limitations of PB.

Democracy in the Twenty-first Century

Democracy spread across the globe during the 1980s and 1990s, reaching diverse places such as Indonesia, Brazil, South Korea, Poland, and South Africa. PB and comparable citizen engagement programs were intertwined with the spread of national-level democracy. In some places, early versions of PB preceded the return to national-level democracy (Brazil, Indonesia), while in other places, reformers adopted PB at the local level in the wake of democratic transitions (Peru, Philippines). The cultural, political, economic, and social diversity of these new democracies demonstrates wide variation in the durability and quality of the new democratic regimes. One prevalent problem across many of these countries is the low quality of democratic practices, with many new democracies being described as practicing "illiberal" or "restricted" democracy, indicating that most citizens could not access political, civil, and social rights that their constitutions formally guaranteed (O'Donnell 1994; Przeworski et al. 1999; Diamond and Molino 2005; Mainwaring and Bizzarro 2019).

Many countries made a parallel commitment to decentralization alongside democratization, delegating service delivery responsibilities and revenues to cities and states (Sellers 2002; Campbell 2003; Giraudy et al. 2019). Reformers across a broad spectrum of the political and policy landscape embraced decentralization, thus opening the door for programs like PB. For example, the World Bank advocated for decentralization to limit corruption and improve service delivery, whereas Leftist political parties, such as Brazil's Workers' Party, advocated for decentralization to give citizens a role in public decision-making.

The combination of democratization and decentralization created an opportunity for governments and civil society activists to reimagine how to incorporate citizens into democratic systems (Genro 1995; Santos 2005). Brazil's Workers' Party led the way, as their newly elected municipal governments developed new programs and policies to move beyond the passive citizenship they associated with representative democracy. But, as this book makes clear, it was not only the Brazilian Workers' Party that deployed citizen participation to deepen the quality of democracy and empower citizens. Rather, governments and international organizations across the globe sought out programs, policies, and institutions that would more actively engage citizens in public decision-making. A proliferation of new deliberative and participatory institutions occurred during the 1990s, 2000s, and 2010s; these institutions were often adopted under the broad frame of "deepening democracy" (Barber 1984; Fung and Wright 2003; APSA Task Force 2012). In parallel, "participatory development" became an important agenda within mainstream multilateral organizations as they promoted citizen empowerment and participation as mechanisms that would improve development outcomes (Nelson and Wright 1995; Fox 1997; World Bank 2003a; Mansuri and Rao 2013; McNulty 2019).

However, beginning in the middle of the 2010s, scholars and policymakers began to note that many of the new democracies were "backsliding" into semi-authoritarian regimes (Levitsky and Way 2010; Levitsky and Ziblatt 2018). For advocates of participatory democracy, like the Open Government Partnership, Participatory Budgeting Project, and the International Observatory of Participatory Democracy, a strong response required expanding the number of participatory venues. Others focused on the importance of basic processes of representative democracy, such as strengthening parties and improving campaign finance rules (Mainwaring 2018). In this book, we advance our understanding of these debates by illuminating the ways that PB may—and may not—raise the quality of democracy and improve people's lives. This book mainly focuses on PB in democratic settings because it emerged and spread primarily in democratic contexts. However, as democracies backslide around the globe and authoritarian regimes prove extremely resilient, we also discuss the use of PB in authoritarian and semi-authoritarian environments, especially in more recent years.

What Is Participatory Budgeting?

PB is an innovative participatory institution that began in the late 1980s as a new democratic decision-making process in Porto Alegre, Brazil.[1] Reformers hoped to use PB to deepen Brazil's new representative democracy by expanding the number of public deliberative forums, increasing the diversity of citizens participating in these forums, and experimenting with different rules to manage participation in these forums (Abers 2000; Avritzer 2002; Baiocchi 2005). Other cities quickly took notice of Porto Alegre's efforts and the purported successes associated with the program. PB subsequently spread across Brazil, Latin America, and the rest of the world based on its potential to help deepen democracy, improve citizens' well-being, and aid political parties in their reelection campaigns (Porto de Oliveira 2017a).

PB programs directly incorporate citizens into public decision-making meetings during which they make decisions regarding the allocation and eventual implementation of a set part of the government's budget. Participants engage in

---

[1] This section is adapted from Wampler 2012.

oversight over the implementation of the selected projects, which then carries into the next year's PB cycle of budget deliberations. In broad brushstrokes, PB programs are designed to bring together residents of a particular area (city, town, sub-district, community) to select projects and allocate capital investment spending (also called infrastructure projects) or social programs, which typically comprise between 1 percent and 5 percent of a given government's budget.

Beyond an operational definition, we think of PB as being based on a set of common principles rather than a specific set of rules (Abers 2000; Santos 1998, 2005; Baiocchi 2005; Wampler 2007; McNulty 2011; Ganuza and Baiocchi 2012; Sintomer et al. 2012; Lerner 2014; Baiocchi and Ganuza 2017). These principles include *voice, vote, social inclusion, social justice*, and *oversight*, all described later in this chapter, and they establish PB's basic parameters that then help to determine more specific program designs and operational rules (Wampler 2012). We find that most PB programs adhere to these five principles, but there is significant variation in how they combine these principles; the variation in commitment to each principle helps to account for different program design and institutional rules. At its core, PB involves opening government budget processes to individuals who need public expenditures to improve their communities. The process tends to work as follows: Governments invite people to attend open forums to discuss their needs. Participants propose projects that are subject to deliberation and voting. Participants then vote to select projects, which the government then implements during the next several years. Most PB programs focus on "brick and mortar" projects, which typically involve making public improvements in areas that lack basic infrastructure. However, some PB programs also include social services (e.g., child care or job training).

PB then makes citizens' voting decisions tangible by implementing selected projects in specific neighborhoods. Many programs have requirements for mandatory implementation of selected projects, which is distinct from other participatory institutions that emphasize citizen input and consultation, rather than citizen decision-making. Simply, one of PB's key innovations is to directly link citizens' decisions in public venues to the implementation of specific projects: People direct governments to carry out projects on their behalf. The original PB programs were binding, with governments pledging to respect citizens' decisions. PB programs are intended to be part and parcel of local governments; PB's advocates hope to generate changes in state–society relations by building new relationships among citizens, CSOs, and public officials.

PB's allure in most places is that it will help citizens and governments practice democracy to solve real problems. The core PB principles—voice, vote, social inclusion, social justice, and oversight—all contribute to reimagining and supporting democracy. PB thus represents "hope for democracy," whereby citizens are incorporated into the *demos* (Dias 2014, 2018). But, PB is also something much more tangible than hope alone, because PB programs direct how governments spend scarce resources in practice. Thus, multiple actors, including governments, CSOs, and ordinary citizens are drawn to PB because it has the potential get things done, and in some contexts, inform development goals. This allure contains multitudes—the core principles promote broad democratic values, while the institutional design is crafted to promote specific policy change.

PB is different from other participatory institutions and social accountability institutions in three ways (see Mansuri and Rao 2013; Fox 2015 for a broader overview of other participatory institutions). First, PB is ongoing throughout the budget process, with public meetings throughout the year. Second, PB empowers citizens to make direct decisions on how to allocate public funds, often from local (subnational) budgets in villages, districts, cities, and counties. Finally, PB participants have the opportunity to monitor how projects are implemented, which creates the opportunity to decrease the likelihood of project-level corruption while simultaneously improving their quality. One crucial institutional advance of PB is that the program rules promote citizen participation at multiple stages of the budget and policymaking cycle (formulation, approval, implementation, and oversight).

The Original PB: The Porto Alegre Model

As noted above, the best-known case of PB is that of Porto Alegre, a city of 1.5 million people in southern Brazil. This experience serves as the original model that inspired PB's diffusion across Brazil and around the world. In this book, when we speak of the "adaptation," and "transformation" of PB, we refer to changes from the Porto Alegre model. The basic tenets of the original PB model include the following:[2]

- The municipality is divided into regions to facilitate meetings and the distribution of resources.
- The municipal government holds meetings throughout the year, covering different aspects of the budgeting and policymaking cycles: distribution of information, policy proposals, debates on proposals, selection of policies, election of delegates, and oversight.
- The government creates a mechanism for evaluating project selection. Each municipality devises its technical format to guarantee that the distribution of resources meets the necessary legal, technical, and political requirements of the overarching legal framework.
- Public deliberation and negotiation take place among participants and between participants and the government over resources and policies.

[2] Adapted from Wampler 2007.

- The government sponsors a "bus-caravan of priorities," though which an elected group of citizens ("PB Delegates") visit all preapproved project sites before the final vote. The visits allow delegates to evaluate the benefits of proposed projects relative to community needs.
- Participants vote on all final projects. Voting can be done by secret ballot or through a public showing of hands. The results become part of the public record.
- A municipality-wide PB council is elected. All regions elect two representatives to this council, which oversees PB and makes final budget recommendations. The council meets regularly with the municipal government to monitor the program.
- After "PB Delegates" approve the final annual budget, the mayor sends it to the municipal legislative chambers for approval. The legislative branch can block specific projects.
- A year-end report is published detailing implementation of public works and programs.
- Regional or neighborhood committees are established to monitor the design and implementation of policy projects.

These rules are designed to produce specific outcomes, such as deliberation, the redistribution of funds to poorer areas, and active citizens. The Porto Alegre model is the prototypical PB process which influenced later iterations around the world.

Under the best conditions, PB programs in Brazil generated positive social and political change. Citizens organized themselves within their communities, presented their demands in public meetings, and worked to secure enough votes to have their projects included in municipal budgets. Once these projects were funded, community leaders engaged in oversight to ensure that the projects were implemented in a timely manner. In 1998, one of our authors observed these dynamics at work during a PB meeting in Porto Alegre. There was a vibrant debate among citizens regarding how to spend the money allocated to their district. Two opposing political camps developed, with one group advocating for a local health clinic. The other group pursued a pedestrian bridge over an increasingly busy road that bisected the community. During the debate, different citizens extolled the benefits of their projects, framing them in terms of the social rights guaranteed by Brazil's constitution. After ninety minutes of deliberation, participants voted: The community elected to fund the health clinic. Government officials then worked across multiple city-level agencies to build the health clinic, which was completed the following year. Importantly, government officials also worked with the group that advocated for the pedestrian bridge to devise small-scale interventions that would improve pedestrian safety in their neighborhood.

This example illustrates how direct citizen engagement shapes the allocation of resources. In Porto Alegre's case, research demonstrates that the PB program allocated additional resources to low-income communities (Marquetti 2003; Marquetti et al. 2008). In addition, comparative studies across Brazil show that the adoption of PB was associated with increased spending on health care, which likely contributed to improvements in infant and maternal health (Gonçalves 2014; Touchton and Wampler 2014).

PB: Transformations and Impact

An expansion of institutional designs has accompanied the widespread adoption of PB. For some governments and their civil society allies, PB is a radical democratic institution empowering citizens to challenge the existing status quo (Genro 1995; Santos 1998, 2005; Avritzer 2002; Baiocchi 2005; Sintomer et al. 2016). For others, PB is a technical tool permitting citizens to signal their preferences to governments (Baiocchi and Ganuza 2017). In some countries (e.g., Peru, Poland), national governments mandate that subnational government use PB, but we find that many subnational government officials are often left to implement PB with few additional resources and little support (McNulty 2011, 2019). For others, implementing PB is part of a broader set of development and governance reforms whereby international donor agencies agree to provide financial and technical assistance on the condition that subnational government adopt PB (Shah 2007). This book grapples with this complex mix of PB program design and operational rules to understand governments' motivations for adopting PB as well as how they adapt the program to suit their needs.

Thirty years after PB's founding, we can now say with certainty that the many early programs in southern Brazil produced the outcomes that politicians and citizens desired, including increased levels of public participation, allocation of resources to poor underserved neighborhoods, increased transparency, and reelection for political parties administering PB (Genro 1995; Fedozzi 1998; Abers 2000; Avritzer 2002; Wampler and Avritzer 2004; Santos 2005; Baiocchi 2005; Wampler 2007; Baiocchi et al. 2011; Gonçalves 2014; Touchton and Wampler 2014; Wampler and Touchton 2019). A large of body of research, employing different methodologies, has produced a generally favorable interpretation of PB's impact on civil society, democracy, and well-being (Abers 2000; Avritzer 2002, 2009; Baiocchi 2005; Baiocchi et al. 2011; Fedozzi 1998; Marquetti 2003; Marquetti et al. 2008; Lüchmann 2008; Romão 2011). In addition, research has also demonstrated that municipalities that adopt PB experience better human development outcomes, such as lower infant mortality, than those that do not adopt PB (Gonçalves 2014; Touchton and Wampler 2014; Wampler and Touchton 2019). Thus, we have a solid body of evidence from Brazil (described in later chapters in more depth) that PB is associated with improvements in the quality of local democracy as well as human development.

Interestingly, PB is in retreat across Brazil, and, as of 2020, among Brazilian municipalities with more than fifty thousand residents, less than forty municipal governments continued to use it (Spada 2020). Furthermore, many of the existing programs are very limited in scope, with few traces of the more radical democratic principles and rules of the original programs. PB experienced intellectual and political retreat as its original supporters in Brazil no longer advocate for it. This produces an interesting conundrum as PB expands across the rest of the world: Brazil is the one country where researchers have systematically demonstrated positive results through PB. Yet, local governments in Brazil are not using PB as much as they did in the 1990s and early 2000s. Part of the reason why may be related to the somewhat contradictory aspect of PB. Although researchers have identified positive outcomes from PB, they have also identified political and policy problems associated with the programs. In other words, researchers can identify positive outcomes being generated by PB, but this doesn't mean that there are only positive outcomes. Specific programs may underperform, and even the best programs may have positive and negative outcomes.

Part of PB's retreat in Brazil is also due to the fact that PB does not *always* achieve its stated goals. When PB programs perform poorly, there is a real risk that citizens' cynicism toward government will increase, their trust will be undermined and governments will not be re-elected. Activists and scholars often point out the poorly run processes lead to "participation fatigue." Moreover, governments may use PB to co-opt community leaders and organizations by introducing processes that provide small degrees of change, but make these groups dependent on the government. Some governments may not adopt PB to promote citizen empowerment at all, but may use the program to funnel community activists into an "invited" space that the government controls (Cornwall and Coelho 2007). Some governments could even use PB as a participatory veneer that hides business-as-usual authoritarian or illiberal practices, leading to what we call the "partici-washing" of PB. In authoritarian regimes, PB has the potential to improve governance, but it may also serve to legitimize regimes with poor records of service delivery, inclusion, transparency, and accountability.

In Wampler's *Participatory Budgeting in Brazil: Contestation, Cooperation, and Accountability* (2007), he identifies two cases (Rio Claro and Blumenau) where the municipal governments adopted PB but did not invest the necessary time or resources to support the program. The poor performance of some Brazilian PB programs discouraged other elected governments from adopting it because PB was no longer seen as a cure-all for democratic and policy ills; mayors stayed away from PB because the costs associated with implementing it were perceived to be far greater than the benefits. In addition, it is plausible that the positive outcomes identified by researchers may not resonate with voters; incremental improvements in health (infant and maternal mortality) or small-scale infrastructure (paving roads, adding waste water piping) may be hard for the average voter to detect. The result could potentially render PB a democratic policymaking process that does not significantly affect citizens' voting behavior.

Other examples of underperforming programs can also be drawn from Peru and Indonesia. In June 2018, residents of Villa María del Truinfo, a shantytown surrounding Lima, Peru, debated how to spend their infrastructure budget through public participatory meetings. The mayor of this district had been removed in a corruption scandal just weeks before the PB process started. The outgoing administrative team took all of their documents, computers, and phones as they departed and left the newly appointed team with no information on how to implement PB. At the first meeting, the new officials from this district told more than one hundred people that they had USD50,000 to spend in 2018. As the process unfolded, however, the municipal officials realized that they had less money than they thought. When the new officials reported their mistake, the neighborhood groups boycotted the subsequent meeting, calling the new team corrupt and inept. Tempers flared and the meeting was postponed. Eventually the government held the meeting and the residents deliberated over the amount originally promised (USD50,000). The process, however, generated distrust and animosity between CSOs and the new municipal government officials. PB programs are not quick, easy fixes that solve basic governance-related problems. When they work poorly, as illustrated here, increased cynicism and distrust about local politics can negatively affect citizens' perceptions about broader issues related to democracy, societal trust, and public deliberation.

Another example of the nuances embodied in PB lies in Indonesia, where participatory programs emerged during the transition to democratic rule in the late 1990s and early 2000s. Building on a small number of successful participatory programs, Indonesia's national government required the country's 400 largest cities to adopt a participatory planning or budgeting process in 2004. However, in a meeting in February 2018, we observed a fundamentally different PB meeting than those in Latin America. Technical planners from the city's urban planning department dominated the discussion and the audience largely consisted of middle-class community leaders. Government officials invited participants from established sector-based organizations (e.g., women, elderly, business) that predated the current democratic regime. One community leader, interviewed after the meeting, spoke defiantly about attending a PB program even though he had not been officially invited to attend. Indonesia's experiences are representative of a broader transformation among many PB programs in the Global South, in which governments actively recruit their political allies as key participants.

All of the above examples illuminate a wide range of PB outcomes: Some programs work well and deliver many benefits to the local population, while others end in infighting, generate cynicism instead of trust, and undermine development efforts. As we show in this book, PB programs around the world are associated with these diverse outcomes—some produce meaningful social and political change while others languish and have few discernible positive effects. Some programs appear to reinforce traditional power structures that marginalize vulnerable groups and confer legitimacy on authoritarian governments. PB thus has the potential to generate change but there are no guarantees. Institutions often bend to internal and external pressures, making similar institutions perform differently due to a variety of factors. In this book, we develop an analytical framework that shows how program design and conditions at the macro- and meso-level strongly influence the outcomes that PB programs generate.

Central Contributions

The book fills a gap in scholarship and practice by reviewing PB's spread and transformation around the world with an emphasis on institutional adaptations and how these adaptations produce variation in PB's impact on social and political change. PB programs share a set of core principles, which we link to distinct waves of diffusion as PB spreads around the world. Different rationales for adopting PB drive each wave of diffusion and influence the adaptations governments make to suit local needs. In this book, we develop theory connecting PB's waves of diffusion to significant adaptations in PB program design. Simply, PB in Poland, Chicago, or rural Kenya in 2020 is quite different from the original PB program in Porto Alegre. PB's institutional design affects the degree to which the programs generate social and political change. We use the significant variation in PB programs to develop a PB typology in Chapter 1. This typology deepens our understanding of how PB processes vary across time and space as well as how the different program types affect the parameters of likely change generated by PB programs.

The book explores the following questions in pursuit of these contributions:

- How has PB transformed during the past thirty years as it spreads around the globe?
- What are the causal mechanisms through which PB programs *may* produce social and political change?
- To what extent have PB programs generated social and political change?

These questions permit us to advance theoretical and empirical debates in five ways. First, we find that PB is not a static institution. Rather, local governments, civil society activists, and international organizations alter core institutional design features to suit their needs. Second, distinct motivations exist for adopting PB, such as deepening democracy, improving accountability, modernizing state-society relationships, and including citizens in allocating small infrastructure projects. Third, PB programs adhere to the five core principles with differing degrees of emphasis. For example, some programs more strongly emphasize social justice, whereas others focus more on oversight. These principles, in conjunction with sequential waves of diffusion, led governments to design new rules, processes, and procedures for their local programs. For example, a move from secret ballots to consultative or consensus-based decision-making processes; a move away from specific rules to promote social justice; a greater emphasis on social inclusion; a shift from municipal (city) level adoption to other levels, mostly to smaller government units (city districts, towns, villages, schools), but sometimes to national or state-level governments.

Fourth, we identify six distinct types of PB program based on these new rules and shifting principles, outlined in Chapter 1. Although local actors transform PB to better meet their local needs, we showcase commonalities that permit us to categorize PB programs into these types. Finally, in Chapter 2, we present a "theory of change," in which we identify the causal mechanisms that are designed to promote social and political change. By explicitly developing this theory of change, we hope to guide researchers, especially those new to the field, as they evaluate PB's impact. We also hope to help policymakers and civil society activists as they try to understand the likely range of changes through PB.

This introductory chapter advances our arguments by describing PB's original design principles with an eye toward distinguishing it from other participatory institutions. PB is distinct from other types of citizen-participation programs— such as Deliberative Polling (Fishkin 2011), community-driven development (CDD) programs (Mansuri and Rao 2013), or community score cards—because PB adheres to the five core PB principles (voice, vote, social justice, social inclusion, and oversight) to create a process to build new institutions and allocate fixed percentages of internal revenue to implement projects selected by participants. Importantly, governments adopting PB privilege different combinations of these principles, which helps to explain the wide variation in the institutional rules.

PB's Core Principles

Voice

PB offers citizens and CSOs the opportunity to voice their ideas and demands in open forums attended by their fellow citizens and government officials. Government officials often convey their spending constraints and inform participants about previous spending decisions. PB thus gives voice to these actors through channels that did not previously exist. In theory, PB demands active participation, which extends the possibility of political renewal by inducing citizens to deliberate with each other and with government officials over public priorities.

Voice developed through PB can multiply as participants carry new information and newly learned deliberative skills into other policymaking venues. PB then helps to build a public sphere, moving public debate beyond political parties and media coverage and extending it to individual citizens and CSOs.

Vote

Vote is another important principle associated with PB because it allows citizens to make specific decisions regarding public spending. This moves PB beyond consultative deliberation and into the realm of state-sanctioned decision-making. This extension of authority explains why PB has attracted the attention of so many ordinary citizens, government officials, and international organizations. In PB, citizens vote to select projects that the government will then implement. In the most successful cases, this is a "binding" decision that the government commits to carrying out. In other cases, the vote is more of a recommendation that then goes to executive and legislative officials for final approval. Having real decision-making authority forces citizens and government officials to work together and make difficult choices regarding how resources are allocated. Voting on these choices also legitimizes spending decisions. The process of project selection maps onto the outcomes associated with PB; changing when, how, and by whom decisions are made alters those decisions and channels them in different directions.

Social Justice

Most PB programs rely explicitly or implicitly on some conceptualization about the importance of "social justice." The original PB program in Porto Alegre explicitly codified social justice through rules that prioritized spending in areas with a high concentration of poor and vulnerable populations. Poor and underserved communities would receive greater resources on a per capita basis than wealthier communities. This is due to the central role of the Workers' Party's radical democratic project of the 1980s, which sought to invert governments' spending priorities (Genro 1995; Villas Boas and Telles 1995; Baiocchi 2005). As PB spreads across the world, the explicit principle of social justice through redistributive spending has receded. Social justice considerations are often discussed during meetings, but most new programs no longer have specific rules to ensure that poorer communities receive greater levels of resources than wealthier communities. Of course, we must bear in mind that some PB advocates work under the premise of expanding voice and vote to traditionally excluded sectors of the population, which potentially gives PB a redistributive component. However, we worry that PB is less likely to achieve tangible redistributive outcomes when the social justice principle is not codified in an explicit set of rules (Wampler and Touchton 2019).

Social Inclusion

The assumption behind PB is that better public policy will emerge by promoting social inclusion, which involves engaging people from a variety of backgrounds and experiences in debate and decision-making about public spending. Thus, who is invited to meetings and who attends is at the core of PB design choices and also has a substantial effect on the quality of PB process and outcomes. Many PB programs seek to expand the representation of traditionally marginalized groups like the poor, women, racial/ethnic minorities, LGBTQ+ individuals, and people with disabilities. Active outreach efforts offer important ways to engage these under-represented groups, as do social inclusion rules, such as quotas for neighborhood delegates. The power of voice and vote is magnified when PB programs include a more diverse range of participants, especially those from traditionally excluded groups, because PB allows *new voices* to be heard in formal, public venues. A meaningful vote attached to PB programs carries the potential to significantly empower these citizens: Individuals from traditionally excluded social and political communities then gain the ability to direct government actions through budgetary decisions.

Oversight

PB programs seek to reform how the state functions by increasing citizen oversight in the hope that increased transparency will improve the provision of public goods. Government officials often use PB meetings to review previous spending decisions and update residents about the implementation status of previously selected projects. Citizens are elected or appointed to oversight committees at the end of a typical PB decision-making cycle; they are given the responsibility of monitoring project implementation over the course of the following year.

Effective oversight requires access to information and resources (time and financial) to undertake the necessary actions as public-works spending evolves. Government projects are generally slow and expensive; understanding their implementation demands some form of training or education about budgets and feasibility studies. Thus, living up to the oversight principle in practice is quite difficult. Participants may find themselves caught between closely aligning themselves with government officials in the hope of generating greater support for PB (broadly construed) and taking steps to hone in on the specific problems with project implementation and budget allocations. This tension—similar to what legislators contend with—requires PB participants to actively support government officials as well as pressure them to improve decision-making and implementation.

In sum, we develop a core set of principles that help classify a process as PB: PB is a policy process that gives voice and vote to participants, includes new actors in policy decision-making, explicitly or implicitly embraces social justice goals, and develops oversight mechanisms for a particular set of public investment projects. In practice, governments and CSO leaders stress different combinations of these principles. For example, some programs more strongly emphasize social inclusion whereas other emphasize oversight. To be considered PB, a program must adhere to all principles, although we recognize that there is extensive variation in the weight that each program provides to specific principles. One goal of this book is to capture the variation across the broader family of PB programs.

Why Is PB Spreading So Rapidly? To What Effect?

Several PB researchers focus on describing its rapid spread around the world. Three books in particular delve in depth into PB's diffusion. Osmany Porto de Oliveira focuses on the vital role of "PB ambassadors," whom he credits with leading the effort to move PB beyond Brazil (Porto de Oliveira 2017a). These ambassadors leveraged existing institutional connections and created new networks to provide information about PB to mayors and civil society activists across the globe. Although the "PB ambassadors" were sympathetic to each other, their efforts were largely uncoordinated as these individuals worked in different institutions and regions as they advocated for PB's adoption. Additionally, as news of PB spread across the globe, government officials became increasingly willing to experiment with the new institutional type.

Second, Peck and Theodore work within the policy diffusion and translation scholarly tradition to explain the spread of PB across the globe. Their book, *Fast Policy: Experimental Statecraft at the Thresholds of Neoliberalism* (2015), treats PB both as a radical democratic experiment that seeks to empower citizens as well as a policy tool that governments adopt. They employ the concept of policy translation to account for how adopting governments translate an existing policy to make it legible in the sociopolitical environment. "Fast policy refers to a condition of deepening transnational interconnectedness, in which local policy experiments exist *in relation to* near and far relatives, to traveling models and technocratic designs, and to a host of financial, technical, social, and symbolic networks that invariably loop through centers of power and persuasion" (Peck and Theodore 2015: xxxi).

Finally, Baiocchi and Ganuza (2014, 2017) argue that PB transformed from a radical democratic project designed to empower citizens to a technical tool to improve basic governance. Baiocchi and Ganuza grapple with how core features of "PB as a technical tool" undermine basic efforts to expand democracy and empower citizens. These authors all seek to explain the spread of PB across the globe, but emphasize different factors driving the program's diffusion. Our book builds on all of these works with a novel approach: We show how the *timing* of PB adoption is strongly associated with the adaptation of basic PB design. We also present a larger number of cases and an expanded theoretical framework. Thus, in many ways, our book builds on these important works and then expands our understanding of PB. Our theoretical contribution is to account for why and how PB programs are adapted as well as to illuminate how these adaptations are likely to produce social and political change.

In parallel to the diffusion studies, researchers have also sought to better understand what outcomes, if any, PB programs produce. A variety of case studies assert that PB participants feel empowered, support democracy, view the government as more effective, and better understand budget and government processes after participating in PB (Santos 1998, 2005; Abers 2000; Avritzer 2002; Baiocchi 2005; Wampler 2007; Baiocchi et al. 2011; Goldfrank 2011; McNulty 2011; Sintomer et al. 2013; Russon Gilman 2016; Su 2017; Cabannes 2018). PB can also theoretically empower historically marginalized groups, such as women or ethnic minorities, by encouraging these groups to exercise voice and potentially wield decision-making power in public venues.

Another consensus from case-study evidence is that participants increase their political participation beyond PB and often join civil society groups following PB processes (Avritzer 2002; Baiocchi 2005; Baiocchi et al. 2011; Goldfrank 2011; Wampler 2015). Many expect PB to strengthen civil society by increasing its density (the number of groups), expanding its repertoire of activities, including brokering new partnerships with government and other CSOs (Baiocchi 2005; Wampler 2007; McNulty 2011; Montambeault 2012). PB proponents also expect the program to improve budget transparency, which may have the effect of increasing government programs' transparency *in general* (Shah 2007; Wampler 2007). Efficient resource allocation at the neighborhood or micro-regional level is another goal inherent in many PB programs (Marquetti et al. 2008; Wampler 2015). PB proponents hope that government service provision will become more efficient through PB's ability to collect information about community needs. Transparency and project monitoring surrounding the program will also decrease waste and fraud as accountability spreads across government contracting and project implementation in other areas. Further, PB proponents expect it to improve residents' well-being through the channels described above. Several recent studies have identified these effects for infant mortality over a relatively short time (Gonçalves 2014; Touchton and Wampler 2014; Wampler and Touchton 2019). Beyond infant mortality, the range of potential impacts could easily extend to other areas, such as maternal mortality, sanitation, education, women's rights, and poverty in general.

Importantly, however, not all cases of PB produce this impact. Some argue that having citizens debate and vote on infrastructure may simply not be worth their time and represents an insincere effort to promote participatory democracy (Albert 2016). Others observe that PB can co-opt citizens to prevent them from making more radical demands for systemic change (Navarro 2003; Junge 2012; Baiocchi and Ganuza 2017). The literature is full of examples from around the world where PB programs do not lead to empowerment and social change (Navarro 2003; Junge 2012; Jaramillo and Alcázar 2013; Allegretti and Falanga 2016; McNulty 2018, 2019; Su 2017). Scholars have also documented PB processes that are plagued with problems like clientelism, elite capture, and corruption (Navarro 2003; Font et al. 2018; Goldfrank 2021; Mansuri and Rao 2013; McNulty 2019; Selee 2011).

In short, many activists and scholars currently have a lot of enthusiasm and high expectations surrounding PB. Others are much warier. Most of our evidence regarding the extent to which PB can and does lead to changes in well-being, civil society, and accountability comes from Brazil and Latin America. We have lots of excellent single-case studies that highlight local changes, but we continue to lack a strong body of analysis that more carefully links PB programs to social and political change. In this book, we caution enthusiasts to give careful thought to what PB is and is not and what PB can and cannot do for communities. Our aim is to better illuminate the diversity of PB experiences and present evidence-based arguments to understand the possibilities and limitations of these programs. In other published works, we use different methodological approaches—single-case studies, site visits, participant observation, interviews, medium and large-N analysis—to identify PB programs that work well and PB programs that perform poorly; we thus draw on more than twenty-five years of research experience with PB and multiple types of data to develop key arguments. In Chapter 2, we develop a clear, well-founded analytical framework that should permit the reader to better identify when, where, and why PB programs produce such varied results.

Advancing the Debate

As the previous section makes clear, PB's spread, evolution, and transformation have given rise to an enormous global literature. Research on PB has followed three distinct evolutionary phases. The first phase involved single-case studies, as scholars attempted to get a better handle on this new democratic innovation. Fedozzi (1998), Santos (1998), Abers (2000), Avritzer (2002), and Baiocchi (2005) led this effort and emphasized the role of civil society as well as PB as a "radical democratic" project. Most studies initially focused on Brazil, but then moved on to other countries and regions as PB was adopted across the globe (e.g., Argentina, Uruguay, Peru, South Africa, Indonesia, the United States, and Europe). For example, we have seen more single-case studies on the United States and several European cities in the 2015 to 2017 period as researchers try to understand the current wave of innovations (Su 2012; Kamrowska-Zaluska 2016; Nez 2016).

As PB evolves, case studies about its transformations have also emerged. There is an interesting and growing literature on who participates (Community Development Project 2013; McNulty 2015; Su 2017), national laws (No 2017; McNulty 2018), and the use of technology in particular cities (Peixoto 2009; Best et al. 2010; Rose, Rios, and Lippa 2010; Miori and Russo 2011; Lim and Oh 2016). Case study research has proven an important first step in generating hypotheses about both process and outcomes associated with PB.

The second phase of research on PB involves medium-N comparative studies, most of which focused on Latin America (Heller 2001; Wampler 2007, 2008, 2015; Baiocchi et al. 2011; Goldfrank 2011; McNulty 2011; Montambeault 2012). These studies developed broader, more generalizable explanations for outcomes associated with PB. Research topics in these studies include variation within and across civil society, government involvement, the role of the legislature, and political opposition. Beyond Latin America, more recent examples of this comparative work extend regional coverage to Europe (Džinić et al. 2016; Sintomer et al. 2016) and Asia (Wu and Wang 2011, 2012; Feruglio and Rifai 2017). Case-study research has generated a great deal of consensus about impacts. However, hypotheses stemming from this research have generally not been tested in large-N studies. Within this second phase of research, scholars began to draw from the diffusion literature to better understand how PB is spreading across the world (Peck and Theodore 2015; Baiocchi and Ganuza 2017; Porto de Oliveira 2017a).

The third phase of PB research involves statistical analyses of a large number of municipalities or countries. One line of work involves analysis of surveys using regression techniques (Wampler 2007, 2015; Johnson 2017). A second line of work involves using municipal-level data to assess how the presence of PB affects social well-being (Boulding and Wampler 2010; Gonçalves 2014; Touchton and Wampler 2014; No 2017; Touchton, Wampler, and Peixoto 2019; Wampler and Touchton 2019; No and Hseuh 2020) or changes in government spending (Hagelskamp et al. 2020). However, large-N work is the most limited of the three types of research due to the difficulty in tracking down reliable and useable data. In fact, Brazil is the only country where large-N, comparative analyses of cities with and without PB have been conducted. These works highlight that the presence of PB programs, when compared to those municipalities without PB, has positive impacts.

Even given this large literature on PB, there is no one source that theorizes PB's principles, processes, mechanisms, adaptations, and outcomes to build the platform for a new phase of research. This book fills that void by developing a conceptual model that helps us understand the varied PB programs and the outcomes that emerge from those programs. It also presents a comprehensive analysis of the evolution and transformation of PB in the last thirty years. Finally, it documents regional experiences with PB in individual chapters.

The seeds of this book begin in 2017 when the authors conducted a "state of the art" analysis on PB for the William and Flora Hewlett Foundation. In addition, two of the authors (Wampler and Touchton) worked with the Making All Voices Count project, housed at the Institute for Development Studies at the University of Sussex, to bring together NGO activists working on PB programs in eight countries in the Global South (http://www.makingallvoicescount.org). These two parallel projects resulted in a rich, up-to-date understanding of PB's transformation as it has spread around the world. This book is also the result of decades of research undertaken by the three authors. Collectively, we have observed hundreds of PB meetings in countries around the world, interviewed hundreds of PB advocates and critics, and participated in international projects, research boards, conferences, and meetings since the mid-1990s. Two of the authors (McNulty and Wampler) published books that used medium-N case study analysis to move beyond the pitfalls of single-case analysis. Wampler and Touchton have also performed large-N survey and observational analyses evaluating PB's performance across hundreds of municipalities. Much of the analysis in the book is based on our own original research, but we have also scoured the literature on PB to bring together the collective insight of researchers from around the world into this one book.

The book makes an important contribution to the growing literature on PB by combining a unique conceptual framework with an empirical analysis of PB's spread and transformation over the past thirty years. As discussed above, much of this existing literature is composed of single-case studies or cross-national comparisons within regions, like Latin America or Europe. Our book is the first cross-national, cross-regional, global overview of the most rapidly expanding democratic institution in the world. There is also a large policy literature on PB, which is primarily empirical and does not build concepts or develop theory surrounding how PB is supposed to work. These strains of literature do not meet and there is a notable lack of theoretical guidance surrounding the program. This book is the first to unify these distinct areas to build theory on PB and provide guidance on the program based on global evidence. Our book takes an important first step to resolving these challenges by carefully examining diffusion and transformation of PB as it spreads from Brazil around the world.

Conclusion

As democracy has both expanded and, more recently, recedes around the world, it is important to understand the potential for public policy to empower citizens and bring governments closer to the people (Levitsky and Ziblatt 2018). However, when it is not working well or is implemented poorly, PB can be detrimental to the goal of deepening democracy. To date, there is no one source that combines careful documentation of the spread of PB with a general theory that explains its evolution and potential impact. Governments, donor agencies, and civil society advocates do not currently have a resource for contextualizing their choices in program design or understanding why distinct outcomes may emerge through PB across different contexts.

We also know that PB today has changed dramatically from its roots in Porto Alegre. This book documents this transformation over time and around the world. Today, PB takes place in villages, metropolitan areas, states/provinces, and at national levels. In addition to municipal officials and local activists, international donors and foundations now actively promote PB's global diffusion. Some new PB processes are highly deliberative, while others have very little debate at all. The variation in PB experiences around the world would be impossible to capture in one place, but we can confidently state that PB programs feature significant differences from one context to the next.

This is also the first book on PB to systematically draw from multiple global regions to build theory, identify trends, and develop expectations for performance. Chapters on Latin America, sub-Saharan Africa, Asia, and North Atlantic PB programs illuminate key similarities and differences across these regions. Another important contribution is an analysis of how governments approach program design and operation, thereby informing our understanding of PB processes in dramatically different contexts.

To better explore these themes, this book provides empirical and theoretical details about PB's evolution, transformations, and impact. Chapter 1 documents the evolution and transformation of PB around the world. Chapter 2 provides an original conceptual model for PB's impact, which captures its potential results, the conditions under which these results emerge, as well as a discussion of the causal mechanisms that drive these outcomes. The remaining chapters explore PB as it has evolved in four global regions: Latin America, Asia, sub-Saharan Africa, and the North Atlantic. Each chapter discusses the way that PB has spread and evolved over time in the particular region, focusing on several country cases that best represent these trends and the particular types of PB that are most prevalent in that region. We offer as much data about process and impact as are available for these country cases; in some places, data are extensive, in others they are not. The book concludes with a discussion that sums up the state of our knowledge on PB as well as the myriad questions that remain to be tackled in future studies.

1

The Global Adoption of PB

Participatory Budgeting is a rapidly spreading and flexible institution found in places as diverse as rural villages in Kenya, the Philippines, Peru, and Indonesia; global cities such as Paris, Seoul, and New York City; and high schools in Phoenix, Recife, and Lisbon. At the broadest level, PB is best conceptualized as a set of core principles that inform program design rather than a specific set of institutional rules. As identified in the Introduction, these principles include voice, vote, social inclusion, social justice, and oversight. The breadth of these core PB principles draws in a wide range of supporters and advocates: Radical democrats, social movement activists, electorally vulnerable politicians, and policy experts located in national ministries and international organizations all find something they like in these principles.

In Porto Alegre, decentralization and a return to democracy offered an opportunity to reimagine participation, with civil society and social inclusion at the forefront of co-governance reforms from the political left. In Chicago, Alderman Joe Moore initiated PB in the ward he represented to revive citizen participation and garner electoral support. Madrid and Barcelona adopted digital platforms to promote direct, widespread input into budget priorities, but largely without regular opportunities for deep deliberation. In the Philippines, the National Department of Budget and Management incentivized cities, towns, and villages to adopt PB in pursuit of transparency, participation, and accountability. For Kenya, World Bank officials helped to implement PB as part of Kenya's constitutional reform and decentralization; they designed PB as a development tool to bring projects to underserved areas and to promote social accountability.

PB now wears many hats, as a radical democratic experiment, as a mandated democratic policymaking process used by national governments to influence sub-national policymaking, as a means for elected officials to build electoral support, as well as a technical policymaking tool, which allows international organizations to promote development and social accountability.

PB programs formally pay homage to the five core principles (voice, vote, social inclusion, social justice, and oversight), but they do so with significantly different emphases. Some programs more strongly emphasize voice and vote, as they seek to improve the quality of local democracy. Other programs stress social inclusion and social justice, with an emphasis on meeting human development goals. Other programs highlight oversight, in the hopes that transparency will produce better use of public resources and improve service delivery. PB's internal

Participatory Budgeting in Global Perspective. Brian Wampler, Stephanie McNulty, and Michael Touchton,
Oxford University Press. © Brian Wampler, Stephanie McNulty, and Michael Touchton 2021.
DOI: 10.1093/oso/9780192897756.003.0002

processes (the "rules of the game") are usually adapted to meet local social, political, and policy needs. PB is not a static institution with a narrowly defined set of rules; government reformers and their allies often alter the basic institutional design to better meet local needs and interests. As a result, there is significant variation in the look, feel, and purpose of PB programs, suggesting a broader "PB family" as well as "sub-families." The Porto Alegre model, described in the previous chapter, has now been eclipsed as governments significantly adapt PB programs to meet local needs.

This chapter develops a framework to account for these adaptations and variations. It explores the political and policy mechanisms that drive innovation, diffusion, adoption, and adaptation. It demonstrates how the sequencing of the diffusion process is strongly associated with specific types of institutional adaptations (Falleti 2005). We draw from the academic literature on institutional isomorphism, and three process-related concepts—*normative, mimetic,* and *coercive isomorphism*—to account for the adoption and subsequent adaptation of PB programs around the world. Importantly, the timing (first, second, or third wave), location (region), and type (e.g., normative, mimetic, coercive) of adoption strongly condition how new PB programs are subsequently *adapted*.

In this chapter, we also recognize the parallel development of participatory governance programs that share similar principles with PB programs, but were not initially identified as PB. During the late 1980s and early 1990s, when PB was being created, communication among potential allies across different regions was difficult—the internet was in its early stages of expansion and phone calls were expensive. The parallel development of similar programs in far-flung places—Philippines, India, Senegal, Bolivia—suggest that the direct participation in policymaking was an important feature of the broader democratization movement. Some of these programs, over time, would mimic PB programs (Indonesia, Philippines) but some of these parallel programs (Bolivia) would maintain characteristics distinct from PB. These programs tend to focus on broader participation in general policymaking, as opposed to PB, which focuses on an excised portion of the budget for citizen-selected projects. Thus, these other programs that are similar to PB may have similar principles, but deploy them in very different ways across the government/policymaking apparatus. As we accumulate data on PB in different contexts, we identify patterns about the range and types of experiences that exist. Using these observations, we build theory to better account for the shifting nature of PB as governments across the world adopt and adapt it.

This chapter ends with the development of a typology that permits us to classify PB programs. We identify six PB types that capture the diversity of cases across the globe: 1) Empowered Democracy and Redistribution; 2) Deepening Democracy through Community Mobilization; 3) Mandated by National Government; 4) Digital PB; 5) Social Development and Accountability; and

6) Efficient Governance. We argue that most PB programs fit into one of these six types, thus allowing us to account for the broad diversity of institutional processes, expectations, and outcomes. One advantage of the typology is that it allows us to identify how clusters of programs under one type are more likely to generate similar outcomes, thus allowing us to generalize from a small number of cases to a larger set of cases (Collier et al. 2012).

Four Mechanisms Driving Policy Innovation

Prior to introducing our typology, it is helpful to review a theoretical discussion of key mechanisms driving policy innovations, diffusion, and adaptation *in general*.

Creation

Policy entrepreneurs take advantage of a policy or political "windows of opportunity" to create new institutions (Baumgartner and Jones 1993). The creation of new institutions at national and subnational levels is more likely to occur during a "punctuated equilibrium," whereby new political actors have political and policy space to design new democratic and policymaking institutions (Baumgartner and Jones 1993). Shifting institutional environments, including decentralization and national-level democratic adoption, create opportunities for local government reformers to experiment with new institutional types. For example, the roots of PB in Brazil are situated in the period of transition to democratic rule from authoritarian rule (Baierle 1998; Abers 2000; Avritzer 2002; Tranjan 2015).

Individual and collective actors, identifiable as "policy entrepreneurs," seek to reform existing governance structures in the hopes of generating political and social change. Kingdon describes policy entrepreneurs as "willing to invest their resources—time, energy, reputation, money—to promote a position in return for anticipated future gain in the form of material, purposive, solidary benefits" (Kingdon 1995: 179). Policy entrepreneurs are motivated by a combination of political, personal, and governance interests to promote new policies (Mintrom 1997). Policy entrepreneurs may come from within the formal political party structures (e.g., Reagan, Gorbachev), be part of a more radical opposition (e.g., Mandela, Lula), or represent the emergence of civil society actors (e.g., Aquino, Havel). New democratic institutions are more likely to emerge in a context where an identifiable group or political party advocates for novel ways of incorporating citizens into public venues. These groups may be from civil society (e.g., social movements, non-governmental organizations (NGOs)), from political society (e.g., parties), or from policy fields (e.g., UN-Habitat). These groups all have a willingness to experiment with new institutional formats to improve process and outcome.

Diffusion

Similar to the creation moment, diffusion also involves the opening of a window of opportunity, during which interested governments are willing to consider adopting new programs. However, the diffusion process differs from the creation moment because the governments involved in the diffusion process are looking *beyond their borders* for innovative policies, programs, and institutions that might help them to solve pressing problems. Governments looking to solve problems often begin by searching the landscape around them (e.g., neighboring towns, states, countries, and regions) to consider the adoption of successful programs in similar contexts. Diffusion is an uncoordinated yet interconnected process leading to the adoption of similar programs (Simmons and Elkins 2004). Innovative programs and institutions spread across countries, regions, and the globe at the behest of NGOs, international funding institutions, political parties, civil society activists, and entrepreneurial politicians.

Previous research identifies three critical factors that make governments more open or susceptible to adopt innovative policies that were initiated elsewhere. First, when government officials are able to identify that they are part of a changing political context (e.g., democratization and decentralization), political reformers will be more open to adopting new policies (Walker 1969; Mintrom 1997; Peck and Theodore 2015). In these cases, governments are willing to adopt new policies but they are not necessarily generating new programs themselves. Second, government officials are initially more likely to look at initiatives undertaken by their neighbors; thus, the spatial proximity to pioneering reforms also helps to explain where governments will look for new ideas (Peck and Theodore 2015; Porto de Oliveira 2017a; Berry and Berry 2018). Both elected officials and CSOs with limited time and resources tend to look for innovative policies in their local regions. Third, government officials or civil society actors use governance and policy networks to gain information about innovations occurring outside their local area (Weyland 2004; Sugiyama 2012; Porto de Oliveira 2017a). Policy networks may include individuals and organizations promoting a specific type of policy innovation that addresses seemingly "wicked" problems. For example, the United Nations and World Bank are international organizations that support policy networks to promote innovation. They work directly with governments to promote and support specific programs, and governments seek their advice and funding when they consider potential programs in a new political moment. Thus, we would expect the diffusion of an innovative program to first begin in the county or geographic region closest to where a pioneering program began, then spread beyond that region through more extensive networks.

Adaptation

The diffusion processes create opportunities for adopting governments to alter the institutions' basic rules, structures, and processes. There is often a "reset" moment when governments adopting diffusing institutions will redesign the institution's basic rules to better address specificities of the local context, while retaining the core ideas or principles of the initial innovation. We draw from DiMaggio and Powell's seminal work on institutional isomorphism to account for institutional similarities and differences as institutions are adopted and then adapted during a diffusion wave. Isomorphism is "a constraining process that forces one unit in a population to resemble other units that face the same set of environmental conditions" (DiMaggio and Powell 1983: 149). Crucially, we expect that the context in which PB is adopted will significantly affect its adaptation. DiMaggio and Powell show that institutions designed to address similar problems will, over time, come to resemble one another because individuals working within these institutions will continue to adapt them to achieve better results; these individuals will seek out information regarding how to redesign their institutions. Implicit in this argument is that institutions are not static; rather, institutional diffusion includes an iterative, ongoing process of institutional adaptation.

DiMaggio and Powell (1983) identify three conceptual mechanisms that capture reformers' motivations for adopting institutions and then influence the scope of institutional adaptation: *normative, mimetic,* and *coercive.* Each mechanism captures reformers' motivations for adapting institutions that achieve a broader, shared goal (e.g., market stability, higher vote turn-out) and also address the specificity of the local context. We expand their conceptual framing to generalize the arguments and encompass the forces surrounding democratic innovations:

- *Normative* pressures are at work when officials believe that there is a compelling ideological and/or moral argument to support the adoption of a new institution. There is often a strong commitment to the core democratic principles associated with the original institution. Under these conditions, we would expect officials to adapt institutions to "realign" the original rules to better match local conditions.
- *Mimetic* pressures are in play when governments adopt new institutions to better align themselves with the prevailing international "best practices." In the face of uncertainty, governments adopt similar institutions in the hopes

that they will gain similar benefits as reported from the best performers. We would expect governments influenced by mimetic pressures to adapt these institutions based on regional norms as well as temporal considerations (e.g., "best practices" at the time of adoption).

- *Coercive* pressures are at work when local government officials are either mandated, strongly encouraged, or induced to adopt the institution. Coercive pressures are more likely when there is a distinct power differential between an actor promoting institutional adoption and a local government where the institutional reform will operate. The more dominant actor could be a political party, a national government, or an international organization (e.g., USAID, the UK's Department for International Development [DFID], World Bank). We would expect governments influenced by coercive pressures to adapt their institutions in ways that reflect the dominant institution's goals and the prevailing international norms around "best practices."

The three categories above are analytically distinct but we acknowledge that there may be overlap in some cases as some governments might be motivated by a combination of these factors. We would expect that a new institutional design would first need to be identified as an international "best practice" before mimetic pressures would lead stronger national (i.e., national government) or international actors to both promote them (mimetic pressures), as well as to insist that their partners adopt them (coercive pressures). Importantly, we find that these analytical categories—normative, mimetic, and coercive—help to explain variation across the six PB types.

Parallel Development of Similar Programs

Comparable institutions, including participatory institutions, may develop in far-flung places as unconnected individuals and organizations devise similar rules to solve similar problems. The concept of parallel evolutionary development best captures this process. Just as animals and plants in distant places of the world develop comparable strategies to contend with comparable challenges, government officials and civil society activists develop processes that are surprisingly similar. In the cases of subnational participatory democratic institutions, parallel "creation" occurred in a comparable context as the first cases of PB, but these cases didn't adopt the "PB" name and brand. During the Third Wave of democracy, broader trends of democratization, decentralization, increased electoral competition, and a widening of civil society help explain the development of new participatory democratic institutions similar to PB (Huntington 1993; Campbell 2003). New democratic institutions proliferated during the Third Wave; of these institutions, PB programs gained the most attention and fame. We do not address the issue of why more governments adopt PB in comparison to other participatory programs but we note that many governments and CSOs across the globe were seeking new ways of conducting politics and PB appeared attractive to an unusually diverse group of actors.

Tracing the Spread of PB

Having described theoretical diffusion processes in general, we can now turn to the creation, diffusion, adaptation, and parallel development of PB specifically.

Creation

Like most new policy programs, PB's creation is best understood in the context of windows of opportunity and policy entrepreneurs. PB emerged in Brazil during a long transition to democratic rule as political outsiders sought ways to reimagine how citizens engage with the state and democratic institutions (Genro 1999; Abers 2000; Avritzer 2002; Wampler 2007; Tranjan 2015). In Brazil, the window of opportunity to create new institutions emerged during its democratization in the 1980s. As the military slowly withdrew from power, government officials and citizens created new institutions and programs to foster citizen engagement in politics and ongoing policymaking processes. In major cities, such as São Paulo and Recife, mayors adopted participatory programs in the early 1980s while the military still controlled the national government (Abers 2000; Wampler 2007; Tranjan 2015). PB's principles and design thus began to take shape in authoritarian environments in Brazil prior to its democratic transition (Tranjan 2015). Local governments took advantage of subnational political windows of opportunity to experiment with new ways of structuring state–society relations. In this sense, PB was part of a larger process in which some government officials and civil society activists sought to build democracy.

Brazil adopted a new constitution in 1988, which allowed for extensive decentralization that greatly expanded municipal-level decision-making authority. Brazilian municipalities gained access to 15 percent of public monies (states spend about 30 percent and the federal government about 55 percent) as well as the responsibility for delivering a wide range of services. These services included urban infrastructure, health, education (a responsibility often shared with states), and social assistance programs. PB thus emerged in a moment of democratization and a municipal-based decentralization process; municipalities were given more service delivery responsibilities and greater resources, creating a historic window of opportunity in Brazil for innovation and change.

As noted in the previous chapter, the city of Porto Alegre is widely recognized as being the birthplace of the specific set of rules associated with PB, though there were other budget-oriented participatory experiences that preceded it in Brazilian cities like Londrina and Recife (Harnecker 1995; Fedozzi 1998; Abers 2000; Tranjan 2015). The Workers' Party (*Partido dos Trabalhadores* or PT) administration in Porto Alegre sought to govern with and for the excluded sectors of the population by "inverting the priorities" of previous administrations, decentralizing the local state, and creating viable participatory channels (Baierle 1998; Larangeira 1996; Genro and Ubiratan de Souza 1997). The mayoral administration created PB in 1989 and placed it at the center of its governing and campaign strategies. Porto Alegre also had a vibrant civil society, including neighborhood associations and social movements (Avritzer 2002; Baiocchi 2005). During the 1980s, PB was born of at least two groups: a democratic socialist political party that wanted to do things differently and an active civil society.

PB gained international fame largely based on the Porto Alegre experience. The Workers' Party leadership exhibited the classic characteristics of policy entrepreneurs—political outsiders who used their surprising electoral victory to experiment with new policies and sought to build a solid base of constituents (Fedozzi 1998; Baierle 1998; Abers 2000; Avritzer 2002; Marquetti 2003; Nylen 2003; Wampler and Avritzer 2004; Baiocchi 2005; Santos 2005; Peck and Theodore 2015). Former mayor Tarso Genro describes PB as a "non-state public sphere" (*espaço públio não-estatal*), arguing that PB is a new type of democratic institution, allowing citizens to engage in deliberative decision making without state domination:

> To construct a non-state public sphere signifies the reversal, the radical reversal, of the process realized under real socialism, in which the State dominated society. It is a civilizing process of the State, a process in which the State becomes a public entity controlled by civil society.   (Genro 1995: 41)

When created, then, PB represented a conscious effort to avoid the state repression of civil society that occurred in the Soviet Union and other socialist settings. Instead, the Workers' Party and many of its CSO allies hoped to build democratic socialism through new state–society interactions. PB was also initially part of a larger process that its supporters hoped would engender a broader transformation of Brazilian political and civil societies. It bears repeating that the original PB experience, that is, the Porto Alegre model, was born out of a radical democratic socialist project.

Diffusion: Isomorphic Adoption and Adaptation

PB programs, based on the Porto Alegre experience, first spread across Brazil, then into Latin America, before moving to other parts of the world, in several waves. Of course, these waves are fluid and there is some overlap across the waves.

The beginning of one wave may start earlier in some regions and begin later in other regions; this delineation of waves is a general guide, not a rigid category, to describe PB's diffusion. Importantly, a process of adaptation accompanied each wave—government officials and civil society representatives experimented with new designs to better align their goals with PB's potential outcomes. Each new wave built on the previous one, resulting in the transformation of new PB programs away from the original PB model. This gives policy designers more options to redesign new programs because they can draw on both older and more recent programs; there is now significant diversity among the world's PB programs. In this section, we draw upon the diffusion approach utilized by Porto de Oliveira (2017a), Peck and Theodore (2015), Sintomer et al. (2016), and Cabannes (2019), although our theoretical interest is more focused on how PB was adapted at the different stages than on its diffusion. We identify three distinct diffusion "waves" that help to explain adoption.

First Wave of Diffusion: Spreading throughout Brazil, 1989 through the mid-1990s

Initially, PB spread quickly throughout Brazil throughout the 1990s, with the Workers' Party at the center of efforts to promote its adoption. A small, outsider party, the Workers' Party's electoral victories in 1989 and 1992 came in large, wealthy municipalities, where they began to experiment with new policy programs.[1] By 1996, thirty Brazilian municipalities had adopted PB and twenty-three of them were governed by the Workers' Party. Three factors best account for why the party promoted PB: a strong civil society base, internal party cohesion, and the presence of policy entrepreneurs who sought to create innovative policies that were not only distinct from their rivals' policies, but also emphasized direct citizen participation, social justice, and transparency (Wampler and Avritzer 2004; Wampler 2007). Adoption was thus driven by a combination of normative pressures, in the sense that some Workers' Party municipal governments strongly supported PB because it aligned with their policy and political objectives. In addition, the Workers' Party's leadership developed the "PT way of governing," that included PB as a core component of their governing strategy (Genro 1999). As such, the PT's national leadership strongly encouraged PT mayors to adopt these programs (Genro 1999; Wampler 2007).

Mayors affiliated with the Workers' Party adopted most PB programs during this first phase. However, by 1996 there were seven PB programs in municipalities

---

[1] PB was only one of several policy innovations spearheaded by the Workers' Party. The Workers' Party stands out within Brazil's multi-party system as a disciplined party that initiated multiple policy innovations, including PB, school fellowships (*Bolsa Escola*), and a minimum living wage program (*renda mínima*) (Sugiyama 2012; Hunter and Sugiyama 2014). Workers' Party governments during this period were willing to experiment with new institutional designs that challenged existing state–society relationships by reorganizing political institutions.

not affiliated with the Workers' Party. The growth of policy networks and spatial proximity best explain this diffusion. As two NGO representatives confirmed in our interviews, NGOs, such as FASE, Instituto Pólis, and Instituto Cajamar, disseminated information about PB's rules and processes to non-PT governments (see also Villas Boas and Telles 1995). Non-PT governments were willing to adopt a new policymaking institution, even though it was closely associated with the PT, because most early academic analyses and policy briefs presented PB in a very flattering light (Villas Boas and Telles 1995).

In sum, PB's diffusion across Brazil included normative adoption as mayors and new governing coalitions sought alternative strategies to govern differently than their predecessors. The examples of normative adoption are most clearly evident in places like Belo Horizonte, Santo André, and Ipatinga, where innovative mayors adopted PB based on the principles and rules associated with Porto Alegre's PB programs (Wampler 2007). However, we also see examples of "coerced" PB adoption, in which Workers' Party mayors, not necessarily committed to PB, were strongly induced to adopt the program (Wampler 2007). Coercive adoption occurred in cities like Blumenau and Rio Claro. In both cases, mayors were not highly supportive of PB but were convinced to adopt it by national party elites and junior partners in local governing coalitions. Finally, in at least one city—Recife—a mimetic process of adoption took place, where a non-Workers' Party government altered an existing participatory program and transformed it into PB in the hope of generating outcomes similar to those reported in Porto Alegre and Belo Horizonte (Wampler 2007).

Key Adaptations of the First Wave (1989 through the mid-1990s)
Governments adapted PB in two ways during the first wave. First, the Workers' Party expanded their commitment to social justice. For example, in 1993, the city of Belo Horizonte created a Quality of Life Index that would become the basis for the distribution of resources through PB (Wampler 2015). Neighborhoods and communities with a lower of quality of life, as measured by availability of public infrastructure (e.g., schools, health clinics), private facilities (e.g., banks), and household income, would receive more resources on a per capita basis than communities with higher scores. The Quality of Life Index allowed PB programs to embed social justice principles in the program design by creating a clear set of rules for differentiating among communities. This became one of the main tools to operationalize the social justice aspect of PB during this period. Although Porto Alegre initially used a simpler index to redistribute resources to poorer communities, Belo Horizonte's creation of a more sophisticated approach suggests a "layering" of new institutional rules onto the Porto Alegre model (Mahoney and Thelen 2010: 15; Montambeault 2019).

Second, Porto Alegre expanded the types of venues and sectors for people to participate in decision-making. They broadened PB to include sectoral-based thematic meetings (e.g., transportation, environment), allowing citizens to participate beyond their specific neighborhood and in broader issue areas. Participants in the environmental sector could deliberate over the adoption of programs or projects that would address a pressing problem, such as a river's degradation or the protection of a natural reserve. In Belo Horizonte, the government created "PB Housing" as a separate program. In this issue-specific program, deliberation and resource allocation focused exclusively on building public housing projects that would become participants' homes (Wampler 2015). This was the first identifiable sector-based PB program, but other places would follow suit, adopting PB in youth programs, housing projects, and schools.

These early adaptations illustrate the ways government officials and their civil society allies created new policies and programmatic rules to deepen the democratic canon and invert longstanding, exclusionary policies (Santos 2005; Mahoney and Thelen 2010; Montambeault 2019). The willingness to experiment is a core feature of PB adoption and adaptation across the globe. From the beginning, government officials and their allies modified PB's existing rules in the hopes of finding ways to better achieve beneficial outcomes. PB is a dynamic institution that permits local officials and citizens to adapt the rules to better address local issues.

Second Wave of Diffusion: Moving beyond Brazil, mid-1990s through mid-2000s

The most significant development during the second wave was the program's adoption *beyond* Brazil, although we note that PB continued to spread across Brazil during this timeframe. PB was promoted by leftist political parties, civil society activists, "good government" reformers and mainstream international organizations throughout this era. The confluence of different actors promoting PB helps to account for the widespread adoption during the second wave as well as the extensive adaptations of the program. During this second wave, PB was recognized as an international "best practice" for combining how governments could simultaneously deepen democracy and improve service delivery within poor communities. During this period, we begin to see a broad set of motivations for why governments adopt PB. Normative, ideological interests drive some governments as they seek new forms of democracy. Less radical governments hope to adopt programs that appear to be working well elsewhere, which corresponds to mimetic adoption. Finally, other governments are strongly encouraged by international agencies or mandated by the national government to adopt PB, which suggests that they are strongly encouraged, or "coerced," into adoption.

Porto de Oliveira's (2017a) work presents an important theoretical and empirical explanation that accounts for PB's international diffusion. Porto de Oliveira identifies individuals and organizations as developing a broad narrative of the new institution's great value (2017a). The broader narrative of PB as a successful democratic policymaking innovation entered the international scene in 1996 when the United Nations Habitat program gave a "Best Practice" award in urban management to the municipalities of Santo André and Porto Alegre for their PB programs (Porto de Oliveira 2017a). This award drew international attention to how a local government institution balanced often cumbersome, time-consuming democratic practices (e.g., participation, deliberation) with the urgency to deliver desperately needed services in resource-scarce environments. PB entered international policy cycles through organizations such as the United Nations and the World Bank at a moment in which national and local policymakers sought institutional and policymaking solutions to improve the quality of many nascent democracies, limit endemic corruption in many states in the Global South, and deliver public goods to poor and marginalized communities (Goldfrank 2012). PB appealed to governments and groups that sought to deepen democracy as well as organizations and groups that identified its potential to improve incremental policymaking processes around the world.

In parallel fashion, PB gained traction among social movements and activists aligned with international leftist and socialist projects. Brazil's Workers' Party, one of PB's key champions, promoted the program beyond Brazil's borders. During the 1990s, Brazil's left created the World Social Forum, which became an important biannual event for activists and social movements affiliated with leftist and socialist ideas (Peck and Theodore 2015). The World Social Forum, held in Porto Alegre for the first three events (2001, 2002, 2003), before a series of other cities, including Mumbai, Nairobi, and Caracas, took over as hosts. Porto Alegre again hosted in 2005 and 2012. At the World Social Forum, leftist activists gained knowledge about PB in Porto Alegre, fueling PB's spread as a normative ideal of the international left (Menser 2005; Peck and Theodore 2015).

Outside of Brazil, several Latin American municipalities led the way in adopting PB: Montevideo, Uruguay, and Caracas, Venezuela, developed similar programs (Goldfrank 2007, 2011). Subnational governments in Peru and Ecuador also adopted PB (Van Cott 2008; McNulty 2011; Cabannes 2014). Leftist governments with strong ties to community organizations led these programs, similar to the Brazilian experiences in Porto Alegre, Santo André, and Belo Horizonte. *Normative* isomorphic forces among ideologically leftist governments fueled this phase of PB adoption across Latin America. For example, the Workers' Party promoted PB across cities in Brazil as part of their efforts to incorporate marginalized populations and civil society into policymaking following Brazil's return to democracy.

In the Global North, PB also began to spread. In Europe, the ideologically leftist Spanish cities of Córdoba (2001) and Seville (2004) were early adopters (Ganuza 2005; Cabannes 2014; Pineda 2004; Proyecto Urbal 2006). In North America, government reformers and leftist activists led the way in the pioneering case of PB in the Toronto Housing Authority in 2001 (Lerner 2014). In South Korea, a local leftist, union-oriented political party had contact with Brazil's Workers' Party and launched the first PB in a small industrial city in 2003 (No 2017). PB became an attractive policy option for many leftist governments because the program's principles corresponded broadly with the parties' ideology of increased participation, social inclusion, and social justice.

International networks and cooperation among government officials provided critical support for the adoption of new policy programs (Porto de Oliveira 2017a). For example, an international policy network funded by the European Union (URB-AL) played a central role in supporting new PB programs. The city of Porto Alegre and a local NGO, Cidade, were key partners in this transition, thus helping to anchor knowledge-transfer to newly adopting cities or those considering PB programs. An NGO based in Ecuador was a key part of the URB-AL process, helping to spread knowledge about PB across the region in conjunction with an urban planner and academic, Yves Cabannes, at the center of efforts to encourage CSOs, NGOs, and governments to adopt PB (Cabannes 2014; Porto de Oliveira 2017a; Cabannes 2019).

The second wave of PB's diffusion involved its mainstreaming into development thinking as a viable democratic policymaking option (World Bank 2003a; Shah 2007). We begin to see cases of mimetic adoption in this era as national-level government officials were influenced by the purported successes of Brazilian PB programs. National-level governments began to require subnational governments to adopt PB to help address a wide range of governance problems.

Most famously, Peru was the first country to mandate universal PB adoption. Peru created a legal framework in 2003 to require all subnational governments to use the program. President Alejandro Toledo, who spent many years as an economist at the World Bank, signed onto this reform effort after officials in the powerful Ministry of Economics and Finance advocated for a national PB law. President Toledo, elected in 2001, had a broad mandate to reform basic governing institutions that would help Peru recover from two decades of civil war, authoritarian rule by President Fujimori, and economic destabilization (McNulty 2011). In this case, however, the PB law emerged in a decidedly neoliberal environment. In 2003, when Brazil's radical democratic experiment was enshrined in Peru's national legal framework, it was adapted into a technical policymaking tool designed to improve decentralized governance. During the early 2000s, the World Bank was attempting to move beyond the initial "Washington Consensus," which was based on the neoliberal tenets of a smaller state, privatization of national companies, greater trade integration, and reduced public spending. The Peruvian example fits into the logic of the second-generation neoliberal reforms, or the "Revised Washington Consensus," in which PB was a technical tool designed to improve policymaking processes rather than a radical democratic project (McNulty 2011; Baiocchi and Ganuza 2017).

The World Bank began to promote PB as a viable policymaking institution during this second wave of diffusion (Shah 2007; Goldfrank 2012). Officials within the World Bank began to conduct research on PB in the early 2000s; the first World Bank study on Porto Alegre's PB was published in 2008 and their first comparative case-study book came out in 2007 (Shah 2007). In addition to the World Bank, other examples of international donors promoting PB include USAID (a branch of the U.S. State Department), which supported El Salvador's adoption of PB programs (Bland 2011). By 2020, PB, or an offshoot named participatory planning and budgeting, was a commonly used programming tool employed within World Bank projects. For example, Kenya's Accountable Devolution Program includes PB as one mechanism to identify development needs and distribute projects across rural, underserved counties.

The introduction of organizations like the World Bank and USAID as major proponents of PB marks a key shift in the program's trajectory (Goldfrank 2012; Mansuri and Rao 2012). These organizations downplayed the original PB models' more radical democratic and social justice components. Instead, they placed much greater emphasis on PB's potential for incremental policymaking and governance. Ganuza and Baiocchi argue that the involvement of these organizations is driving PB toward becoming a technical policymaking tool (2012, 2017). The radical democratic principles that made PB a "school of democracy" in Brazil had largely disappeared. Major international organizations supported programs that included the technical aspects of PB's incremental policymaking but did not include key rules that promoted social justice.

Key Adaptations of the Second Wave (mid-1990s through mid-2000s)
Four major adaptations to the original Porto Alegre PB model emerged during this timeframe. The first major change was that national governments began to require subnational units to adopt PB. Peru (2003) and the Dominican Republic (2007) were at the fore of this shift (McNulty 2011, 2019). Mandating PB significantly alters local politicians' incentives to be involved in the programs; PB becomes a top-down effort driven by the national government in this context rather than a part of a local project to reform policy. Mandating PB became a way for national governments to promote the strengthening of democracy as well as additional transparency processes in policymaking at the local level. From the original two cases of PB in Latin America, this adaptation was widely diffused during the third wave of adoption.

Second, governments began experimenting with different ways to incorporate citizens into the PB process during this era. For example, governments in Córdoba and Seville, Spain, developed a mixed form of participation—CSOs and NGOs directly appointed some participants, while other participants came from the general population. In Indonesia, governments invited citizens to participate. This reflects governments' turn away from the "open participation" rule-set of the original PB program and toward a system of incorporating citizens and organizations that governments already know and work with. This obviously lowers the varied costs associated with recruiting people to attend meetings, but it creates a potential problem in that governments may be using PB to reach out to their political allies and ignore their critics. By shifting emphasis on who gets to participate (which largely means that the government is responsible for recruiting/ inviting participants), there is now a greater likelihood that PB will be an "invited space" whereby government allies are the most likely participants (Cornwall and Coelho 2007).

A third major adaptation of the second wave was the shift to consultative decision-making in project selection and away from binding decision-making. This shift meant that governments accepted citizen input but they did not necessarily make a firm commitment to implement the citizens' chosen projects or programs. This was evident in the Dominican Republic and Spain. These PB programs emphasized the importance of citizens' voice in deliberation, but minimized citizens' voice in final project selection. This adaptation in conjunction with the "invited participation" issue, identified in the previous paragraph, creates a policymaking environment in which government supporters are the most likely to engage in these public venues; they are less likely to directly contest and disagree with government officials. Thus, the combination runs the risk of creating a "toothless" PB process whereby governments and their allies dominate these processes with little to no push-back from citizens.

Finally, governments began to de-emphasize social justice criteria as the basis through which citizens would use PB to distribute resources in this era. Many cities did not include specific social justice rules in their programs, especially those that we categorize as the results of coercive and mimetic adoption processes. The lack of rules that govern resource distribution means that PB programs that are more recently adopted are more likely to replicate existing patterns of allocation rather than creating new forms of allocation. Although it is possible that PB programs without specific social justice rules will increase spending in traditionally under-funded and poor communities, this change in spending is increasingly contingent on direct government support rather than drawn from PB's core design features.

In sum, the combination of adaptations during the second wave of adoption suggests that PB became unmoored from its radical democratic principles. There was a simultaneous taming of the most democratic aspects of the program as well as a push to make it a well-structured policymaking institution. Some leaders adopting PB were inspired by the more radical democratic features of the original program, but other governments were more interested in PB as a policymaking tool.

Third Wave of Diffusion: PB's Rapid Spread around the Globe, mid-2000s through 2020

The international adoption of PB increased during the third wave of diffusion as governments in Europe, North America, Africa, Asia, and Australia adopted and adapted PB to meet their political, social, and governance needs. During this period, we find normative adoption led by leftist-oriented governments and civil society groups (e.g., Participatory Budgeting Project or the International Observatory of Participatory Democracy) as they sought to promote new forms of citizen engagement. We also have a major push toward mimetic adoption as a growing number of governments sought to adopt PB, which was becoming part of the international "tool kit" of democratic policymaking tools (Dagnino and Panfichi 2006; Fung and Wright 2003; Peck and Theodore 2015; Baiocchi and Ganuza 2017). Importantly, we also find that coercive adoptions increase during this third wave of diffusion, which is attributable to the rise of PB as a central part of the international policy reform agenda. Thus, two factors differentiate the second and third waves of diffusion: By 2006, PB was a widely recognized international best practice, which meant that centrist, moderate governments were willing to adopt it because it wasn't a massive overhaul of existing systems. The second major shift was that international organizations began to insist that their partners, often local governments in Global South countries, must use PB as one component among greater reform efforts.

The pace of PB adoption quickened during the third-wave period due to the work of organizations like the World Bank, the European Union, the Participatory Budgeting Project, the International Observatory of Participatory Democracy, Empatía, and the Open Government Partnership; these organizations provided resources, personnel, and technical assistance to help governments adopt these programs (Porto de Oliveira 2017a). The aforementioned groups represent a wide range of policy and ideological positions, suggesting that PB had become well-entrenched in international policy and political communities as a viable institution to solve a myriad of problems.

During this period, we see normative, mimetic, and coercive forms of adoption; the motivation behind policy adoption is strongly associated with the type of adaptations that PB programs experienced. When normative commitments to democracy motivate governments, they are more likely to emphasize rules that promote democracy, community mobilization, and building trust. When improving governance motivates governments, their adaptations are more strongly associated with the principles of efficiency, transparency, and government effectiveness rather than social justice. During this third wave (mid-2000s through 2020), the most common form of adoption was coercive, as more national governments required subnational governments to have PB (Dominican Republic, Poland, Indonesia) or governments were induced to adopt PB by major international organizations (Kenya, El Salvador). The World Bank's involvement heavily influenced PB's adoption in sub-Saharan Africa, where governance and social accountability teams from the World Bank worked with in-country World Bank professionals to promote PB as a means to achieve transparency and improve service delivery (World Bank 2003b, Shah 2007). In the words of Baiocchi and

Ganuza, PB thus transforms into a governance "technique" or "tool," moving away from its more democratic roots (2017). Logically, this shift makes sense because the World Bank does not directly promote democracy, focusing instead on citizen empowerment, social accountability, and transparency as means to achieve social and political change.

During this third wave, PB spread across Africa and Southeast Asia, often at the behest of international organizations, most importantly the World Bank. The World Bank was directly associated with the adoption of PB in Mozambique, Kenya, Ethiopia, Uganda, Indonesia, and Russia (Shah 2007; Dias et al. 2019). The World Bank's promotion of PB was part of a "best practice" suite of reforms—we characterize this as mimetic adoption because World Bank officials sought to promote best practices (Goldfrank 2012). But the story gets more complicated when we consider these practices from the perspective of government officials who are being "strongly encouraged" to adopt PB, thus suggesting more subtle forms of coercion. Within the Global South, dual pressures are present: Many local governments are interested in adopting PB because it is identified as a best practice, but these governments are also strongly encouraged by national government or international organizations to adopt PB. Thus, it is a combination of mimetic and coerced adoption. National governments mandate that local governments implement these programs. International organizations have the power and authority to "strongly insist" that recipient countries adopt their policy recommendations because their programs carry essential development funding, which governments rely on to deliver services and build capacity. In 2017, the World Bank began to require that citizen participation be included in all its development projects, which meant that countries must adopt some sort of citizen engagement if they want to receive external funding (World Bank 2020). Although World Bank-sponsored projects can use other participatory programs, PB is a common option because it touches on the key aspects of participation, policymaking, budgeting, and transparency.

We most clearly see the normative adoption of PB in the older, better-established democracies of the United States, Canada, and Europe during this third wave of diffusion. Governments in this region are not influenced by international organizations in the same ways that many countries in the Global South are. In the United States and Canada, civil society activists drove PB adoption to draw attention to the benefits of these programs. The programs in the United States and Canada place a stronger emphasis on democratic renewal as government officials and civil society activists try to move beyond the constraints associated with representative democracy. In many cases, a noted bias in representation and policy outcomes fosters a sense that democratic institutions are atrophying and require reform to engage, incorporate, and serve the broader population. PB represents an attempt at inclusive reform and engagement through direct, deliberative democracy; theoretically, these processes will produce policies and solve problems that better reflect public preferences and priorities.

Our research also reveals examples of governments adopting participatory programs that they label PB, but where PB's core principles (voice, vote, oversight, social justice, and social inclusion) are only minimally present. These types of projects suggest mimetic adoption because governments are not embedding these principles in key institutional design features, but are trying to associate a local program with the positive "PB brand." Thus, we hypothesize that mimetic-driven adoption, when there is limited local "political will" to support PB, is likely to produce more limited results than when PB programs are driven by normative pressures. The Paris PB program is noteworthy for adopting PB in 2015 and devoting a significant amount of resources to it—roughly USD125 million for citizens to allocate each year (Arhip-Paterson and Fouillet 2018). This level of spending was far higher and much more extensive than in comparable cities such as Chicago and New York (Russon 2016). And yet, a close examination demonstrates that the Parisian PB process does not promote extensive deliberation or citizen decision-making. Rather, Paris's PB largely depends on an online process in which citizens and community groups can register their proposals. Although the adoption of digital democracy is at the cutting edge of democratic innovations, we find that this normative goal does not include aspects of more radical democratic projects that seek to empower the most marginalized members of the population and it does not include in-person deliberation as a mechanism for social transformation.

Finally, we also see subnational PB adoption in authoritarian environments during this most recent wave. The most prominent cases are in China and Russia (Wu and Wang 2011; Cabannes and Ming 2014; Wu 2014; Cabannes 2019). In China, government officials and a small group of NGOs advocated for the adoption of PB as a means to improve local governance. Chinese PB programs share some of PB's broader principles—greater citizen involvement in deliberation, increased oversight, and an effort to expand social inclusion. However, China's overarching sociopolitical environment moves the program far from PB's roots as a radical democratic process. In Russia, the World Bank worked closely with regional and municipal governments to implement PB programs. The programs in the more rural areas had a stronger emphasis on basic infrastructure development and building social accountability. The programs in the urban areas focused on building community and trust. In this book, we mostly focus on democratic country case studies, but we do explicate some cases of PB in authoritarian contexts in Africa and Asia and return to this issue in the conclusion.

We continue to lack systematic analysis on the quality and scope of PB principles (voice, vote, oversight, social justice, and social inclusion) in practice in authoritarian national contexts, but two points stand out. First, it is possible that governments can effectively use PB programs in authoritarian environments to improve governance without any sort of movement toward multi-party democracy or the expansion of rights. These improvements come through giving public officials better access to citizens' demands, which then allows governments to prioritize which projects they invest in. In addition, it is also possible that generating local oversight can create internal accountability mechanisms that permit high-level officials to better monitor the activities of lower-level officials. This may help to generate greater legitimacy for the government because lower-ranking government officials are motivated to provide policies that are beneficial to the communities that they oversee. Within authoritarian regimes, PB very much resembles Baiocchi and Ganuza's description of it as a "technical policymaking" tool.

Second, we note that the principles associated with PB and the accompanying program design elements began to take shape at the end of military rule in Brazil prior to its democratic transition (and in parallel processes in Indonesia). Local governments took advantage of small political windows of opportunity to experiment with new ways of structuring state–society relations (Trajan 2015). In this sense, PB was part of a larger process in which some governments and civil society activists sought to build democracy. Thus, we recognize the possibility that PB may be part of a citizen-empowerment process of more deliberative, open decision-making, which could serve as a step toward democracy, even if the overall context in which it is adopted is not democratic. However, the limited research currently available on PB in authoritarian regimes in China and Russia does not indicate that PB is expanding citizens' civil, political, or social rights (He 2011; Wu and Wang 2011; Cabannes and Ming 2014; Wu 2014).

Key Adaptations of the Third Wave (mid-2000s through 2020)
Two key design adaptations took place during the third wave of diffusion. The first was a shift to PB at the sub-municipal or district level. This adaptation allows lower-level government officials to experiment where city-level officials may have been unwilling to do so. There is no set program design strategy for sub-municipal PB. For example, Toronto initiated PB in a public housing authority (Lerner 2014), whereas Chicago adopted PB in a single ward. New York City's PB began in four city council districts, the program in Vallejo, California, was linked to a municipal bond, and Boston's PB was exclusively youth-focused. This adaptation allows for interesting experimentation around program design that can be altered to pursue very specific outcomes. It is noteworthy that all of the aforementioned projects sought to emphasize social inclusion, suggesting that these adaptations were broadly normative.

Second, the expanded use of technology in PB represents another key transformation in the third wave of diffusion. This adaptation follows the dramatic decrease in the cost of technology, in terms of both hardware and software. Of course, PB was created in the late 1980s, prior to the digital revolution. During the third wave, government officials across the world sought to take advantage of lower costs by creating new means of incorporating technology. This included using technology to deliberate (e.g., Empatía and its European PB programs), using an online system to propose projects (e.g., Paris, Madrid), using technology to map projects and future needs (Surakarta, Nairobi), and using an online platform to select projects (Madrid, Paris).

Parallel Developments of Similar Institutions

As noted earlier, policy and political institutions that are strikingly similar to PB emerged prior to and during these three waves of diffusion (Heller 2001; Selee and Peruzzotti 2009; Melgar 2010; Rifai 2017). These programs emphasized citizen participation, direct engagement of citizens in budget-related processes, social inclusion of excluded individuals and groups, oversight, and social justice consideration. Some morphed into programs that are now called PB and others did not.

To best understand these parallel developments, it is useful to recall that the core principles underpinning PB can be traced back to important debates about participatory democracy in political theory circles and later policy circles, especially in Europe. In other words, the principles and ideas associated with PB were not new. Key ideas about participatory democracy circulated among political theorists in the 1700s and 1800s. Jacques Rousseau nodded to the importance of direct democracy in his work on the social contract and these ideas are reflected in movements such as the Paris Commune in the late 1800s. A century later, in 1962, the Students for a Democratic Society in the United States published the Port Huron Statement, which was a call for greater involvement of citizens in participatory democracy venues. By the time that PB emerged in Porto Alegre, leftist activists and labor movements around the world had advocated for participatory forms of democratic arrangement for more than one hundred years.

It was novel, however, that these ideas became grounded in the international development lexicon in the 1980s and 1990s. NGOs like Oxfam International and donors like the Ford Foundation began working with local partners around the world to implement participatory planning techniques, such as participatory rural appraisals. At the same time, the Third Wave of Democracy began to spread into Latin America and Asia and leftists and civil society activists began to use these principles in their means of governing. Several brief examples from the Philippines, Indonesia, Senegal, India, and Bolivia illustrate these parallel developments. In three examples, the Philippines, Indonesia, and Senegal, we see the early programs transition into formal PB programs.

For example, in the Philippines, the "People's Power" movement led the return to democratic rule in 1986 with the ouster of the dictator Ferdinand Marcos. A 1991 decentralization law then gave cities greater authority. In Naga City, a newly elected government came to power in the early 1990s and adopted principles (e.g., direct citizen participation, oversight) similar to those associated with PB (Melgar 2010). Nearly two decades later in 2010, these Naga City government officials would serve as part of a reformist presidential administration and implement a PB program that was led by the national government (Magno 2013). The roots of PB in the Philippines are thus deeply entrenched in the specific sociopolitical configuration of the country. Yet, the government also drew from international experiences to take advantage of new rules and processes that were not part of the original cases in Naga City.

The World Bank also led one of the most ambitious village-level participatory programs in Indonesia during the late 1990s (Gibson and Woolcock 2008; Barron et al. 2011). The development of Community-Driven Development in Indonesia and the Philippines was based on principles similar to PB—citizens deliberate in public venues and are then directly involved in deciding how public resources will be allocated. These programs also included specific oversight mechanisms (Gibson and Woolcock 2008; Labonne and Chase 2009, Barron et al. 2011). The program gained momentum following the 1999 ouster of the longtime dictator, Suharto, and eventually expanded to all seventy-four thousand Indonesia villages around the rubric of participatory planning and budgeting. In addition, some Indonesian cities implemented a city-level PB program in 2002 based on ideas and principles gathered by activists during a junket to the Philippines.

In Senegal, the rural community of Fissel adopted a PB-like program in 2002 (Gaye 2008; Porto de Oliveira 2017a). The adoption of PB in Senegal is associated with a decentralization process that began in 1996 and increased local governments' involvement in public spending. This process also increased attention on such issues as citizen participation, social control, and transparency. More specifically, Fissel's program advocates the following principles: social inclusion and participation, equity, accountability, transparency, sustainability, efficacy, and civic engagement (Gaye 2008). Fissel is a somewhat exceptional case in that it adopted a PB-type program without strong ties to the international development and political communities. Other Senegalese cities began to adopt PB programs in the 2010s as well, but this was often done in conjunction with international donors and development agencies.

In some countries, however, the participatory programs did not evolve into formal PB programs. For example, in Bolivia, the 1994 Law of Popular Participation codified participatory development planning processes in all municipal governments in the country (see Blanes 2000; Maydana 2004; Albó 2008; McNulty 2019). The law emerged as a response to an economic crisis that had hit the country in the late 1980s and was billed as a second-generation structural reform effort. The participatory process outlined in the law formalized neighborhood organizations which could participate in development planning and propose development projects to the municipal leaders, who then debated them and determined what to fund.

A citywide oversight committee, made up of members of these same organizations, then monitored the project spending to hold their officials to account. However, participants do not select projects directly and do not allocate a fixed proportion of the budget. These programs use deliberation as a way to inform citizens' project proposals, but the government has no requirement to fund any of these projects. Thus, Bolivia's programs are distinct from the Brazilian programs, but are clearly within the same family of reform.

The Communist Party of India-Marxist (CPM) won the 1996 governor's race in Kerala, a state located in India's southwest (Heller 2001). The CPM launched the "People's Plan Campaign" to democratize policymaking processes at the village level (panchayat). To accomplish this goal, the government mobilized an already active civil society and devolved significant financial resources to the villages. The Kerala Planning Board reports that upwards of 2.5 million people participated in the village-level meetings in 2000. Furthermore, Heller (2001) reports that between 35 percent and 40 percent of the participatory programs' resources were directly allocated to the villages. "A remarkable result of the campaign has been the mobilization of local resources, both in the form of financial and labor contributions. That citizens are parting with their time and income to contribute to local government initiatives suggests that institutional reform has created new incentives and opportunities for local action" (Heller 2001: 143). The "People's Plan Campaign" never formally adopted the name "Participatory Budgeting." A subsequent government, from a different political party, discontinued the participatory program. Yet, we consider the Kerala program as belonging to the category of programs that are "PB-like" because it shares many of the same principles—citizens gain voice, exercise vote, engage in oversight, and the programs encourage social inclusion and social justice.

In sum, governments in far-flung places across the globe adopted programs based on principles similar to those in Porto Alegre. They faced a series of challenges similar to those in Brazil and had similar "windows of opportunity" that allowed them to produce new programs. Initially, these programs were not branded or labeled "PB," but in some places, like Indonesia and the Philippines, a shift occurred as their proponents began to call them PB in international venues. This shift to make their programs more like PB suggests mimetic adaptation because government officials were motivated to alter their rules to be in better alignment with international norms. At the same time, these new PB experiences have much greater differences in institutional design than they do in the core organizing principles, reflecting the range of opportunities available to governments at the time of adoption rather than differences in core principles. We now present a typology of PB that allows us to better illuminate how the timing and sequencing of adoption affected how local governments adapted the rules to meet policy and political needs within their local context.

Typology of PB Programs

In this section, we distinguish among different types of PB programs using five criteria. Four of the criteria are directly related to the core principles (vote, voice, social inclusion, social justice, and oversight) and a fifth factor focuses on the implementing agents' motivation for adopting PB. Typologies help classify similar programs with the goal of (a) generalizing from a small number of experiences to a greater number and (b) setting expectations regarding what we should expect from existing programs (Collier et al. 2012). However, it is important to keep in mind that typologies are useful for analytical purposes and never neat in practice. In reality, specific programs may share characteristics of more than one type and real-world examples may overlap. Although we recognize some programs may have characteristics associated with more than one type, we classify PB programs based on their most dominant characteristics.

This typology builds on two noteworthy examples of similar efforts where researchers developed either a typology or a taxonomy of PB programs. Sintomer, Röcke, and Herzberg (2008, 2016) developed a typology based on European cases, focusing on differences in participation as the key distinguishing features that separate PB programs. This approach is useful because it considers how variation in institutional design affects who participates as well as what participants do within PB. Because their approach is limited to European cases, their typology does not capture three of the six types that we develop here. Cabannes and Lipietz (2018) developed a taxonomy of PB programs based on three competing logics that form distinct clusters, or types, of PB cases: Political (or Radical Democratic), Good Governance, and Technocratic. Their article advances our understanding of PB because it acknowledges how adopting governments are motivated by very different reasons to experiment with a PB program. We move beyond this taxonomy to include a broader number of cases that can better capture the diversity of experiences.

We distinguish our typology from these other approaches by closely aligning it with PB's core principles as well as emphasizing key actors' motivations for adoption. The degree to which the following five factors are present in each program to create the typology: "Participant engagement," "internal decision-making process," "resource allocation," "degree of local control over resources," and "actors driving adoption." Variations across these criteria help us to distinguish among different PB programs. We develop many examples of these types in Chapters 3, 4, 5, and 6.

"Participant engagement" captures the degree to which PB is open to all citizens and the means through which citizens are recruited to participate in PB. When the process is open to a greater range of citizens, we hypothesize that there is a greater likelihood for including a diversity of voices during key deliberations. Conversely, when governments selectively invite citizens to participate, we hypothesize that debate will be more constrained because the principal participants are government allies or a target audience. This criterion thus taps into the extent to which citizens can exercise *voice*. It also taps into the extent to which local governments are able to successfully promote *social inclusion*, particularly regarding the participation of individuals and groups that generally have limited access to political decision-making processes.

The "internal decision-making process" addresses how citizens exercise a vote in the PB process. More specifically, it first captures whether decisions are reached through a specific vote or through consensual deliberation. We hypothesize that decision-making processes that permit a secret ballot are more likely to represent the interests of more marginalized communities. We also hypothesize that consensual decision-making limits the independence of citizens from government officials. This criterion thus taps into the form and intensity of *vote*.

The "resource allocation" criterion captures whether the programs specifically allocate resources to traditionally underserviced and poor communities. We hypothesize that programs that include specific mechanisms to ensure that resources are allocated to poorer communities will more likely advance social justice considerations. Conversely, we hypothesize that programs that do not include specific social justice mechanisms are much less likely to ensure that poorer, disadvantaged communities receive resources. This criterion taps into the *social justice* principle.

"Degree of local control over resources" refers to the extent that implementing governments have both the administrative authority and financial resources (tax revenues) to implement projects selected by citizens. We hypothesize that greater local control over finances as well as greater availability of resources and state capacity will incentivize governments to allocate their resources to PB programs; when governments have sufficient flexibility they are willing to create a broader role for citizens in the policymaking process. Conversely, when governments have limited resources, they are likely to allocate few resources to PB programs. The implication is that when resource-poor governments adopt PB, they may be unable to implement many PB projects because they lack the basic state capacity and resources to do so. This criterion thus taps into the *oversight* principle because it is based on the degree of local control over resources as well as the ability of citizen-participants to monitor program spending. Of course, this moves beyond the oversight principles to reflect the extent to which local governments have the capacity to implement projects discussed and selected by citizens.

Building on the earlier section of this chapter, the "actors driving adoption" criterion captures the motivations (normative, mimetic, and coercive) that drive governments' decision-making and the level of adoption (e.g., municipal, subnational, national). We hypothesize that as the intensity of norm-driven local support increases, so too will the likelihood that the government will allocate the necessary political, administrative, and financial support for PB. Conversely, when the program is driven by mimetic or coercive pressures, there is a greater likelihood that the programs will be narrower in scope. This criterion also moves beyond the core principles as it captures the actors who are most strongly promoting the adoption of the program.

These five factors form the basis for a typology of PB cases, summarized in Table 1.1. Although we can analytically distinguish among the five factors, it is important to note that they are not fully independent from each other. Rather, the factors interact to produce different outcomes. For example, when governments recruit their allies to participate (voice), when they use consensual decision-making (vote), and when there are no formal rules around redistributive politics (social justice), it becomes far more likely that the PB program will represent the government's core interest. In turn, these types of programs are unlikely to produce either the deepening of democracy or the foundations for accountability. Conversely, when governments successfully recruit a broader range of participants (voice), when they use a secret ballot (vote), and when there are formal rules around redistributive politics (social justice), it becomes far more likely that the PB program will produce outcomes that promote democracy, accountability, and human development.

Based on the aforementioned criteria, we can thus identify six types of PB and their key distinguishing features:

- Empowered Democracy and Redistribution
- Deepening Democracy through Community Mobilization
- Mandated by National Government
- Digital PB
- Social Development and Accountability
- Efficient Governance

Empowered Democracy and Redistribution

Key distinguishing features include participation open to all, binding decision-making through a secret vote, and rules that require that greater resources to be spent in poorer, under-resourced communities. These PB programs are the most radical because they are designed to encourage the participation of poor communities and also seek to distribute greater allocations of public resources to these communities through the PB program. These programs seek to empower new actors that are engaging in politics and ensure that resources are spent to address their needs. The adoption of these programs is driven by normative considerations as local governments are highly motivated to dramatically alter how local politics works. Key examples include the pioneering cases of Porto Alegre, Belo Horizonte, and Recife, three mid- to large-sized cities in Brazil.

Table 1.1. Typology of PB global programs

PB type	Participation	Decision-making	Resource allocation criteria	Local control of resources	Actors driving adoption
Empowered Democracy and Redistribution	Open to all; sub-districts further localize participation	Secret ballot; binding decisions	Poor communities receive more funding	Moderate to high	Normative; municipal-led
Deepening Democracy through Community Mobilization	Open to all; sub-districts further localize participation	Mixed voting methods; binding and consultative processes	No fixed rules; general support for social justice.	Moderate to limited	Normative; led by municipal and sub-municipal
Mandated by National Government	No fixed rules—depends on local officials' interests	Varied; depends on local officials' interests	No fixed rules	Unfunded financial mandate	Mimetic and coercive; national-led
Digital PB	Online	Online; often focuses on pre-selected menu	No fixed rules	Moderate to high	Normative and mimetic; municipal-led
Social Development and Account-ability	Often invited	Consensus-based	None	Minimal	Coercive and mimetic; led by international and national actors
Efficient Governance	No fixed rules—depends on local officials' interests	Limited; consultative processes	None	Moderate to high	Mimetic, technocratic governments seeking efficiencies

Source: Authors.

Deepening Democracy through Community Mobilization

Key distinguishing features include participation open to all, an emphasis on social inclusion of politically marginalized groups, varied voting methods that lead to semi-binding decisions, and a stronger emphasis on building community through deliberation. Although the programs are inspired by the ideological values of the original PB cases in Brazil, they don't have specific social justice rules because of local political considerations. In the North American context, many of the programs are at sub-municipal levels while in the European context, implementation is most often at the municipal level. Examples include New York City, Chicago, Toronto, Córdoba, Seville, and Mexico City.

Mandated by National Government

Key distinguishing features include a national requirement that subnational governments must use PB as part of their annual budget process. National governments may provide technical guidance that helps subnational governments implement these programs, but this is often minimum. National governments often do not provide additional resources to help subnational governments implement projects selected by citizens. In most cases, national governments appear to be driven by mimetic considerations; when PB became an international "best practice," national governments were willing to adopt it in the hopes that they could improve basic governance. Key examples include Peru, the Dominican Republic, Poland, Indonesia, and South Korea. It is plausible that over half of all PB cases are mandated by national governments.

Digital PB

A key distinguishing feature is that most participation is conducted online. Citizens propose and vote on projects through online processes; some programs also include deliberative venues that permit an exchange of ideas and information of the existing programs. Parallel to the online programming, there may also be off-line participation opportunities to propose policies and vote. At the core of digital programs are efforts to include greater numbers of participants and overcome the high opportunity costs associated with participation in most face-to-face PB programs. A combination of normative and mimetic forces appears to influence governments to adopt digital programs. Their normative interests can be seen most strongly in their innovative uses of digital platforms; in some ways, they are creating new ways to engage citizens. But their motivations are also influenced by the mimetic adoption—these digital programs work within the general umbrella concept of PB, with an adherence to its core principles. Key programs include Paris, Madrid, and Barcelona.

Social Development and Accountability

Key distinguishing features include an emphasis on human development outcomes (e.g., Sustainable Development Goals), the use of consensus-based decision-making, and the active involvement of external development agencies in promoting PB. A notable change within this typology is that participants and governments are both highly interested in producing specific policies that can positively affect local human development. In addition, there is also a strong emphasis on transparency, which is supposed to increase oversight and accountability. In terms of motivations, most programs are "coerced" by international development organizations. PB is now an international gold standard, which means that international agencies such as the World Bank, USAID, and DFID are more likely to insist on its adoption as part of broader governance reform. Although subnational governments may be normatively predisposed to support PB, we believe that the relative strength of the international agencies means that the adoption of these programs is coercive. Key examples include Kenya, Mozambique, and El Salvador.

Efficient Governance

Key distinguishing features include an emphasis on using citizen participation as a mechanism to improve spending efficiencies in order to make better use of taxpayer revenues.[2] There is a strong emphasis on transparency, as government officials seek to demonstrate to the broader public that they are working to use public resources more efficiently. Mimetic motivations drive the adoption of these programs, as adopting governments seek to align their practices within international best practices. In these cases, adopting governments primarily seek to improve service delivery through citizen consultation. Key programs can be found Germany, Poland, and, to a lesser extent, France and South Korea.

Like all typologies, this is an analytical tool that helps us describe and better understand the numerous PB programs around the world. In practice, some PB programs may not fit neatly into a type, but may cross the boundaries of two types. For example, South Korea and Poland mandate that subnational governments adopt PB, but these programs also have characteristics associated with the

---

[2] We draw heavily from the excellent work of Sintomer, Röcke, and Herzberg (2016) to better understand the motivations and functioning of the Efficient Governance type.

Efficient Governance type. However, we classify them as Mandated because the programs' core characteristics are more closely related to the Mandated type than to the Efficient Governance type. The added benefit of this typology is that it helps to organize a broad number of cases into specific types that then allows us to better understand the patterns and groupings of PB adaptions; this typology links PB's core principles, the diffusion process, and design characteristics to provide a useful framework to understand the rapid pace of change. In Chapter 2, we are also able to hypothesize about the potential changes that we should expect from the different types.

Conclusion

PB continues to spread around the world, changing in interesting and important ways. The adaptation of PB to better address the local context and political interests of governments and/or civil society activists is a hallmark of PB's evolution over thirty years. Early PB cases were municipal-led programs in which leaders tried to invert the political priorities of local governments; these cases are represented by the Empowered Democracy and Redistribution type. Between 1995 and 2020, governments significantly adapted PB in fundamental ways. For example, PB is now housed at the sub-municipal level (Toronto, New York City, Chicago); it is mandated by national governments (Peru, Poland, Indonesia); it uses consensus-based decision-making (Kenya, Mozambique); and promotes online participation (Paris and Madrid). In this chapter, we develop a typology of PB programs that classifies programs based on their adherence to the core set of PB principles, defined in the introductory chapter. This classification scheme enables us to provide a more comprehensive understanding of wide variation.

Our research demonstrates that there is no single impulse driving adoption. Rather, we can identify three mechanisms that best account for the different motivations for government adoption of these programs: normative, mimetic, and coercive. As we explain in Chapter 2, the range and breadth of social and political change expected from these programs can be linked in part to the motivations associated with their adoption. We find that radical democratic principles motivated governments in the pioneering cases of PB; we would expect that these governments will more heavily invest in programs that promote social inclusion and social justice. In other cases, governments adopt PB as they are seeking to learn from the international community; they want to adopt programs that improve how the state functions as well as improving state-society relationships. These mimetic motivations are important because they signal that governments are interested in some type of reform, although they may not be willing to take the more radical steps of delegating authority to citizens. Finally, many governments are strongly induced to do so by their international partners.

Based on the typology, we identify four distinct groupings of PB adaptation. First, PB entered wealthier democracies through the lens of Deepening Democracy through Community Mobilization. In these cases, centrist, or center-left governments adopted PB as a means to promote social inclusion and overcome citizen apathy, especially among more marginalized groups. Importantly, many of these groups were inspired by the Porto Alegre PB program, but they were unable to adopt the specific redistribution rules due to the local political context. Second, we find most cases of Social Development and Accountability to be in the Global South, especially in resource-strapped countries. This particular type is driven by international organizations (e.g., World Bank, USAID), which seek to use small-scale projects to improve development outcomes as well as to lay the foundations for accountability.

Third, we find greater variation in where PB is being Mandated by National Government, but a commonalty across these countries is that the national government seeks to induce local governments to alter their policymaking process through national directives. Finally, we also find that the Efficient Governance and Digital Participation types are most likely to be found among the wealthier democracies. For the former, government officials adapt PB to help them modernize their policymaking processes, often using consultative processes. We find that Digital Participation is most likely to be among wealthier countries, as governments have additional resources and administrative staff to implement these types of programs.

PB has the potential to transform people's lives. However, as it has been diffused we also know that many programs will have a limited impact because government officials and their civil society allies have few incentives and few resources to promote dramatic change. In Chapter 2, we develop a theory of change that more explicitly identifies the macro and meso conditions that establish parameters of change. We also theorize the links between the type of PB program and the parameters of change that we might expect from each one.

2

Theorizing PB's Effects on Individuals and Communities

PB began as a radical democratic policymaking process linked to a broader political project whose architects hoped would empower citizens and lead to significant social and political transformation. PB's advocates believed that they had found an institutional process that would deepen democracy and improve citizens' well-being. PB's popular appeal, therefore, is based on the fact that it combines the broader goals of deepening democracy with the mundane, technocratic process of incremental policymaking (Genro 1995; Santos 2005; Shah 2007). The opportunity to generate social change particularly appealed to reform-minded leaders in many parts of the Global South, where millions lack access to public goods, such as education and health care, and also live with poorly functioning democratic institutions.

As PB spreads around the world, researchers and practitioners are documenting a variety of ways that it changes individuals and communities. Researchers continue to gather evidence from across the globe that, in some cases, connects PB to positive and important changes such as shifts in public spending, an increase in civil society activities, enhancements in accountability, and improvements in well-being. However, it is crucial to emphasize that, in most places, researchers have either not found strong effects from PB or lack compelling data to evaluate PB's impact. Further, there is some evidence that PB can erode trust in government, generate cynicism, or lead to other negative effects on communities, which means that we should be cautious about naively extolling PB's virtues. Therefore, we know that PB produces positive outcomes in some contexts, but the evidence also demonstrates that it can produce weak or negative effects on communities in other circumstances.

There is a large scholarly literature on PB, including hundreds of articles, books, and chapters as well as an extensive literature produced by NGOs, CSOs, and community-based organizations. However, the broader academic and policy fields continue to lack a theoretical framework that identifies the causal mechanisms that produce social change. This lacuna is particularly salient as scholars explore broad numbers of cases located in different global regions. This chapter begins by summarizing the potential outcomes that PB programs can generate, as documented in ongoing research. Our framework first shows how change occurs at the individual level (among citizen participants, civil servants, and elected

Participatory Budgeting in Global Perspective. Brian Wampler, Stephanie McNulty, and Michael Touchton,
Oxford University Press. © Brian Wampler, Stephanie McNulty, and Michael Touchton 2021.
DOI: 10.1093/oso/9780192897756.003.0003

officials). The model then demonstrates that change also occurs at the community-level in three key areas: accountability, civil society, and well-being. Following this review of the potential outcomes generated by PB, the second part of the chapter identifies the macro and meso factors that condition these outcomes. Therefore, this chapter builds theory surrounding PB's causal mechanisms and provides a framework for expectations regarding where PB is most likely to have meaningful, positive impacts. We argue that this "theory of change" must be kept in mind when PB proponents design, implement, or support PB processes to capitalize on its potential in the short and long runs. In the final section of this chapter, we link this theory of change to the six PB types presented in Chapter 1 to establish the parameters of change most likely to be produced by each type of program. We expect that that there will be wide variation in PB outcomes across the six types.

Theory of Change

Our theory of change describes potential social and political outcomes associated with PB. We present an evidence-based overview of the capacity of PB to generate these outcomes and the factors that condition possible outcomes in three areas: stronger civil society, greater accountability, and improved well-being. The empirical evidence that we present in the regional chapters that follow help us to build our theory and illustrate key arguments.

Before explaining our conceptual model, however, several caveats are in order. The conceptual model presents an abstract theoretical process that is never neat nor linear in practice. The model explicates a causal process with multiple independent variables but, in reality, these variables continuously interact and the processes driving change are iterative. Further, in some aspects, a variable can be both the end (outcome) as well as the means to that change. For example, the civil society sector in a particular country is an explanatory factor (meso-level) that helps to explain variation in outcomes, but can also be part of an outcome that the PB process produces. More concretely, in most cases, having a denser, more engaged civil society is a positive factor that often improves the quality of PB. In turn, PB generates further advances in strengthening civil society. We recognize that this formulation could be construed as tautological, but we argue that co-governance institutions like PB are best understood when scholars show how citizens and CSOs affect and are affected by the new institution. Figure 2.1 below presents this framework graphically.

We begin our analysis with a discussion of the outcomes produced by PB, based on a broad review of the evidence. We posit that change begins at the individual level and then, potentially, aggregates up to community levels. We hypothesize that individual-level change has spillover effects that change aspects of their communities.

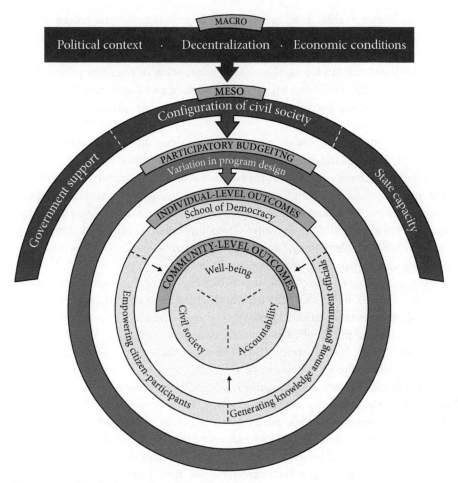

Figure 2.1. PB: Conceptual model of change

Individual-level Outcomes

Participants and public officials may change their attitudes and behaviors as they gain access to information, engage in new forms of deliberation, exercise their vote, and monitor implementation. We discuss the changes that have been documented by researchers in terms of three key actors in the PB process: citizen-participants, elected officials, and civil servants.

Citizens: Engaging, Deliberating, and Empowering

Extensive studies have shown that PB programs have the potential to *educate* citizen-participants through the dissemination of budget and policy data, engage them in *deliberative* "schools of democracy" within and beyond PB, and *empower* them to demand greater access to basic constitutionally guaranteed rights (Avritzer 2002; Nylen 2002, 2003; Baiocchi 2005; Wampler 2007; Lüchmann 2008; Pinnington et al. 2009; Baiocchi et al. 2011; Romão 2011). When PB processes do reach their potential in terms of social inclusion—that is, engaging people from a variety of backgrounds and experiences in debate and decision-making about public spending—a broad set of community members benefit from these outcomes.

A multi-pronged process generates individual-level changes in attitudes and behaviors. Through the PB process we can identify distinct ways that citizens' attitudes and behaviors change at the individual level, but we must be cognizant that more significant change is more likely to occur when several of these processes occur simultaneously and reinforce each other. We briefly turn to three areas—knowledge-building, learning about the inner workings of democracy (i.e., a school for democracy), and empowering participants—that best capture how and why PB can drive individual-level change.

First, increasing citizen-participants' policy and budget knowledge can build a base of information that sharpens their understanding of the policymaking process, and prepares them to better present their own interests in a public format as well as to engage public officials in more policy-oriented ways (Wampler 2007; Pinnington et al. 2009; Lerner 2014). Gaining policy-related knowledge often permits citizens to more actively work to promote their own interests. Gaining an understanding of how a complex state is designed (national, state, and local governments or the division of authority across sectors) allows citizens to direct their demands to appropriate public offices. For example, in 1998, government officials held a meeting at Porto Alegre's city hall where they provided detailed information regarding how the local state was organized as well as the different sources of revenue (e.g., local taxes, federal transfers). We have seen similar processes at work in Peru and Kenya. This learning process supported citizens' within PB but, perhaps more importantly, it can also help citizens more broadly as they engage different parts of the state beyond PB.

Second, PB will often act like a "school of democracy" whereby citizen-participants engage with other citizens inside and parallel to official programs (Baiocchi 2005; Pinnington et al. 2009; Lerner 2014). Citizens learn to deliberate, gain knowledge about how governments function, access specific information about budgets, and begin to engage in democratic practices. PB participants also learn about citizenship and their political rights, which theoretically activates them beyond the program. Citizens may change their attitudes and perceptions of local government when they are directly involved in these incremental policymaking processes. In turn, citizens often gain a better understanding of the constraints that governments face, especially in terms of the difficult trade-offs that government officials often have to make. In these circumstances, citizens gain the necessary skills to engage in more democratically oriented deliberations with other citizens as well as with community organizations. Finally, in places that bring a diverse group of community members together to deliberate, citizens also meet and interact with people from different backgrounds.

We have observed this happen around the world. For example, In April 2010, university professors held a meeting in Belo Horizonte where they provided a history of political organizing and participatory governance in Brazil. The objective was to work with community leaders to improve their mobilization efforts so that their communities would be better prepared to work within the participatory process. In 2014, Wampler and McNulty also observed city council members in Vallejo, CA talking to constituents about using PB to make tough choices about their very limited budget after the city declared bankruptcy in 2008.

Because of this education process, PB programs often incentivize individuals to work within CSOs, which subsequently induces citizens to engage their own communities differently (Baiocchi et al. 2011). Citizens and community leaders often discuss PB processes, project proposals, and implementation status in their communities, therefore linking non-participants to their community organizations as well as to the PB process. Case-study research has shown that PB participants increase their political participation beyond PB and join civil society groups following exposure to PB processes (Avritzer 2002; Wampler and Avritzer 2004; Wampler 2007; Baiocchi et al. 2011; Touchton and Wampler 2014; Lerner 2014; Hagelskamp et al. 2016).

Finally, PB can empower individual participants because it allows them to exercise democratic rights in a formal policymaking institution (Wampler 2007; Cabannes 2019). PB allows citizens to more actively exercise rights that are formally guaranteed under their country's constitutional framework. Democratic practice often allows citizens to use the rights they bear as members of the polity by deliberating and voting in public forums. Democracy can then gain support when citizens "practice" democracy through functional PB programs. This may increase trust of their fellow citizens as well as government officials. Working within PB could also increase perceptions of the legitimacy of democratic processes.

Importantly, there are considerable differences at the individual level along class, racial/ethnic, and gender dimensions that significantly affect how participants engage in broader PB processes. Basic social cleavages affect, first and foremost, who is likely to attend a meeting as well as how participants deliberate and vote during meetings. For example, women often make up a large percentage of participants in many Latin American and African processes, but they tend to have a smaller role in comparison to male participants, during key decision-making stages (Abers 2000; Baiocchi 2005; McNulty 2015; 2018; Ng 2015). With regard to class, some programs explicitly seek to incorporate poor and politically marginalized communities by creating specific "pro-poor" social justice rules designed to draw these citizens (Marquetti et al. 2008; Wampler and Touchton 2019).

We recognize the importance of these micro-level characteristics (gender, class, race, etc.) and consider them more explicitly at the meso level—configuration of civil society—as well as at the macro level—political context and economic conditions.

Elected Officials: Opening Access and Gathering Information

PB often induces elected government officials to alter how they exercise authority and engage the public. Individual-level change occurs when elected officials directly engage with citizens and community groups through the auspices of PB. First, government officials benefit from gathering information directly from community members, which then improves these officials' basic knowledge surrounding communities' needs (Public Agenda 2016). PB provides a forum where government officials can seek input from citizens about community needs and use that information to better target programs and projects within and beyond PB. Government officials also seek assistance with project implementation and oversight through PB, mobilizing community members as their eyes and ears to report waste, mismanagement, and fraud. Finally, PB provides a model for government officials to work with CSOs and citizen-leaders to co-govern in general, not just within PB. Expanding policy networks across civil society and community leadership provides a platform to work together on other issue areas and in other forums to sustain PB and improve governance. This is especially relevant for elected officials whose electoral incentives align with PB goals of promoting civil society and mobilizing marginalized populations in pursuit of development. Early reports from Kenya's experience suggest that PB produces at least some of these impacts, with citizens and community-based organizations working together to complete projects and reporting implementation delays to government officials (World Bank 2017). In Indonesia, government officials regularly meet with community leaders in the PB meetings to get a better idea of their general and specific demands.

Thus, PB may alter the ways government officials operate in other areas beyond PB, as well as how elected government officials calculate their interests, which may then produce social change. Elected officials gain important knowledge about citizens' preferences and needs. Not all officials desire this input, but those who do listen to citizens' preferences and needs can positively alter their behavior, change their priorities, and use PB to legitimize their decisions. In the United States, this information and process has also been credited with these officials' re-election (Public Agenda 2016). We posit that elected officials are more likely to invest the time and resources to ensure that PB works well when they believe that PB can affect their re-election opportunities. Of course, it becomes much less likely that they will dedicate the resources necessary to create vibrant PB programs capable of change if these officials calculate that PB will only have a marginal effect on their re-election efforts.

Civil Servants: Gathering Information and Realigning Administrative Processes

PB often induces elected civil servants and bureaucrats to alter how they engage the public, organize internal decision-making processes, and implement projects. Two broad types of civil servants are often involved in PB. We see civil servants who are engaged with organizing PB meetings, recruiting participants, and working directly with the public throughout the process. We also see more technically oriented civil servants, such as accountants, civil engineers, and medical professionals, involved in the process. We note that individual-level change among these civil servants occurs through two processes.

First, change occurs when these civil servants gain access to new information (Albert 2016). This mostly involves direct engagement with citizens, through which the public officials gain a better understanding of people's key needs and demands. It also occurs through site visits in which public officials visit the communities involved in PB, allowing the civil servants to better understand their complexity. This is particularly important in informal settlements and shantytowns where there is tremendous variation in neighborhood layout and basic infrastructure. For the more technically oriented civil servants, working in these informal settlements often requires a reboot of how they engage in the public. Service delivery and project implementation processes may be altered as a result of the new information.

Second, changes among civil servants also occur as they often modify internal administrative practices to ensure that projects are implemented (Albert 2016). If the traditional model is based on receiving projects from mayors, governors, and legislators, the new model is based on receiving project proposals from citizen-participants. The projects may be quite different than they are used to receiving, which requires technical staff members (e.g., engineers) to alter how they design and implement projects. During the implementation phase, civil servants often need to work closely with community leaders to explain the reasoning behind different implementation decisions, which also changes how civil servants serve the public.

Finally, we recognize that the relationship among civil servants, citizens, and elected officials can be quite contentious (Albert 2016; Foroughi 2017). Civil servants administering these programs provide the frontline response to participants who demand greater access to public resources. Many civil servants are thus placed in the difficult position of trying to balance the high expectations often associated with adoption of new programs with significant implementation constraints. The presence of contentious relationships helps remind us that there is a lot at stake for the different actors involved in the process—participants need access to public goods, politicians seek to develop a program that can advance their electoral ambitions, civil servants seek to advance their agencies and careers. Underlying the contentious activity is a basic power imbalance between the state and citizens, mainly of whom are poor and politically marginalized.

This section demonstrates that social change begins at the individual, or micro, level. The adoption of a PB program creates the opportunity for the people involved in PB—citizens, government officials, and civil servants—to change their attitudes and behaviors. Of course, we also know that the breadth of individual-level change will vary significantly across PB programs for reasons that are described in more detail below. And, in many cases, these changes are rare. For example, there is a large literature that documents civil servants using PB to co-opt or manipulate participants and participants getting frustrated with low quality meetings that lead them to stop coming (Wampler 2007; McNulty 2011; Albert 2016; Foroughi 2017). Here, our main argument is that individual-level change *can be* aggregated to communities around them. Finally, we highlight outcomes in areas that have already been observed while recognizing the possibility of outcomes across a broad spectrum that have yet to be recorded in practice. Thus, we summarize the known universe of PB outcomes but acknowledge that there may be many more beyond civil society, accountability, and well-being and among different actors.

From the Individual to the Community

PB programs generate broader impacts when individual-level changes in attitudes and behaviors are combined to produce change at the community level. We identify three areas where we are most likely to see change: civil society, accountability, and well-being. We note that PB promotes accountability and civil society through the entire program, rather than via specific development projects. By this we mean that although it might be possible to link specific infrastructure projects (e.g., access to a health clinic, a new well) to some elements of accountability or civil society, most improvements in community-wide accountability or civil society would occur because of a new forum for co-governance, a new focus on transparency, and a newly empowered population—not because of any specific project. Small improvements in well-being are indeed tied to local projects, but, there, too broader improvements are tied to PB programs' diffuse set of impacts across entire communities.

Civil Society

Adopting PB has led to stronger civil societies in many places around the world. We conceive of a stronger civil society along two dimensions. One includes "density," which generally refers to the number of CSOs in a given community (Putnam et al. 1994). Stronger civil society sectors can lead to increased advocacy, improved public policy outcomes, and increased social capital. The second dimension includes the repertoires of action—what these CSOs actually do (e.g., mobilization, organizing protests, engaging in social audits, participating in formal public venues, internal democracy). Thus, what CSOs are capable to doing within and parallel to PB matters considerably to how PB programs will function. In some places, the accompanying democratization of civil society will modify basic state–society relations at the local level (Avritzer 2002; Baiocchi 2005; Baiocchi et al. 2011; Goldfrank 2011).

Hordijk (2005), Baiocchi (2005), Baiocchi and Ganuza (2017), and Touchton and Wampler (2014) demonstrate that PB is associated with an increase in the number of CSOs operating in areas where governments use PB. Furthermore, Françoise Montambeault (2016) finds that, under certain conditions, participatory institutions can change the nature of state–society relations at the municipal level in Mexico and Brazil (see also Baiocchi et al. 2011). McNulty's (2013) work in Peru shows that, under some circumstances, PB can lead to increased funding and technical assistance skill-building for non-profit organizations. All of these studies document measurable outcomes that emerge in civil society due to PB.

Several examples of PB around the world illustrate these changes. For instance, Lambayeque, Peru, a small town on the country's northern coast, adopted PB in the early 2000s. CSOs came together for the first time to form a consortium of organizations to identify local priorities and advocate for them in PB forums. CSOs were also behind the initial push toward PB in Indonesia. In 2000, following the fall of the dictator Suharto, Indonesian civil society activists travelled to the Philippines to learn about their participatory programs; these activists sought to build new programs to increase the power and authority of citizen participation. In Indonesia, CSO activists sought to expand the role that citizens might play in new democracies. These activists partnered with a local government in Surakarta to launch the country's first city-level, PB-type program. This program placed a strong emphasis on the role of citizens and CSOs in the new participatory processes because CSO activists were a key part of the design process. As in these examples, PB is thought to produce a stronger civil society by increasing CSO density (number of groups) and changing their repertoires of action, such as expanding the range of CSO political activities and promoting policy-oriented partnerships with governments.

Accountability

PB can also promote changes in accountability by altering state–society relationships (Shah 2007; Wampler 2007, 2008; Baiocchi et al. 2011). By this, we mean that PB alters how citizens engage public officials as well as how public officials engage citizens. Accountability is a relational concept in which ongoing interactions between citizens and government officials affect how governments utilize public authority and public resources. PB affects this accountability relationship in several different ways. Initially, citizens voice their policy demands in a public forum, thus signaling their key needs to government officials. Some of these specific demands may be included in the budget, but are also part of a broader exchange of information which government officials will use to better inform their policy agenda.

PB's oversight mechanisms can play an important role for accountability. PB programs frequently include some sort of formal oversight institution such as a committee. These committees, when working well, can limit waste, fraud, and incompetence in project implementation. In turn, community members are more likely to hold governments to their promises to deliver services using their tax revenue and to perceive governments as legitimate. Individuals and firms are then more likely to comply with local tax regulations. For example, in Belo Horizonte, Brazil, community leaders are elected to an oversight committee, which then monitors each infrastructure project. The committee has several responsibilities, including approving the formal bid, ensuring that the correct materials are used, certifying that the project is built according to the contract, and finally, verifying that the project is complete to facilitate final payment. In the Vera Alta Cruz *favela*, an oversight committee monitored remodeling of a public health clinic to ensure that the project would be done properly (Wampler 2015). Committee members were aware that the public investment in their community was rare and so they wanted to make sure that the project was completed according to agreed-upon plans.

When not working well, oversight committees are much less likely to improve accountability. In Peru, oversight committees are notoriously weak, rarely meeting or visiting project sites after the PB process formally ends every year in July (Grupo Propuesta Ciudadana 2009; McNulty 2019). In some places, the government officials do not provide the information that the committee needs to perform its function. Members of these committees, typically volunteers from CSOs, do not receive funds to offset their travel costs, so it can be expensive for them to travel to project sites to check on the work. This partly explains the poor performance of PB in Peru.

One reason that social accountability through participatory institutions is possible is that transparency initiatives, such as Freedom of Information Acts, are also emerging around the world. There is a growing body of social science research that demonstrates that greater transparency helps citizens place an additional check on government officials (Fox 2015). Subnational governments are now required to make budget and project information public through their websites and reports. In turn, the PB process provides another forum for this information to be shared.

Government officials are now shining a light on budgets and policymaking processes, which creates a strong incentive for them to ensure that government revenues are being used properly. Governments may focus, for example, on increasing tax revenues to expand their available resources. Or, they may focus on creating efficiencies to make better use of public revenues. PB's public engagement and oversight mechanisms raise incentives for governments to make better use of scarce resources, especially when elected officials stake some of their political capital on the process. Government officials in the Brazilian city of Vitoria da Conquista adopted PB but then realized that they also needed to raise revenues to pay for the additional projects. They embarked on a public campaign that encouraged residents to request receipts when they purchased any goods. The idea behind this campaign was that the business issuing the receipts would then have to pay the required sales tax to the municipal government. Ultimately, such efforts raise awareness around the importance of responsibility to pay taxes, which should subsequently increase government revenues (Touchton, Wampler, and Peixoto 2019).

Well-being

PB can alter individual and community well-being by channeling investment to public works and social programs that directly improve ordinary citizens' lives. For instance, implementing PB projects routinely expands public services to underserved areas (Marquetti 2003; Wampler 2015). Participants can thus learn that pursuing public goods through collective decision-making processes is beneficial, which increases accountability among governments and perceived legitimacy among citizens. Both governments and organized groups are quick to publicly hail the programs, which then reinforces perception of good governance and strong outcomes. These more plentiful, higher-quality public goods can improve individuals' health, education, and employment as they use public services in each policy arena.

The literature provides evidence that PB can strengthen the provision of public services in practice, particularly in Brazil. For instance, a World Bank study (2008) assessing PB in Brazil finds a strong, positive association between PB and access to water services; this is an issue of particular importance to people living in informal settlements because they often lack direct access to basic public infrastructure. This is an excellent example of how PB can address the infrastructure deficit faced by poor communities. Several studies in Brazil also find that PB is associated with higher spending in health-related areas and lower levels of infant mortality, which also has a clear class dimension because infant mortality affects poorer families at much greater rates than middle- and upper-income families (Gonçalves 2014; Touchton and Wampler 2014; Wampler and Touchton 2019). Based on these articles, we infer that PB is linked to higher spending in public health care because poor citizens participating in PB rely on the public health system. There is ample evidence that some of PB participants' principal demands are to build new health clinics, reform those already in use, and provide resources to support hiring additional personnel (e.g., nurses, community health agents). This heightened focus on health, we argue, sets the conditions for lowering infant mortality because it spurs governments to invest more resources in health care.

Beyond health clinics, PB programs alter the basic dynamics of state–society relations for health service delivery. The constant interaction between community leaders and government officials allows for the exchange of information: Community leaders provide information about community and individual problems, which then allows government officials to respond to residents' needs. This information is as basic as identifying who is pregnant in the community (in order to transport expecting mothers to prenatal doctor's visits) to identifying larger problems such as open sewage, which can lead to a variety of diseases. Beyond Brazil, however, it is not clear if this is happening—we need much more research on these outcome variables to understand if PB conducts health information from communities to governments.

In general, we know that not all PB programs achieve this or many other goals described above (Wampler 2007; McNulty 2011, 2018; Goldfrank 2011, 2021; Vincent 2012; Albert 2016; Sintomer et al. 2016; Dias, Enríquez, and Júlio 2019). The evidence above shows how PB *can* strengthen civil society, increase accountability, and improve well-being under certain conditions (Avritzer 2002; Santos 2005; Baiocchi 2005; Wampler 2007; Baiocchi et al. 2011; Lerner 2014; Touchton and Wampler 2014; Touchton et al. 2017; Cabannes 2019). Yet, in many cases, PB programs do little to advance civil society, accountability, or well-being, and may even lead to troubling results, such as citizens' participation fatigue, increased public cynicism, or new venues for corruption (Wampler 2007; Goldfrank 2011; McNulty 2011; Albert 2016). We argue that macro and meso factors condition the range of possible outcomes associated with PB. The following section develops these conditioning factors in greater depth.

Conditioning Factors

Here we identify macro-level factors, such as the national political context, the decentralization of political and policy authority, and the economic conditions, that help to structure the PB process and its results (See Figure 3.1). Then, we discuss the meso level, which includes specific factors that directly support a localized participatory ecosystem, including the existing configuration of civil society (density and appropriate political repertoires), government support, and state capacity.

We argue that variation across macro and meso levels best explains variation in how and when PB produces change in civil society, well-being, and accountability. For example, we would expect that two similarly designed PB programs located in very different macro contexts would produce significantly different outcomes. A democratically elected government working closely with civil society partners in New York City faces very different challenges than a democratically elected government in Nairobi or Mexico City. The factors that condition outcomes exist along a spectrum and it is unusual to find PB programs operating under circumstances where all of the factors that are theoretically most conducive to PB are present. Nevertheless, we expect programs to perform better when they are embedded in environments with more conditioning factors that facilitate positive outcomes.

Macro-level

Three macro factors strongly condition whether or not PB programs generate social and political change: the broader political context, the extent of decentralization, and local economic conditions.

Broader Political Context

The broader political context, specifically regime type, matters greatly for PB performance. PB is more likely to generate the community-level impacts, as discussed above, in democratic contexts. Government officials in democracies have stronger electoral and governance incentives to incorporate citizens' voice and vote into specific policy changes. In turn, citizens are more likely to exercise their rights, including voice and vote, when they are situated within a broader democratic ecosystem. Of course, democratic institutions are relatively new in many places adopting PB, which helps explain why PB advocates identify the program as a key means to "democratize democracy" (Santos 2005).

At the broadest level, the democratic context usually includes legal protection of civil, political, and human rights, which affects how people participate, deliberate, and monitor their governments. Basic legal and political protections surrounding freedom of speech, assembly, and the protection of CSOs' autonomy from direct state interference all theoretically promote a wide range of beneficial outcomes. Rights protections are important because citizens need to be able to freely critique government officials; citizens' voice, vote, and oversight abilities are fundamentally constrained if citizens operate in the public sphere under threat of reprisals. For example, women and ethnic and racial minorities have greater access to basic civil and political rights, it is more likely that they will participate in PB processes.

The sequencing of PB adoption and a national-level democratization process is another significant factor that affects the type of PB that governments adopt. The time between a democratic transition, for example, and the adoption of PB affects the "window of opportunity" that is available for governments, CSOs, and citizens to pursue radical social and political change (see Chapter 1). In countries that have relatively new democracies, such as Brazil, Indonesia, Mexico, Peru, South Africa, and South Korea, a strong emphasis on building democratic norms, values, and practices provided fertile ground to encourage democratic reformers to expand PB's boundaries. In Brazil, for example, the transition to democracy during the 1980s included a strong emphasis on generating "the right to have rights," whereby individuals came to identify themselves as rights-bearing members of the polity (Dagnino 1998). Governments adopting PB thus conceptualized it as a school of democracy, in which citizens would first learn about their rights and subsequently exercise them. PB was thus initially one key channel that would later expand the boundaries of the new representative democracy.

In contrast, more established democracies (such as those in Western Europe, the United States, and Canada) place a greater emphasis on renewing the social contract by revitalizing their democratic roots. In the United States, for example, PB advocates sought to incorporate individuals who were not likely to participate in elections or other public events. In New York City, this means that a concerted recruitment effort significantly increased the number of immigrants, Latino, and Hispanic participants in PB (Su 2016).

Interestingly, governments in authoritarian and semi-authoritarian regimes are increasingly adopting PB. This is a relatively new phenomenon and there is very little research on PB's effects in these contexts. For example, PB now exists in China, Cuba, Russia, and Uganda. We do know that PB in authoritarian contexts is quite different from the PB described in Chapter 1 (Cabannes 2018; Dias 2018). Governments in authoritarian contexts tend to adopt PB as a public policy tool to improve governance outcomes and increase the efficacy of public spending. In these countries, governments are not elected in free and fair multi-party elections, but they do have constraints on their spending. Thus, PB may prove most useful as a means to include citizens in tough spending decisions. Governments in authoritarian contexts may seek to improve citizen well-being, but do not also pursue the outcomes that are associated with democratic systems (accountability and a stronger civil society). Much more research is needed to evaluate PB's effects as it is adopted in authoritarian and semi-authoritarian contexts around the world. The existing evidence suggests that PB will likely have more positive effects in democratic contexts, even in new democracies. These positive effects have been now documented in places such as Brazil, the United States, and Portugal, all of which have democratic regimes. But we lack a body of evidence that has more systematically evaluated PB's impact in semi-authoritarian and authoritarian environments.

Decentralization

Decentralization plays a crucial role in PB experiences because most PB programs are adopted at municipal, village, and district levels. Decentralization offers government officials and citizens greater degrees of local spending authority and a greater local budget to allocate through PB. Subnational governments need to have resources, capable staffing, and the legal authority to implement subnational participatory programs like PB. There is no way that subnational PB processes, and the decisions that emerge from them, can be meaningful without effective fiscal and administrative decentralization. Decentralization is a requirement even in top-down, mandated processes because local governments and citizens need opportunities to make decisions about their subnational government's spending. Decentralization also creates an opportunity for subnational governments to access new resources and create participatory institutions like PB in the first place.

Reformist governments in decentralizing systems often have a window of opportunity to invest additional resources in PB because no specific political group or bureaucratic unit "owns" these resources. For example, constitutional reforms accompanied decentralization in Brazil (1988), Indonesia (1998), Peru (2002), and Kenya (2010). An emphasis on participation accompanied decentralization in all of these cases, creating the political and policy conditions that favored PB adoption. In turn, new, larger local budgets incentivize the citizen and CSO participation that is necessary to sustain PB processes.

Economic Conditions

The national and local economic conditions significantly affect the degree to which local governments have the capacity and resources to implement PB in a way that generates the outcomes documented above. PB programs allow citizens to intervene directly in government spending, producing a close relationship between governments' available resources and citizens' ability to exercise decision-making authority. Simultaneously, public resources must be available so that governments can delegate authority to citizen decision-making forums; PB programs lose their distinctive characteristic of allowing citizens to select specific projects when public resources are absent. Moreover, governments are more likely to withdraw or limit PB program funding as resources become scarce. In contrast, governments are more likely to invest in PB when resources are plentiful.

In general, the availability of additional resources permits government officials to dedicate more funding to PB during periods of economic growth. Government reformers adopting PB can avoid difficult political struggles with entrenched bureaucrats or legislators in these cases; rather, reformers can side-step disagreements and allocate new resources to PB programs. The Philippines under President Aquino (2010–16) is an excellent example of a reformist president overseeing the allocation of hundreds of millions of dollars through PB.

In wealthier countries, it is uncertain if PB will have the same impacts. Public investments in wealthy countries (e.g., resources, staffing time, etc.) may be sufficient to improve quality of life. For example, it is possible that PB-based public investment in middle- and upper-middle-class neighborhoods would improve overall quality of life, for example by affecting how residents use public space. However, PB might simultaneously have little effect on more basic indicators of well-being, such as infant mortality or access to education, because basic access to health and education are already established. It stands to reason that PB's effects on well-being may be much greater in poor neighborhoods in wealthy countries, where PB-related public investments can initiate virtuous circles of reform, causing basic health and education to improve. In sum, previous levels of performance across different issue areas will likely condition the type of programs that countries adopt and the goals that these PB programs pursue. The cost of implementing small infrastructure projects in Chicago, New York City, or Paris is much higher than in Nairobi or Lima. Moreover, investing USD1 million will have a much greater impact in these low-income settings than in the wealthier cities. Thus, "moving the needle" on social policies is often easier when social conditions are very poor; small policy projects can have big impacts in areas surrounding well-being. Impacts in other contexts may be extensive, too, but those impacts depend on the program goals and associated program type.

In sum, the broader sociopolitical and economic context (macro-level) in which PB is adopted and embedded will condition its impact across a wide variety of outcomes. Variation in the political context, the degree of decentralization, and the underlying economic conditions influence PB's performance in different ways and subsequently channel PB's influence. More concretely, this means that we would expect the outcomes generated in Paris to be quite distinct from those in Kenya or Indonesia. We expect countries with higher state capacity and greater resources (e.g., France, Germany, and the United States) would more efficiently complete a greater number of projects, but that these projects' overall impact on poverty and well-being may be lower because these countries already have high-performing public services. Of course, their impact on other areas, such as efficient service delivery, may still be quite high. On the other extreme, we would expect that low-income countries with limited resources and low state capacity (e.g., Mozambique) would struggle to implement projects, but that the limited number of successfully implemented projects might make a significant difference in well-being. A third group of middle-income countries (e.g., Brazil, Indonesia, Mexico) is positioned between the two extremes; middle-income countries often have sufficient resources for at least some redistribution to poor, rural places. In these middle-income countries, some local governments may also have enough of their own resources to implement a broad range of projects that impact many citizens' lives.

Meso-level

Three key factors most strongly condition the extent to which PB programs generate social and political change at the meso level. These include government support, configuration of civil society, and state capacity.

Government Support

Strong, active support from top government officials is an important part of PB's success because they help to mobilize the local state to support the PB programs. One of the most important ways to show this support is the degree to which governments are willing to work with CSOs and citizens to "co-design" the PB process. When governments willingly incorporate citizens during the design phase, it is more likely that PB's "rule set" will better reflect the joint needs of public officials and citizens. During the ongoing participatory meetings, active government support is also necessary to recruit participants, hold meetings, engage with a wide range of citizens, and encourage a combination of focused and broad discussion. Internally, top government officials need to organize the necessary administrative support to hold PB meetings and other processes. Beyond these types of workers, it is also necessary to ensure that technical policy experts—civil engineers, budget, and procurement specialists—are also involved at two stages: an initial proposal stage and the implementation phase. When technical experts realign their work to support PB, there is a greater likelihood that these programs will have a more significant impact. Thus, mobilization of state capacity, based in the efforts of both elected officials and career civil servants, is a vital part of the process.

The importance of supportive leadership can be seen through the experiences of two cities in Peru, where the design and political context is the same. In Lambayeque, a city in the north of the country, in 2005, the mayor at the time (Yehude Simon) was a strong supporter of participatory democracy and asked his team to implement the process in a way that encouraged robust participation. As a result, some very interesting projects emerged. In that same year in Ayacucho, the mayor made it clear that he would not listen to the participants' recommendations and they stormed out without a vote. Interviewees who had been there alleged that the mayor mostly approved projects for his supporters and party members through clientelistic networks.

The level of resources allocated to PB is often a decision made by the local government. There is a strong correlation between the breadth of PB's impact and the level of resources allocated to the program (Wampler 2007; Goldfrank 2011; Cabannes 2014; McNulty 2019). When PB programs have more sizable resources, they are more likely to implement more projects as well as larger, more expansive projects. Higher levels of resources make people's participation more meaningful because their participation has a greater impact. Conversely, when governments dedicate fewer resources to PB, we would expect the overall impact to decrease because there are weaker incentives for people to participate, which means that the impact on civil society, accountability, and well-being will also be weaker. Stronger government support for these democratic, incremental decision-making processes is vital. This support is even more important when a national government mandates PB. The specter of "unfunded mandates" means that many governments may not support the robust implementation of PB programs because it requires short-term resources (personnel, staff time) and medium-term resources (for building projects selected by citizens); if national governments don't provide additional resources to local governments, PB programs may only exist on paper.

Several factors may induce government officials to allocate greater resources to PB. First, political competition through representative elections theoretically induces politicians to invest in activities that citizens support to win their votes; PB simultaneously appeals to citizens for the voice and vote they gain in policymaking processes. A minimal level of political competition among parties appears to be an important element in creating vibrant PB programs because it induces parties to respond to citizens' demands. Politicians and political parties position themselves as policy entrepreneurs, seeking to attract voters by demonstrating the breadth of their proposed reforms.

However, weak parties and weak party systems in most countries in the Global South make it very difficult for ordinary citizens to identify which reformers and parties are responsible for new forms of citizen engagement. This means that political reformers often have a hard time claiming credit for their reform efforts, diminishing politicians' and parties' potential interest in a new political project that delegates authority to citizens. In sum, political competition may motivate politicians to devote more resources to PB but conflicting interests may also reduce their interest in doing so.

Political ideology is a second factor motivating politicians to devote more resources to PB. Ideologically leftist political parties (e.g., Workers' Party in Brazil; PSOE in Spain; ANC in Durban, South Africa; Communist Party in Kerala, India) initiated the earliest PB programs in their respective regions. These parties used PB as a political platform through which to signal their interest in changing the social, economic, and political status quo. Parties also used PB to seek other citizens' votes by signaling their efforts to expand democratic practices.

Executive–legislative relations are a third area that affects politicians' degree of support for PB. A contradictory feature of many PB programs is that authority is often first concentrated in the hands of a fairly strong executive (e.g., mayors and governors), who then delegates resources and decision-making authority to citizens. Executives' significant involvement helps to explain why political reformers are at the center of efforts to adopt PB—these executives dedicate precious time and political capital to PB in the hopes of generating desired social and political changes. Most PB programs also require strong leadership from public officials to promote the delegation of authority because governments are central to organizing PB.

Elected legislatures, such as city councils and state legislative bodies, play an oversight role in PB programs, checking government officials' and citizens' decisions. They can also check the types of policies citizens select, as well as monitor policy implementation. However, the potential drawback of legislative and mayoral oversight is that politicians may begin to use PB as a channel through which to bolster their electoral support. We should note that many legislators oppose PB because they view it as a threat to their position in a representative democracy; the argument is that popularly elected legislators have greater legitimacy to make decisions surrounding public resources than unelected citizens. Elected legislators often believe that a core part of their responsibility is to make policy and allocate resources in a way that represents constituent interests. In many legislators' views, PB usurps some of that authority and places unqualified citizens in control of resources. As a result, executive support for PB is often greater than legislative support.

Existing Configuration of Civil Society

Variation in the existing density of civil society and CSOs' broader political repertoire also helps to explain differences in outcomes generated by PB. In this sense, civil society is both cause and consequence of PB's impact. We recognize that this part of the argument might appear tautological because we also identify an expansion of civil society as an outcome of PB. Our answer to the conundrum is that PB outcomes must be understood in relation to local starting points. We should not expect PB programs to produce the same changes in civil society when they are established in environments with very different civil society configurations. For example, when PB is adopted in an environment with an existing robust civil society, we would expect that the program would broaden citizens and CSOs access to public deliberation and public decision-making. When PB is adopted in an environment with a very limited civil society, we would expect that PB would play an educational and mobilizing role to better induce citizens and CSOs to work together in public processes. The existing configuration of CSOs can also determine how many historically marginalized groups are participating. Because PB programs are inserted into existing state–society relationships, we must therefore account for the configuration of civil society in the initial founding moment as well as during the outcome phase.

Greater CSO density before PB is implemented can promote more vibrant programs. This is because established CSOs have clear incentives to organize their followers to attend meetings as well as recruit new members. Greater CSO density can also broaden the range of citizens and communities actively represented in PB processes. In addition, greater numbers of participants can place pressure on government officials and allow supportive government officials to defend PB programs. We do not want to fetishize the number of participants in PB programs, but a greater number of participants helps to legitimize PB processes because non-participating citizens and political leaders often use the number of participants as a visible, easily verifiable way to gauge the relative importance of participatory processes.

An additional way that civil society conditions PB is through the range of activities that established CSOs already pursue and can use PB to accomplish. CSO leaders who already act as community organizers are often at the center of dense webs that link physical neighborhoods, religious centers, schools, daycares, and broader social movements. These leaders are well-positioned to use this role to advocate for policies through PB. In this scenario, community leaders add to their skillsets and marshal their networks to engage government officials and civil servants through PB.

Existing trust between government and CSOs can also condition the outcomes from PB once it is implemented. PB is a co-governance institution, in which government officials and citizens must work together to solve pressing problems. Government officials (elected, appointed, and civil servants) must learn how to engage citizens in formal deliberative processes and informal discussions that surround PB programs. Citizens, too, must learn the art of engaging public officials without being co-opted by governments. Previously established social trust between citizens, civil society, and governments allows for forging stronger partnerships through PB, which increases the likelihood of vibrant programs.

In sum, the configuration of civil society affects the vibrancy of PB programs. We should expect a larger role for government officials when civil society is weak. In contrast, we should expect community leaders and citizens to play a larger role when civil society is more robust. Civil society's starting point helps influence the type of PB program that government officials can implement. This also means that "civil society" outcomes are directly linked to their starting point. We should not expect that PB will engender a completely new, vibrant civil society; rather, the initial starting point will set the parameters of social and political change.

State Capacity

State capacity is another meso-level factor directly related to PB outcomes. The local and national states' capacity to implement specific, citizen-selected projects influences PB's long-term sustainability; governments must have basic administrative capacity and resources to organize PB effectively and to implement selected projects. Researchers, activists, and NGOs need to carefully consider the capacity of a state to implement projects as well as its available resources to fund project implementation.

Extensive research has documented that participants in many PB processes prioritize "pro-poor" projects, such as those that target the community's most disadvantaged areas (Marquetti 2003; Marquetti et al. 2008; Wampler 2007). But project selection is just the first phase. It is crucial that these public works projects are implemented after they are selected. However, it is difficult for subnational governments in many Global South countries to spend their budgets because their internal financial systems are weak. This is very common in Peru and Brazil, for example, where governments at every level fail to execute 100 percent of their annual budgets. In the Philippines, under the auspices of their PB program, it was difficult for rural villages to access the necessary technical expertise (e.g., engineers) to help design bridges and drainage systems. Thus, the implementing government needs training and resources to establish the different steps of the PB process in contexts where PB is new or mandated by national governments. An educated civil service sector that has been trained about PB's goals and the potential outcomes will also help to develop and oversee a more participatory form of PB programing. This condition is also important when governments contract with organizations to execute projects during PB's implementation stage.

Sufficient funding for civil society training and infrastructure projects is crucial. Usually, the amount of money allocated through PB is small relative to the overall subnational (and national) government budget. National budgetary requirements can also impede the effectiveness of the PB process in places where subnational governments rely on national budget transfers. For example, Peruvian government officials often report that the national government budget process makes it very hard to undertake PB on an annual basis. The national investment project database is difficult to use and the national government will not fund infrastructure projects after PB approval until several costly feasibility studies (often not included in the original budget) are complete. Further, annual budget projections often do not align with final budget transfers. These complications have led many Peruvian citizens to lose faith in the government's ability to respond to their demands. The Philippines had a similar experience in which a presidential administration rolled out PB for small towns, but a key difficulty was aligning local and national bureaucracies to implement projects. The inability to implement many agreed-upon projects hampered the Philippines' PB program, thus limiting the scope of the impact as well as potentially undermining citizens' support for PB.

In sum, meso-level factors significantly condition outcomes surrounding PB. Government support, configuration of civil society, and state capacity play different roles within PB processes and influence performance in a more targeted way than the macro-level environment. Meso-level factors vary across subnational regions and municipalities and thus show wide variation both within and across countries, making it difficult to generalize more broadly about PB performance at the meso level, but easier to leverage other municipalities' experience to identify locations where PB programs are likely to generate better results.

Variation in Program Design

As Chapter 1 documents, there is now wide variation in PB programs and their institutional design. Going beyond external conditioning factors, PB program designs and operational rules are internal factors that directly influence outcomes. Digital PB (Paris, Madrid), Housing PB (Belo Horizonte), Participatory Planning and Budgeting (Indonesia), and PB in city schools (Phoenix, New York City) are all variants within the broader family of projects that are considered to be PB. The core principles of PB, discussed in the introductory chapter (voice, vote, social justice, social inclusion, and oversight), are included in PB programs through specific design choices made by local governments and, sometimes, their civil society partners. The selection of specific PB rules and the broader program design reflects the founders' values as well as what they hope to accomplish. Institutional design thus matters as specific rules affect program outcomes (Goldfrank 2011; Rifai 2017; Sintomer et al. 2016; Wampler and Touchton 2019).

Between the creation of PB in 1989 and 2019, we identify four design areas in which there is considerable variation across PB programs. These include the level (or scale) for which PB is adopted, the presence of an explicit social justice requirement, rules that regulate who can participate, and the oversight authority extended to citizen-participants. Importantly, these aspects condition the outcomes and transform PB over time. We note that some institutional design rules are developed through co-design processes that bring together citizens, CSOs, and public officials, whereas in other cases, the basic rules are decided without much citizen engagement. Even in the cases where there is co-design, the rules become part of a broader set of PB institutions that affect how they function. Thus, when we conceptualize difference in PB design, it is as a meso-level factor that provides the overarching structure that people then work within. This discussion focuses on the ways in which these choices condition outcomes. In the conclusion of this book, we return to these variations and discuss how they have shifted over time.

Scale

PB began as a municipal program but now operates at all levels of government around the world, including neighborhoods, schools, villages, cities, metropolitan regions, counties, provinces/states, and in national agencies. PB's scale can affect outcomes in several ways. For example, it affects the level of resources that citizens allocate as well as the size of deliberative forums. Citywide participation increases the likelihood that citizens will have access to sufficient resources to generate meaningful impact. Conversely, the level of resources is likely to be much smaller when PB is implemented at the village level, which will then result in smaller-scale projects. However, we need to recognize that smaller-scale projects can also generate meaningful change. For example, paving a road or building a simple pedestrian bridge may cost a lot less in rural communities than a similar project in a city, but the impact on people's daily lives and livelihoods may be greater than in the city.

Social Justice Requirement

The earliest PB experiments in Brazil included a "social justice" requirement, which directs governments to increase spending in geographic areas that are underserved and under-resourced. Research suggests that evaluating proposed projects using a formal social justice requirement, such as the Quality of Life Index discussed in Chapter 1, is associated with improvements in well-being over time (Wampler and Touchton 2019). The broader lesson is that when social justice is explicitly included as a rule, or at least as a guiding principle, there is a greater likelihood that the PB program will produce social change in poorer communities.

Social Inclusion

Relatedly, a key variation in PB programs around the world is social inclusion, or the issue of who is invited, recruited, or encouraged to participate in the process. In some communities, any community member is invited and encouraged to come. Active outreach is conducted to get people who tend to be disengaged from politics into these forums. This is true in New York City, for example, where innovative outreach strategies are employed, such as knocking on doors to invite people and giving out information about PB meetings at subway stations. Thus, some programs seek to promote social inclusion by paying careful attention to who participates. However, in other cases, government officials make little effort to encourage people from diverse backgrounds to participate. Or worse, since governments try to fill the room with their supporters and partisan affiliates. Finally, some programs prefer to invite representatives from CSOs to participate in meetings. These processes tend to have much lower numbers of people who participate in PB.

Voting Rules

The Porto Alegre model used the secret ballot as the means for citizens to select PB projects. If there was only enough funding for one project, then the winner would be whichever project received the most votes. If there was enough funding for multiple projects, then citizens may have multiple votes; the projects with the greatest number of votes were selected. One of PB's recent, significant transformations is that consensus-based decision-making is now used to select projects in many settings—there is no formal vote, but there are extensive deliberations that guide participants toward project selection. Different voting rules, such as a show of hands or "dot voting," where participants have multiple votes, occur in other programs. Different PB design choices regarding voting can open processes to historically marginalized populations. Examples include quotas for leadership positions (e.g., requiring that a certain number of seats are reserved for women) and waiving a national citizenship requirement, which allows all residents to vote. Some operational rules engage individual citizens (open meetings), while others encourage or even mandate CSOs' participation but exclude the public (closed meetings). Anecdotally, it seems that programs that incorporate citizens directly, such as in the Brazilian PB model, will engage more people overall than those in places, like Peru, that restrict participation to representatives from CSOs.

Oversight

Rules and design will also include choices about oversight and monitoring mechanisms. At the earliest moments of the policy cycle, governments provide information on the level of resources available for project selection. This fosters formal and informal discussions about revenues and sectoral distribution of public resources. Once projects are selected, citizens may be involved in monitoring contract bidding to ensure that the scarce resources allocated to their projects are used properly. In addition, many PB programs have implementation committees that directly oversee the creation of physical infrastructure. Citizens can verify the quality of the work being done if the projects are relatively simple and commonplace. Thus, PB has the potential to initiate a broader understanding of how public resources should be spent. Presumably, more effective oversight leads to improved accountability as well as stronger civil society and enhanced well-being.

Hypothesizing Breadth of Political and Social Change by PB Type

The typology developed in Chapter 1 is also useful to establish expectations regarding potential outcomes associated with each type. In this section, we identify a preliminary range of likely outcomes that each type will produce. These outcomes are also affected by the conditioning factors (macro- and meso-level) identified above. Importantly, we see strong associations between the macro-level context and the type of program governments adopt. In broad brushstrokes, for example, we most frequently see the Empowered Democracy type emerge in new democracies, where civil society activists and government reformers push for the inclusion of rights-based social inclusion and social justice. Deepening Democracy types are more likely to be found in older, more-established democracies that are struggling with apathy and social exclusion; these programs are promoted by progressive/leftist CSOs and political reformers who are trying to revitalize the promise of democracy rather than building democracy from the ground up. The Social Development and Accountability type is more likely to be found in the Global South because international organizations promote the combination of "supply-side" changes (e.g., transparency, efficiency) and "demand-side" changes (citizen empowerment and basic participation in public process). We find Efficient Governance in wealthier democracies where civil servants and local governments lead the process. Finally, we find Digital PB types mainly in wealthier cities, primarily in the Global North and middle- and upper-income countries. The one PB type that is most common across all regions is Mandated by National Government, which we see in Latin America (Peru, Dominican Republic), Europe (Poland), and Asia (South Korea and Indonesia).

Empowered Democracy and Redistribution

These PB programs have their roots in more radical forms of democratic renewal, often with the explicit intention of allocating additional resources and services in poor and underserved communities. Of the six types, we expect to see the strongest community-level outcomes: These programs make strong commitments to more radical forms of democratic participation and deliberation *and* they have specific social justice rules that promote redistribution. We would also expect that these programs would promote accountability more than other PB types because Empowered Democracy and Redistribution programs feature relatively active participation among citizens, coupled with governments' voluntary commitment to reconfigure how they engage with citizens, participants, and community groups. In addition, we would expect that these programs would revitalize and strengthen civil society because they reward broad mobilization, especially within poor communities. Finally, we would also expect that these programs would improve well-being because their rules make explicit commitments to allocate greater resources to poor communities. Of course, this type is associated with the original PB cases in Brazil due to the explicit inclusion of rules that require additional spending to occur in poorer, underserved communities.

Deepening Democracy through Community Mobilization

Many PB programs have their roots in efforts to revitalize existing democratic processes; these programs emphasize the inclusion of marginalized communities as well as rebuilding trust between city residents and government officials. The lack of explicit rules that require the programs to allocate greater levels of spending to poorer communities is an important difference between this and the Empowered Democracy and Redistribution type. There may be normative, implicit, or moral claims within these programs to promote social justice, but there are no specific requirements for allocation of greater resources to poorer communities. We would expect these programs to strengthen accountability because they focus on generating new forms of state–society engagement. Second, we would expect these programs to revitalize and strengthen civil society because they reward broad mobilization, especially within traditionally marginalized communities. Thus, we would expect similar accountability and civil society outcomes associated with the Empowered Democracy and Redistribution type. However, we would expect much weaker gains regarding well-being because the Deepening Democracy through Community Mobilization type lacks an explicit requirement allocating PB projects to poorer communities.

Mandated by National Government

These PB programs are based on constitutional or legislative requirements that subnational governments adopt PB. National governments often provide limited technical assistance to these programs, which means that subnational governments face the challenge of implementing PB without the necessary professional capacity and administrative structures. In addition, many of these programs are also hampered by being "unfunded mandates," which means that resource-starved subnational governments are supposed to adopt PB in the context of no additional resources. Subnational elected governments may have few incentives to adopt PB, and they may therefore not invest their valuable and scarce time and energy to establish vibrant PB programs. Local CSOs may not be interested in investing their time in a participatory program mandated by a distant national government. Thus, our expectation is that most PB programs mandated by national governments will produce limited results, although there may be exceptional cases that may produce more robust outcomes. More specifically, we hypothesize that nationally mandated PB programs will not produce significant gains across civil society, accountability, and well-being because disinterested governments and a marginalized civil society will not work together within PB to produce vibrant PB programs.

Digital PB

These PB programs are generally more efficient at incorporating large numbers of city residents into online participatory decision-making processes. These programs may have an off-line component, but participation in face-to-face meetings is generally not required. Across the three outcome areas, we expect that Digital PB programs would generate some changes in accountability, but we do not expect to see many meaningful changes in civil society or well-being. First, we hypothesize that these programs can strengthen accountability because government officials voluntarily commit to new forms of citizen engagement. Governments are thus more likely to provide transparent information and the necessary administrative support to both induce citizens to participate as well as to make participation a positive experience. But, we also hypothesize that most Digital PB programs will not strengthen civil society because these programs often lack deliberative processes to allow for learning across CSOs; Digital PB programs also lack incentives to encourage robust community engagement, which means that online participation is much more likely to be individual-oriented. The limited effort to strengthen CSOs restrains the expansion of accountability in these programs. This is because government officials do not necessarily have a strong partner in civil society in these contexts; there are no organized groups focused on PB that can demand that the government adhere to its legal, policy, and political commitments. Finally, we do not expect well-being to improve through Digital PB because most projects do not require that citizens address key challenges facing poor communities.

Social Development and Accountability

Countries in the Global South tend to adopt this PB type at the behest of international organizations, such as the World Bank, USAID, and DFID. These PB programs are generally adopted in sociopolitical environments that are plagued by high levels of poverty, limited experience with accountable democratic institutions, low state capacity, and relatively limited civil society engagement. Thus, these programs emphasize building the foundations for democracy and accountability, strengthening civil society, and investing in development-related projects. In general, we expect to see some political and social change across all three outcome areas through these programs, but the degree of change is fundamentally different and weaker than the outcomes we expect through the Empowered Democracy and Deepening Democracy types. On the one hand, we expect change through Social Development and Accountability programs in places where these are groundbreaking experiences at the local level. Adopting democratic policymaking processes for the first time at the local level will likely generate change because people and governments are working together in public venues in unprecedented ways. Thus, the mere presence of PB is likely to promote some change when the programs represent new ways of managing state–society relations. However, we also expect the change to be more limited than in other contexts because the underlying macro- and meso-level conditions are characterized by limited public resources, weak state capacity, high societal demands, and partially accountable governments. Thus, the breadth of change for these programs is likely to be much smaller than in the Empowered Democracy and Deepening Democracy types.

We expect that Social Development and Accountability programs are laying the foundations for new forms of social accountability. This requires creating new relationships among government officials and citizens in the context of a fragmented state and often fractured civil societies. For many governments, states, and CSOs, this is the first time that they are being asked to jointly participate in public decision-making processes. These programs also create an opportunity to expand civil society because citizens are often encouraged to mobilize to participate. In many cases, PB program administrators attempt to develop civil society (rather than just mobilizing an existing civil society to come to meetings). Finally, we would expect to see improvements in well-being through these programs because they are often geared toward small-scale development projects. We thus see the potential for the programs to produce meaningful improvements in well-being at the local level, but we do not know the extent to which these may scale up for larger impacts. We note that it will be very difficult for researchers to systematically engage in large-N data analysis to test hypotheses in this area due to the uneven quality or general absence of data.

Efficient Governance Programs

These PB programs gather citizen input to help government officials make more efficient use of public resources. These programs focus on increasing citizens' budget knowledge as well as the real limitations governments face when they allocate scarce resources. We would expect to see shifts in accountability through these programs but limited or no changes regarding civil society or well-being. We would expect that these programs would expand accountability because the government will open its financial books and policymaking process to citizens. However, given the limited expansion of authority to citizens and the lack of incentives to mobilize, we would expect these programs to produce very limited strengthening of civil society. Similar to the Digital Participation type, the expansion of accountability is limited in this PB type because it does not promote civil society's development into an organizational space that can hold governments accountable. Finally, given this program type's focus on efficiencies, we would expect few ground-breaking shifts in well-being. If the proponents of the Efficient Governance type are correct, then we should see better (and more efficient!) use of public resources, which may have the effect of incrementally improving service delivery. These programs have the potential for important changes, to be sure, but these changes fall far from PB's more radical roots that were associated with "an inversion" of spending and policy priorities.

In sum, we expect to see significant variation in the political and social outcomes that different PB program types produce. This section develops a future research program to test these expectations. We expect programs that are most similar to the original PB programs in Brazil (Empowered Democracy and Redistribution) to produce the most robust outcomes for poverty reduction and strengthening democracy. In contrast, we expect to see much more limited results for poverty reduction as governments adopt PB with program designs and operational rules that de-emphasize in-person deliberation, binding decision-making through secret votes, and pro-poor policy allocation. Still, these distinct program types may produce robust outcomes in a wide variety of different areas that are not connected to poverty or democracy. Regardless of specific rules, mandated PB programs will likely have fewer localized political incentives for performance, which will make it less likely that local governments will invest the necessary time and energy to make PB a vibrant democratic institution capable of transforming lives.

Conclusion

This chapter presents an original theory of change that captures the causal mechanisms connecting PB processes to political, social, and economic outcomes. Our framework also identifies the factors conditioning outcomes surrounding PB and its potential impact. Then, we are able to hypothesize the potential outcomes based on the type of PB (as introduced in Chapter 1). Several important insights emerge from this exercise. First, research has demonstrated that PB can change communities (Baiocchi 2005; Baiocchi et al. 2011; Sintomer et al. 2016) and well-being (Gonçalves 2014; Touchton and Wampler 2014; Wampler and Touchton 2019). However, this evidence is primarily drawn from a few countries or cases. We want to reiterate that much more research is needed to fully understand PB's potential impact in the thousands of places around the world where it now exists. Second, we know that context matters for obtaining positive outcomes through PB. We identify several macro- and meso-level factors that will condition the eventual results that emerge from any PB experience. Third, individual actors (e.g., CSO leaders or elected officials) also matter greatly. Reformers and decision-makers make important choices about rules and program design that condition the outcomes as well. The repertoire of these choices has changed over time, a point that we elaborate in Chapter 3.

Finally, it is important to reiterate that high-quality PB processes fostering social and political change do not always emerge; in some regions, we would expect the emergence of high-quality programs to be the exception rather than the rule. Researchers have not found strong effects from PB in many cases and lack compelling evidence surrounding PB's impact in others. PB may even erode perceptions of legitimacy in some cases where PB is used as a veneer to cover clientelist or authoritarian processes. These observations lead us to be cautious in singing PB's praises without evidence to support the claims. It is clear that PB can produce positive outcomes in some contexts, but also that these contexts may not be as common as PB advocates hope.

Drawing on our theory of change and our PB typology, the book now shifts to an analysis of a wide variety of PB experiences that exist around the world. The following chapters explore PB as it spread from Latin America (Chapter 3), to Asia (Chapter 4), North America and Europe (Chapter 5), and Africa (Chapter 6). We detail both the waves of diffusion and adaptation as well as the outcomes that have been documented in all of these contexts. Each chapter provides evidence and an overarching justification for case selection to more fully illustrate what PB looks like in the dozens of nations in which it now takes place. This takes the form of short overviews of key country cases, with evidence drawn from elite interviews and participant observation in each global region. We draw on existing literature and situate it within our analysis for other countries where participant observation was not possible. The result is a series of mini-cases that demonstrate how governments adapted PB in the key cases to fit their needs.

3

Where It All Began

PB in Latin America

Latin America is the birthplace of PB as well as the region where it first spread rapidly and widely. In 1989, the Workers' Party created PB in several cities, including Porto Alegre, Brazil, as a radical democratic project that would help to invert the government's spending and policy priorities. PB quickly spread around Brazil and then to hundreds of Latin American cities. Today, PB exists in almost every country in Latin America—in towns, districts, metropolitan areas, and states. According to the Latinno database, at least fifteen countries in Latin America have experimented with or continue to use PB as a tool for engaging citizens in decision-making, including Argentina, Brazil, Colombia, Costa Rica, Guatemala, Mexico, Panama, Peru, and Venezuela. The *Participatory Budgeting World Atlas* estimates that PB takes place in more than three thousand cities in South America alone (Dias, Enríquez, and Júlio 2019). Most of these countries have a legal framework that either permits or requires cities and states to use PB.

In many Latin American countries, the adoption of PB took place as part of broader democratization processes, which provided a window of opportunity for democratic innovations. This is true of the original PB in Porto Alegre, the world's first national PB Law in Peru, and a post-conflict reconstruction process in El Salvador. Policy entrepreneurs from different ideological backgrounds imagined PB as a tool that could solve context-specific problems, such as the need to engage citizens in a new democracy (Brazil), the need to keep politicians accountable to residents (Peru), or a desire to build trust among citizens and local government officials (El Salvador). Concurrent to democratization, there was also a regional push to decentralize, which provided additional opportunities for subnational governments to experiment with new democratic and policymaking processes. The chapter highlights how reformers are drawn to PB as part of their efforts to solve various governance-related quandaries in these decentralized state contexts.

Because of its widespread prevalence, there are too many PB programs in Latin America to document in this chapter. Programs vary in terms of location, goals, and outcomes. Rather than attempting to cover all countries, we instead focus on four: Brazil, Peru, El Salvador, and Mexico. We focus primarily on Brazil and Peru for two reasons. First, they represent the groundbreaking and earliest cases of two PB types in the region: Empowered Democracy and Redistribution and Mandated by National Governments. Much of the information that we have about impact

Participatory Budgeting in Global Perspective. Brian Wampler, Stephanie McNulty, and Michael Touchton,
Oxford University Press. © Brian Wampler, Stephanie McNulty, and Michael Touchton 2021.
DOI: 10.1093/oso/9780192897756.003.0004

comes from the Brazilian cases due to its PB programs' longevity and Brazil's collection of a broad range of data at the municipal level. From Peru, we also have considerable data on impact, though much of the analysis suggests impacts are quite limited.

Second, this book's authors have spent many years (decades, in fact) conducting original research in these two countries. McNulty began research on PB in Peru in 2002 and has conducted more than two hundred interviews with key stakeholders. Wampler first attended a Brazilian PB meeting in 1998, and has attended more than a hundred and fifty participatory meetings in Brazil and interviewed over two hundred activists and governments officials. Touchton learned about PB in Brazil and Mexico during his dissertation fieldwork in 2006 and began researching it in earnest in 2010.

In addition to Peru and Brazil, we also document the cases of El Salvador and Mexico to illustrate the adaptations that emerged over time, as detailed in Chapter 1. El Salvador is an excellent example of the Social Development and Accountability type and Mexico illustrates the Deepening Democracy through Community Mobilization type. We recognize the widespread adoption of PB by cities in Uruguay, Argentina, Ecuador, the Dominican Republican, Colombia, and Venezuela but we choose to focus on Brazil, Peru, El Salvador, and Mexico because they represent broader trends in the region (see Dias, Enriquez, and Júlio 2019 for more).

The chapter highlights three central findings. First, although PB emerged as a radical democratic project, it has lost its social justice emphasis, as evidenced in the Peruvian and Mexican cases. It evolved into something more akin to a policy tool to engage citizens in local government decision-making; few places are explicitly using PB to advance redistribution goals through rules and design decisions (Baiocchi and Ganuza 2017). Second, Latin America is also the place where reformers first started experimenting with national laws. Although this top-down process is not producing strong outcomes, PB advocates in other regions of the world have learned from these experiences to adapt their own processes to increase the likelihood of success. Because of its extensive adoption in Latin America, we also see normative and mimetic pressures leading to its adoption in places like Mexico and El Salvador. Third, Latin America is the region with the most comprehensive analysis of social and political impact, which shows many cases where PB did have a verifiable and positive impact (Baiocchi et al. 2011; Gonçalves 2014; Touchton and Wampler 2014; Wampler and Touchton 2019). However, this extensive research also includes many cases in which researchers were unable to identify any impact at all (e.g., Wampler 2007; McNulty 2011; Goldfrank 2011; McNulty 2019). As we explain below, there are a wide variety of outcomes across the region, from high performers who appear to be meeting many program goals to underperforming programs that do not appear to have any impact. Data from the region provides much of the basis for the model of change presented in Chapter 3. Table 3.1 above presents a regional summary of PB, its key variants, and its diffusion over time.

Table 3.1. PB in Brazil, Peru, Mexico, and El Salvador

PB type	1989 to mid-1990s	Mid-1990s to mid-2000s	Mid-2000s to 2020
Empowered Democracy and Redistribution	30 Brazilian municipalities	250 Brazilian municipalities and one state; Dozens of Latin American cities in Venezuela, Uruguay, Peru, and more	
Deepening Democracy through Community Mobilization		Mexico City begins PB (2001–05)	2010 revived in Mexico City and spreads to 30 municipalities and one state; 40 Brazilian municipalities in 2020
Mandated by National Government		Approximately 2,000 Peruvian municipalities and regions (2003)	Approximately 160 municipalities in the Dominican Republic (2007)
Digital PB		Belo Horizonte, Brazil	
Social Development and Accountability		28 municipalities in El Salvador	16 municipalities retain PB in El Salvador
Efficient Governance			

Source: Authors.

Empowered Democracy and Redistribution

Brazil

The Workers' Party (*Partido dos Trabalhadores*, or *PT*) and its civil society allies developed PB during the 1980s and early 1990s during the re-establishment of Brazil's democracy (Harneker 1995; Abers 2000; Avritzer 2002). As discussed in earlier chapters, PB as we know it today began in Porto Alegre 1989 when the mayor, the municipal government, and local CSOs, invited citizens to participate in discussions regarding how to spend scarce municipal resources (Baierle 1998; Fedozzi 1998; Abers 2000; Avritzer 2002; Baiocchi 2005; Lüchmann 2008).[1] The

---

[1] During the same time period, other municipalities developed similar budget-related participatory programs (Tranjan 2015). Examples include Londrina (state of Parana) and Recife (state of Pernambuco), suggesting that Porto Alegre's PB developed in a broader context of institutional renewal and creation.

experience proved successful, and, over time, the municipality opened the process to broader public participation. PB was born.

Porto Alegre's PB quickly became known as the most successful program and this experience emerged as the model experience in Brazil, as described in the Introduction. PB spread rapidly around the region from this point due to the role of policy entrepreneurs and the allure of the various norms embedded in this project, such as increased citizen participation, citizen-based decision-making, and transparent governance (Porto de Oliveira 2017a). The social justice emphasis in the original PB in Porto Alegre continued for at least two decades in Brazil, giving rise to the Empowered Democracy and Redistribution model. Yet, the number of cities using PB in Brazil has actually declined to fewer than forty by 2020 and the social justice emphasis has now faded (Spada 2020).

The Workers' Party electoral victory in 1988 occurred in a broader context of simultaneous democratization and decentralization, which provided a window of opportunity for PB after the Brazilian military stepped down in 1985. CSOs pressed for greater access to public processes. The 1988 Constitution, often labeled the "citizens' constitution," incorporated participatory elements in several innovative ways. These innovations included allowing municipal and state government to experiment with new participatory institutions (Avritzer 2002). Since its inception in the early 1980s, the Workers' Party's agenda had emphasized social justice and participation; policy entrepreneurs developed PB to help achieve these goals.

PB in Porto Alegre, namely, the Porto Alegre model, described in the Introduction, occurred annually and relied on open local assemblies where delegates were elected to represent their interests in a series of meetings sponsored by governments. During these meetings, government officials shared information and participants developed project proposals. Through the emphasis on social justice, the Porto Alegre process stressed the redistribution of resources to poor areas in the city. Over time, Brazilian mayors adapted this model and created new programs, sometimes employing innovative technologies (Avritzer and Navarro 2003; Wampler 2007; Lüchmann 2008). For example, some government officials added a thematic track to expand the number and types of public venues in order to encourage people to deliberate over a wider range of issues. However, the core commitment to empowerment and redistribution remained.

Due to the active role of the Workers' Party, PB quickly spread around the country. Workers' Party mayors began to implement the process, some due to their normative commitment to the principles and others due to pressure from party leaders (Genro 1995, 1999; Wampler and Avritzer 2005; Wampler 2007; Goldfrank 2011). Non-Workers' Party mayors began to adopt PB as well, especially as NGOs in the Porto Alegre metropolitan region began to offer technical assistance. By 1996, thirty municipalities undertook PB annually, twenty-three of which were governed by PT mayors. By 2004, over two hundred and fifty Brazilian municipalities had voluntarily adopted PB at some point (Wampler and Avritzer

2005; Wampler 2007). An enormous literature on Brazilian PB programs thus developed to try to document and explain different facets of these programs.[2]

Importantly, PB was never a static institution. Rather, policy entrepreneurs often adapted it to better address thorny political problems (How to increase social inclusion? How to promote social justice?) and incremental policymaking processes. Many of the founding cities (e.g., Porto Alegre and Belo Horizonte, which adopted PB in 1993) continued to adapt the process to increase participation and ensure social justice. For example, the city of Belo Horizonte created a Quality of Life Index to ensure that neighborhoods with greater needs would receive more resources per capita (Wampler 2015). Brazilians also created thematic and sectoral PB. For example, Belo Horizonte created "PB Housing" to develop public housing for participants. In Porto Alegre, the government created a "policy thematic track" that encouraged participation across communities to address key issues (environment, transportation).

As PB spread, the Brazilian state of Rio Grande do Sul scaled up PB to the state level, where it was used to make decisions about state budgets; this foreshadowed debates about mandating PB through national laws and in different levels of government (Goldfrank and Schneider 2006; Legard and Goldfrank 2020). In 1998, the Workers' Party's Olívio Dutra, the mayor who initiated PB in Porto Alegre, rose to the position of governor of this state and initiated a statewide process that built on their success at the municipal level. In these processes, the government invited citizens to municipal- and regional-level plenaries to elect delegates to represent them in state meetings. These delegates then developed a list of funding priorities (Goldfrank and Schneider 2006). Thus, these delegates represent their areas in statewide meetings that primarily follow the original PB model. However, the budget in Rio Grande do Sul is much larger (an estimated nine times larger than Porto Alegre's) and hundreds of thousands of people participated in some years (Goldfrank and Schneider 2006).

In the late 1990s and early 2000s, some cities also started adopting online PB, or "e-PB," including Belo Horizonte which now has one of the largest e-PB processes in the world (Wampler, Touchton, Spada 2019). Considered successful due to the fact that it has engaged at least 10 percent of the Belo Horizonte electorate, research on the process has shown that outreach is important (in this case email served as an effective tool) and moderated discussion boards improved the deliberative process (Peixoto 2009; Sampaio et al. 2011; Coleman and Sampaio 2017; Peixoto et al. 2019).

---

[2] For more on PB in Porto Alegre and Brazil more generally, see Abers 1998, 2000; Avritzer 2002; Baiocchi 2005; Baiocchi, Heller, and Silva 2011; Fedozzi 1998; Fung and Wright 2003; Heller 2001; Lüchmann 2008; Nylen 2003; Wampler 2007. See Porto de Oliveira 2017a and Sintomer et al. 2013 for more on the diffusion process.

Over time, PB's role as a radical democratic project lessened and it became one of many democratic policymaking institutions implemented by Brazilian mayors. Ben Goldfrank's work (2018) notes that in some Brazilian cities PB later became part of the status quo and mayors turned to new ways to innovate in the realm of citizen participation. Françoise Montambeault (2019) documents another example of this gradual change in Belo Horizonte, after the Workers' Party fell out of power and subsequent leadership became more pragmatic and diversified their citizen empowerment options.

Of course, discussion of the creation of PB is impossible without the mention of its quiet recession in the very place it began. To the great disappointment of the thousands of advocates and activists who designed the world's first PB program, the Porto Alegre mayor's office suspended the process in 2017. But PB's central importance to the government decreased as early as 2004, when the Workers' Party left office (Wampler 2007; Melgar 2014). In Porto Alegre, we conceptualize PB's heyday as being from 1990 to 2004, followed by a slow decline from 2005 to 2015, with its elimination in 2017. The governments governing Porto Alegre from 2005 to 2016 were not strong supporters of PB, but maintained the program due to civil society's support for it as well as because it was part of Porto Alegre's international brand. Simon Langelier (2015) attributes the decline and eventual end of PB in Porto Alegre to three factors: 1) the rise to power of an anti-participatory, right-wing political party; 2) the eventual disillusionment of civil society actors; and 3) the lack of a legal framework to guarantee the process on an annual basis.

More broadly, a 2012 PB census found that only seventy PB processes continued to exist in cities with populations over fifty thousand and a 2020 census found less than forty cases in Brazil (Spada et al. 2012; Spada 2020). Spada (2014) elaborates, noting that when the Workers' Party rose to national power, especially with the election of Lula in 2002, participatory policies began to focus on national-level participatory programs, such as policy conferences and councils. Local-level programs, such as PB, became less important (Spada 2014). At the same time, mayors were looking for newer local-level innovations and PB lost its appeal. Thus, Brazil is also a case that demonstrates how PB can end when it is perceived as a partisan project, when expectations are not met, and when citizens experience participation fatigue.

PB's presence in Brazil for over three decades gives researchers the best opportunity to assess whether and how PB makes a difference in people's daily lives. Brazil has tracked data on this process for thirty years making its data relatively rich and accessible, which lends itself to large-N analyses. We therefore know a great deal more about PB's effectiveness and ability to meet the stated goals of this democratic innovation in Brazil than anywhere else in the world. We find evidence of social change at individual and community levels (in line with the theory of change presented in Chapter 2) across the areas of accountability, civil society, and well-being.

First, changes in individual attitudes about efficacy, trust, authority and democracy are well documented in Brazil (Nylen 2003; Baiocchi 2005; Cameron, Hershberg, and Sharpe 2012; Wampler 2007, 2015; Baiocchi and Ganuza 2017). Much of this work focuses on changes in participants who attend meetings, propose projects, and vote on funding. For example, a number of researchers studying Brazil have found that PB can change attitudes of citizens who participate (Avritzer 2002; Wampler and Avritzer 2004; Baiocchi 2005; Wampler 2007; Goldfrank 2011). Research also demonstrates that PB altered participants' support for local democracy, their sense of empowerment, their perception of government or government efficacy, and their basic knowledge of budget and general government processes (Baiocchi 2005; Wampler 2007; Marquetti et al. 2008). Montambeault (2016), in a comparison of PB in Brazil and Mexico, finds that PB can also lead to improved citizenship practices among participants, which can lead to an improved sense of belonging. Thus, a variety of case studies assert that PB participants feel empowered, support democracy, view the government as more effective, and better understand budget and government processes after participating in PB.

Research demonstrates that government officials can change as a result of PB as well. For example, Wampler's (2015) work in Belo Horizonte finds that PB led government officials to innovate in terms of solving local problems. The theory and design of PB provides government officials, both elected and appointed, additional interactions with citizens, which provide opportunities for them to hear and respond to citizens' needs. These interactions create new sources of knowledge, which creates the opportunity for government officials to act differently.

Victor Albert's (2016) work offers a cautionary perspective to findings about participation. In his observations of PB in Santo André, Brazil, Albert richly documents the interactions between government officials and citizens. On the one hand, PB brought these actors together in a forum that would otherwise not exist. In one meeting, Albert documents that poor residents had the chance to explain to the mayor that their neighborhood lacked adequate services. However, Albert also watched as government officials often ignored both the participants' pleas for more attention to their issues and their proposed projects. His work reminds us that just having people in the room at meetings does not always lead to quality interactions. Albert's and Wampler's findings illuminate the contradictory nature of many PB programs, which vary considerably from one municipality to the next—PB creates opportunities for more citizen–government interactions, which may generate improvements in service delivery (narrowly) and state–society relations (more broadly). And yet, these interactions may also reinforce existing power differentials between governments and citizens. By this, we mean that some governments may use PB as a governing and electoral vehicle in which they receive citizen input but do not then delegate authority to citizens to promote a co-governance process.

Research on PB in Brazil provides a wealth of data on participation. Between 2000 and 2003, Porto Alegre averaged thirty-five thousand participants per year

(Wampler 2007). The World Bank estimated that 19.8 percent of city residents reported having attended a meeting (World Bank 2008). Participation in Belo Horizonte, a city with a slightly larger population than Porto Alegre, surged to forty-three thousand in 2001, when they changed to a biannual cycle (large mobilizations every other year), and they averaged nearly thirty-seven thousand participants from 2001 to 2010 (Wampler 2015). We also know that women tend to participate in strong numbers as both participants and leaders of the process, especially as the process gained strength over time (Wampler 2007). The same patterns exist with the least-educated and poorest citizens (Baiocchi 2005; Nylen 2003; Wampler 2015).

Brazil also uses several innovative design practices to promote social inclusion. In *São* Paolo, Brazil, from 2001 to 2004, the Workers' Party incorporated affirmative action principles into the process to target socially vulnerable populations, such as Afro-Brazilians, elderly, youth, members of the LGBTQ+ community, indigenous groups, the homeless, and people with disabilities (Hernández-Medina 2010). The government set up an election process by which participants who represented these segments needed fewer votes to become delegates, not through quotas (Hernández-Medina 2010). Research from Brazil also shows that outreach efforts matter in terms of these outcomes. A recent study in Brazil found that non-partisan Get Out the Vote campaigns can also increase participation in PB (Peixoto, Sjoberg, and Mellon 2019).

Research on Brazil has identified three areas where we are most likely to see community-level change through PB: civil society, accountability, and well-being. First, PB in Brazil strengthened civil society by increasing its density, that is, increasing the number of groups and creating new partnerships (Baierle 1998; Abers 2000; Avritzer 2002; Baiocchi 2005; Baiocchi et al. 2011; Touchton and Wampler 2014). PB also provides new channels for new partnerships with government and citizens or CSOs, particularly when government officials are committed to the process (Baiocchi et al. 2011; Touchton and Wampler 2014). Wampler (2007) documents two cases where civil society and supportive mayors worked together to institutionalize participatory democracy. Importantly, CSOs' repertoires of action (cooperation and contestation in successful cases) explain the more successful partnerships.

The extent to which these changes emerge depends in large part on the preexisting nature of civil society in the local (or subnational) context in which PB is introduced (Wampler 2007). Baiocchi, Heller, and Silva (2011) make this important point when delving into the role of civil society in cities with PB and those without PB. They find that PB deepens democracy when CSOs can organize independently and develop their own demands. Their work shows that a deep understanding of the nature of civil society before PB is implemented is the best way to conceive of the potential for results. This finding also suggests that in some cases with extremely weak civil society sectors, reform efforts may be more productive if focused on other aspects of democracy, and not PB. As Baiocchi, Heller, and Silva (2011) write, "local context was critical to shaping outcomes" (145).

Second, there is also a substantial body of evidence from Brazil that show that better-performing PB programs improve accountability (Abers 2000; Avritzer 2002, 2009; Baiocchi et al. 2011; Wampler 2007, 2015). New relationships can emerge that are less adversarial and more collaborative when states and society work together more effectively (Montambeault 2019). In some cases, participants and government officials develop new shared interests. For example, in Brazil, Wampler (2007) finds that when government officials follow PB rules, improved horizontal accountability does emerge. And, vertical accountability mechanisms also improve when civil society and government work together. This finding is echoed by Baiocchi, Heller, and Silva's (2011) comparison of four PB processes to four comparable cites without PB in Brazil. In the PB cases, CSOs were able to effectively hold elected officials to account, especially in areas with relatively strong civil society sectors before PB was introduced.

There is some additional early evidence that PB improves rates of tax collection, which is strongly associated with accountability. If PB is improving citizen's accountability to their local governments, we would expect government officials to be able to collect existing, on-the-books taxes and that citizens would be more likely to pay local taxes. Touchton, Wampler, and Peixoto (2019) compare Brazilian municipalities with PB to those municipalities without PB. They demonstrate that, holding all else equal, municipalities with PB collect nearly 40 percent more in local taxes.

Finally, research in Brazil demonstrates the degree to which PB can improve citizens' well-being. For example, in an early study of PB in Porto Alegre, the World Bank (2008) found that PB led to improved access to water services, which improves citizens' daily lives but can also have a broader effect on health due to improved sanitation. This preliminary evidence provided support for the assertion that PB could help to improve well-being, often through redistribution of resources to poor communities (Marquetti et al. 2008; Goldfrank 2011; Goldfrank and Schneider 2006). The redistribution of resources is an explicit goal of the Porto Alegre model, and several studies have documented meeting this goal for many years. For example, Marquetti (2003) demonstrates a redistributive effect of capital investment and public goods and services in Porto Alegre from 1992 to 2000. Armando Rendon Corona (2006) carefully links this outcome to the way projects are scored in the evaluation process.

However, these studies covered a relatively short period of time, which means that other factors could have improved access to water, and focused on a single, exceptional case, making it hard to determine whether these results are generalizable beyond Porto Alegre. To move beyond the limitations of that work, researchers began to use large-N studies to evaluate PB's impact. Most significantly, Gonçalves (2014) and Touchton and Wampler (2014) identify improvements in citizens' well-being (see also Boulding and Wampler 2010; Touchton et al. 2017). With data spanning twenty years, Touchton and Wampler (2014) find that PB programs are strongly associated with greater municipal spending on health care and sanitation and lower infant mortality. The effect is greater in programs that have been in place longer and where Workers' Party mayors are in power. There is no consensus on how long it may take for effects surrounding well-being to appear, but initial work suggests that reductions in infant mortality can happen over a relatively short time (Gonçalves 2014; Touchton and Wampler 2014).

The above research compares municipalities with PB to those without PB. However, additional research evaluates differences in PB's impact among municipalities that all use PB. For example, Wampler and Touchton (2019) administer a unique survey to 114 Brazilian municipalities that each have PB but differ in program design and operational rules. A key finding is that those municipalities with specific social justice rules have lower rates of infant mortality than municipalities whose PB programs lack specific social justice rules. These rules alter project selection and, more broadly, alter the public discussion about how public resources should be allocated. There are two key lessons that we draw from this study and the broader debate. First, it was better for Brazilian citizens to live in a municipality that adopted PB than somewhere that did not adopt PB. Second, it was even better for citizens' well-being if their PB program adopted specific social justice rules than if it did not adopt them. More broadly, a key lesson is that institutional design (differences in scale, voting rules, decision-making authority, and social justice) have an important impact on outcomes.

In sum, there is a large literature about PB in Brazil, much of it suggestive, if not definitive, regarding PB's potential impact. The preponderance of positive outcomes conditioned by a variety of factors related to local context leads us to posit that the empowered democracy type of PB, with its emphasis on social justice, may be the type that produces more robust democratic and development outcomes. Future research will need to develop this line of reasoning further.

From Empowered Democracy to Mandated by National Government

As noted in earlier chapters, PB in Brazil quickly became known in international circles as paradigmatic of the wave of participatory development processes that gained strength during the 1990s. In 1996, the United Nations awarded Brazil's PB programs with its prestigious "best practice" award, thus drawing attention to PB, which in turn encouraged other governments across Brazil to adopt it. Leftists and international development professionals flocked to Brazil to learn more about this innovative engagement mechanism and PB advocates presented the Brazilian experience in several international conferences. In the mid-1990s, officials from the World Bank and UN Habitat also began conducting research on and promoting

PB. This helped PB spread around Brazil and across Latin America throughout this decade (Goldfrank 2012; Baiocchi and Ganuza 2017; Porto de Oliveira 2017a). Cities in Argentina, Uruguay, Ecuador, Peru, Colombia, and Mexico all began to experiment with PB in their local contexts in the late 1990s and early 2000s. Because of PB's normative appeal to these officials, most of them adopted some version of the Empowered Democratic and Redistribution type, although the emphasis on social justice and redistribution also began to slowly wane in many places.

For example, some Peruvian municipal leaders attended conferences in the 1990s, heard about the experience in Brazil, and decided to implement the idea in their own cities. Participatory planning and budgeting took off in the late 1990s in Ilo, a port town in the south of Peru (López Follega et al. 1995). In Villa El Salvador, a shantytown outside of Lima, elected leaders from the United Left began to undertake participatory planning in the early 1990s (see Bracamonte et al. 2005; Remy 2005). In 1999, they launched a formal participatory budget process that continues today. Another example emerged in the mid-1990s, when the first indigenous mayor of Cotacachi, Ecuador, began to promote participatory development processes including PB (Van Cott 2008). The city's first PB experience took place in 2001 and was also quickly recognized by international observers as successful. As one municipal official notes, "Participatory budgeting is the main strategic tool for realizing the vision and mission of the new municipality of Cotacachi, based on intercultural dialogue and the search for consensus between the people and municipal authorities" (Saltos 2008: 6).

As PB took hold across the region, debates began to emerge about how to create a sustainable process that would not die out when elected leaders who supported and initiated the process eventually left office. One way to address this issue lay in advocating for constitutional frameworks or laws in cities and nations that codify PB in the policymaking process, which would be one form of coercive pressure. The interest in more formally institutionalizing PB is one factor that led to the world's first national PB law in Peru.

Peru

In 2003, the Peruvian government passed the world's first national law mandating PB in all subnational governments around the country (for more, see McNulty 2011, 2012, 2013). Many of the advocates for this reform studied the Porto Alegre experience or heard about it in conferences. Peru's Participatory Budgeting Law (Law 28,056, passed in 2003 and reformed in 2009) mandates that all subnational governments—meaning regions (similar to states/provinces), provincial capitals (like counties), and municipal districts (similar to cities/towns)—undertake PB annually. However, as the first example of a national law, PB in Peru has been mostly disappointing to the original reformers as well as participants. This case provides a good example to examine the factors that can intervene in PB to reduce its potential impact.

Peru's national PB law emerged as part of a sweeping decentralization reform passed by Congress in 2003 during an intense moment of democratic transition. The country had just experienced ten years of authoritarian rule under Alberto Fujimori (1990–2000), who had centralized power into the Executive and wielded power in extremely corrupt ways. A growing social movement made up of citizens and activists demanded decentralization and transparency after years of anti-democratic policies and the release of videos of a key Fujimori advisor bribing national politicians. Thus, the fall of Fujimori alongside citizen disgust with corruption provided the window of opportunity to develop this innovative law through mimetic pressures.

Several policy entrepreneurs promoted the project. President Alejando Toledo (2001–06) campaigned on a promise of decentralization, democratic reforms, and neoliberalism. Toledo was a Stanford University-trained economist who had also worked at the World Bank. During the redrafting of Peru's Constitution, Toledo supported the inclusion of PB as a democratic policymaking process that would align with his policy and political agenda. In addition, several leftist congressmen who had implemented PB or similar participatory programs in their cities when they served as mayors strongly advocated for participatory budgeting and planning to be included in the constitutional reforms. Interestingly, these leftists found an unlikely ally in the technocratic Ministry of Economics and Finance (MEF) and the head of the National Budget Office, Nelson Shak, who drafted and advocated for the PB Law (as opposed to the decentralization reform language that stressed citizen participation in planning in general). Top officials in the MEF hoped that PB would control spending and keep government officials accountable (McNulty 2011).

Peru's PB Law states that the MEF will oversee the process and provide instructions to all subnational governments regarding the specifics of PB. The original participatory budget law outlined eight phases, later collapsed to four, that local governments would be required to use during their year-long planning cycle. First "participating agents" (representatives from CSOs) are invited and trained. Then, local governments and the participant agents hold workshops to train participants regarding how to develop project proposals. A technical team is also formed, usually consisting of civil servants and CSO representatives to review and rank proposals. Another meeting takes place where the top-rated proposals are presented and a final vote is taken. The final phase consists of setting up an oversight committee, made up of CSOs, to monitor spending and progress on prioritized projects.[3] Thus, this form of PB places considerable emphasis on

---

[3] Three additional decrees (Supreme Decrees 097-2009-EF, 142-2009-EF, and 131-2010-EF) also relate to and clarify aspects of the process.

inviting representatives from civil society and not all residents in a neighborhood, which is a key departure from the Porto Alegre model. A second shift away from the Porto Alegre model was to use a technical team to evaluate and rank the projects, which is similar to PB in the Philippines and Indonesia. Finally, the entire process is set up as a transparency and accountability tool, not a social justice initiative. Thus, PB in Peru has few of the attributes of the Porto Alegre model when it comes to social justice and inclusion.

There are some cases of PB working relatively well in Peru. For example, when PB first started in Cusco in 2004, the mayor began to use it to fund a soccer stadium, a typical populist move. However, after pressure (and a threat of a boycott) from civil society activists, including labor activists who had a history of working with the local government, the mayor agreed to link the PB projects to the strategic development plan in the following year. After that, PB in Cusco began to fund educational projects, among others, and is still considered one of the most successful in the country. More recently, in a wealthy district of Lima—Miraflores—the local government has committed to a well-organized online voting process for their PB program. Again, this process is considered to be relatively successful in that it is one of the first processes in Peru to successfully hold voting online (Leon 2010).

However, PB has become a formality in most of Peru (McNulty 2011, 2019; Remy 2011; Lopez Ricci 2014; Prodescentralización 2017). Representatives of CSOs complain that approved projects get held up in bureaucratic processes or canceled when governments change (McNulty 2011). Authorities hold forums and present projects for approval without robust debate or deliberation. Participants are often disillusioned about the process, noting in interviews with McNulty that many of the citizens do not actually deliberate about projects and that votes are perfunctory. For example, in 2018 McNulty observed several PB meetings in Pueblo Libre, a middle-class urban district in Lima. The municipal officials mostly presented to the participants—first the details of the previous year's budget, then a list of projects that participants had proposed. The technical team ranked the projects and the only vote was to approve the top five projects. There was no deliberation about the projects before voting. The bulk of the decision-making took place behind closed doors. Thus, few in Peru argue that PB is solving societal political, economic, or social problems. Importantly, even given the limitations in Peru, few argue that it should not exist; rather, advocates consistently note in interviews that the process must be improved in order to truly engage residents in public policy decisions. In general, we have limited research regarding the impact of PB in Peru in terms of changing individuals or communities. To the best of our knowledge, no large-N research on individual-level attitudinal and behavioral changes exists regarding PB in Peru. However, extensive interview research and observations by McNulty suggest that participants have learned much more about government and public budgeting since the process was introduced in 2003. Many participants are now proficient in writing project proposals and study local project budgets more regularly. On the other hand, PB has not effectively improved community outcomes. When compared to Brazil, a wide body of research suggests that changes at the community level are *not* systematically emerging in Peru. McNulty's (2019) work specifically tests the hypothesis that PB in Peru is leading to improved indicators of municipal services, corruption, clientelism, and accountability. There is no evidence that leaders are more accountable, for example, primarily because the oversight committees are extremely weak in most cities and towns. Civil society is notoriously weak in Peru, and the PB process has done very little to change this. PB has also not changed patterns of corruption and clientelism in the regions and cities, and people's trust in their municipal officials has not improved at all since the law passed (McNulty 2019).

In terms of well-being, most evaluations also find that PB is not improving Peruvians' quality of life. For example, when testing the relationship between PB and water and sanitation service provision, Jaramillo and Alcázar (2013) undertake a large-N statistical analysis of spending and find that PB has little to no effect on coverage or quality of water. When studying the effect of PB on agricultural policy, Jaramillo and Wright (2015) come to a similar conclusion. In fact, they argue that PB is leading to even *less effective* local government services (Jaramillo and Wright 2015). The World Bank (2010b) analyzed several years of participation, and finds that, in general, participants vote for "pro-poor" projects. However, because many of the approved projects are not implemented in a timely way, these projects do not have the social impact that we have seen in Brazil.

Nor do these projects empower women. Diana Miloslavich Túpac (2013) undertook a comprehensive gender analysis of the participatory budget process, analyzing investment projects from 2008 until 2011 in all areas of the country. Miloslavich Túpac finds that the percentage of projects that are geared towards improving the lives of women in the regions and municipalities was less than 1 percent of all projects during the 2011–14 period.

We also know that, unlike Brazil, women's organizations and community groups that represent indigenous and ethnic minority communities do not participate in large numbers. For instance, Amazonian and Afro-Peruvian communities participate at lower rates than the rest of the population, even in areas where they are concentrated (Romero and de Assis 2016; McNulty 2019). There are two exceptions to this. First, Peruvian women do participate in larger numbers in wealthier urban district processes, when compared to regions, rural areas, and poor neighborhoods of urban areas (McNulty 2018). Second, anecdotal evidence also suggests that some municipalities with particularly progressive leadership have incorporated women in interesting ways. For example, in San Juan de Miraflores, a poor district in Lima, there is a Women's Federation that meets regularly to make a list of the project demands for the municipal PB (Van Cott 2008; McNulty 2011). When Susana Villarán was mayor of Lima, she dedicated one million Peruvian soles (roughly USD300,000) to projects that focused on gender empowerment. Although the funding was quite limited, it is the only time that a separate fund for gender projects was set aside. When Villarán left office, the city closed down the fund. However, these examples are relatively rare occurrences in Peru's PB landscape, and generally emerge due to the commitment of a leader in a city or region. The data on participation in Peru suggest that the mandated design and/or the decision to invite CSOs and not individual community members to participate may be restricting participation.

Again, PB does work better in some towns and regions than others (McNulty 2011; Montecinos 2014; Portillo and Jacinto 2018). Research has shown that PB tends to engage more people and be more effective in areas of Peru that have committed officials leading the process (McNulty 2011; Montecinos 2014). This suggests that in contexts where national governments mandate PB, it works best in places where leadership is committed to the principle of citizen participation, as in other country contexts where it is not mandated by the national government.

The findings from Peru—mostly disappointing—strongly suggest that mandated PB generates fewer positive outcomes than the empowered democracy type. Mandated PB programs are often adopted for good reasons, namely the desire to keep PB sustainable and/or the decision to implement accountability measures in places with long histories of corruption. However, subnational governmental officials have too little buy-in because national officials mandate the process. Additionally, the local sociopolitical context is not always conducive to positive outcomes. Thus, the existing body of work on mandated PB, though admittedly limited, suggests that it is hard to make subnational elected officials conduct truly participatory PB processes that lead to concrete community-level changes.

Social Development and Accountability

El Salvador

As PB matured and spread across Latin America and the globe, international organizations promoted PB as a best practice. Today, PB is increasingly identified as a "tool" or "technique" that international organizations, such as the World Bank and USAID, use to promote better governance (Goldfrank 2012; Baiocchi and Ganuza 2017). PB in El Salvador, which USAID originally funded, is a good early example of this phenomenon and shows how mimetic pressures led to at least one PB program in Latin America.

In El Salvador, following the civil war, it was clear that reconstruction would demand improved local governance and enhanced citizen engagement (Arnson 2001). In this post-war reconstruction context, USAID began to fund "democracy-strengthening" programs. The Democratic Local Governance Activity (DLGA), implemented by RTI International, took place from 2002 to 2005. They established PB in twenty-eight municipalities (out of approximately three hundred) (RTI International 2000; Bland 2011, 2017). RTI chose the municipalities, which represented a mix of urban and rural governments, as part of a selection process used by USAID that incorporated governments with a demonstrated interest in participatory practices (Bland 2011). Many municipalities were already familiar with participatory governance because post-war reconstruction efforts also stressed participatory governance, such as town hall meetings and participatory planning processes for projects funded by the Social Investment Fund for Local Development (FISDL). Thus, several municipalities in the country had relatively extensive experience with some form of participatory process by the time RTI formalized the PB program (Bland 2011).

Gary Bland (2011) describes the design of the PB processes in the following passage:

> The PB development process, which required from eight to twelve months to complete, began with considerable preparation and diagnosis of the municipality, led by a project team assigned to each locality...A "participatory diagnosis" followed this preparatory stage. The diagnosis entailed a series of territorial workshops at the neighborhood and canton levels for identifying critical projects for inclusion in the budget. With DLGA support, municipal officials then convened a municipality-wide assembly to define the vision and objectives of PB and further discuss local priorities...Decisions were reached by forging consensus, not through a formal voting process. DLGA's local technical teams conducted project feasibility studies and helped examine the departmental and national-level framework for proposed projects to promote successful implementation...[citizen advocacy groups] brought representatives of local organizations together with council members to oversee implementation, though some were stronger than others...The final product was a multi-annual participatory strategic and investment plan for each municipality. The plan identified all programs and projects considered technically feasible, prioritized them as determined in the meetings, estimated costs for each, and budgeted for each item (identifying future resource streams as needed) for the short, medium, and long term. (868)

There is very little research about the impact of PB in El Salvador. However, the case does offer an interesting finding about PB after donor support ends since, in 2005, USAID pulled its external support. Gary Bland, working for RTI, returned to El Salvador to document PB in 2009 and 2016, wondering if the initial investment in PB would generate enough interest and support that the programs would continue after the discontinuation of funding. Bland (2011) found that in 2009, 32 percent (nine out of twenty-eight) of the municipalities still used PB although they no longer received external support. By 2016, 57 percent (sixteen out of twenty-eight) of the municipalities had PB practices, in rural and urban areas with mayors and officials from both left and right (Bland 2017). Generally speaking, this means that only three in ten municipalities initially used PB when external funds dried up, but this increased to six in ten over time. This suggests that the ideas and processes associated with PB remained a part of the policy debate, driving subsequent governments to ultimately return to use PB. The reasons for this relative success in sustainability are not entirely clear. Bland (2011) notes that those municipalities with higher scores on their "Basic Criteria" index, which measured compliance with the methodology, were most likely to have a more sustainable process. This case does provide some good news for advocates of donor-led processes, suggesting that they might last over time.

Deepening Democracy through Community Mobilization

Mexico

In other places in Latin America, PB advocates increasingly viewed this institution as a way to deepen democracy in a region where democratic gains were increasingly few and far between, and not only as an efficient tool for budget decisions. The emphasis on social justice began to wane, although PB was still viewed as important for strengthening democracy. This is best illustrated by the rapid spread of PB in Mexico. The adoption of PB in Mexico emerged in the broader context of democratic reforms that developed within "development planning" programs during the competitive authoritarian regime of the Institutional Revolutionary Party, or PRI (Selee 2011). The PRI reformed the constitution in 1983 and 1997 to allow citizen participation mechanisms in municipal (municipal development planning councils) and state governments (Benton 2016). In the late 1990s and early 2000s, when the PRI was falling from power, Mexico also passed several laws that stressed transparency, accountability, and participation in general and, more specifically, in budgeting processes. National CSOs worked with government officials to open up the government as the country moved to a more competitive democracy at the turn of the century.

One of Mexico's first formal PB process took place in 2001 in Mexico City's Tlalpan Borough as part of the Party of the Democratic Revolution's (PRD) efforts to bring democracy closer to the people. Local CSOs were also decisive in this work. The process started to expand to additional districts in the city, but ended in 2005. The process began again in 2010, and the municipal government then codified PB in the Citizen Participation Law of the Federal District, which has been updated regularly since. The law states that the Legislative Assembly of the

Federal District must allocate 3 percent of the budget through PB. Originally, this was mostly an effort by the PRD, working with civil society activists at the local level, as part of a leftist political platform.

According to Sanchez (2013), Mexico City's PB process takes place in two steps during the year: 1) information about the process is distributed, proposals for projects that solve some community problem are solicited, and then a technical team makes preliminary viability assessments of the projects; and 2) citizens engage in consultations and voting. Both in-person voting (called *mesas*) and online voting are now possible. Mexico City's Electoral Institute is tasked with overseeing the voting. Any resident of the area can participate (see also Valverde Viesca 2017).

Several CSOs monitor the process in Mexico City annually, forming an "observation network." For the 2016 process, they report that 13,265 projects were submitted and 1,764 were approved; the majority of the projects were public works ("*obras*") or addressed crime (Instituto Electoral del Distrito Federal 2016). Their evaluation suggests that voting took place successfully in most areas, but the quality of information about projects given before voting was of limited quality. Maria Montoya Aguirre (2017) and Alberto Escamilla Cadena's (2019) work both argue that the process is not transparent and suffers from clientelism. Furthermore, around 3 percent of the population engaged in the process, which is similar to the number of participants in other cities.

PB has slowly spread to other parts of the country, and García Bátiz and Téllez Arana (2018) estimate that by early 2016 more than thirty cities and almost 27 percent of the country's population has some form of PB in their community.[4] As of 2014, PB was taking place in cities all over the country, including Mexico City, the states of Jalisco and Sonora, as well as in cities like Guadalajara, Tlaquepaque, Zapopan, Chalco, Ecatepec de Morelos, Toluca, Tepic, San Pedro Garza García, and Santa Catarina (Aguirre Sala 2014). Many programs are short-lived and only last a few years. Further Cejudo et al. (2019) argue that the numbers of participants in meetings that do exist and continue tends to be low, as there is not a "culture of citizen participation" (Cejudo et al. 2019: 97). Françoise Montambeault (2016) documents PB processes in Netzahualcoyotl (Neza) and León, finding that PB is not able to overcome persistent clientelism in Neza, but it does in León, partly due to institutional design choices and partly due to different sociopolitical contexts. Specifically, the nature of civil society and political competition proved determinate in explaining the outcomes generated by PB.

Some innovations have occurred as PB spreads around Mexico. In 2015, the state of Jalisco, led by a governor from the PRI, began to use PB in their state

---

[4] See http://mpcmx.org/ for information about citizen participation mechanisms in Mexico, including PB. See also García Bátiz and Téllez Arana (2018) for a discussion of its spread around the country.

budget-making process. By the end of 2016, 26 percent of the population over twelve years old in Jalisco had participated in some way in sixty-six municipalities.[5] The state has used innovative outreach and engagement mechanisms to ensure such widespread participation, such as a digital platform called *Vamos Juntos*. This relatively new process has been hailed as an example of PB that has reached a large group of citizens, partly due to the numerous workshops that are taking place around the state and the digital platform. As of this writing, however, it is too soon to say if this project is sustainable or will have lasting impact.

In 2014, the municipality of Cananea approved a Fund for Regional Sustainable Development (or Mining Fund) to distribute extractive rents to communities surrounding a copper mine (Cejudo et al. 2019). With World Bank support, the municipality recently decided to employ PB to determine how to spend its mining revenues. This was the first case of a city using PB to determine spending of its mining fund in Mexico, and advocates hoped that it might spur other cities to do the same. After one year of the process, however, the World Bank finalized its assistance and the mayor left office. According to our interviews with evaluators, his successor decided to not continue PB and the experience ended after only one year. This is one example that illustrates how vital political support is to the success of PB (see also García Bátiz and Téllez Arana 2018).

Both the El Salvador and Mexico examples demonstrate how leaders have innovated and experimented with a variety of PB types as this particular participatory institution spread around the region. A commitment of some domestic leaders to PB's values and norms motivated many of these cases while donors pushed forward others. These cases also demonstrate how much more there is to do in terms of evaluating PB's impact, even in this region. Few studies have assessed the outcomes that have emerged from most PB cases beyond Brazil and there is much more research that can be done in this region.

Comparative Analysis

Much of the data regarding the impact of PB comes from Latin America, and, more specifically, Brazil. Case studies, comparative longitudinal, and large-N analyses demonstrate that PB can impact individuals and communities in positive ways. However, these outcomes do not always emerge. One lesson from this region is that PB is more likely to empower individuals, change civil society, improve accountability, and lead to changes in the community's well-being when Empowered Democracy programs emphasize social justice as part of the process as well as when government leaders are committed to creating robust processes in

---

[5] See their metrics on the government's web portal for more data: https://vamosjuntos.jalisco.gob. mx/informaci%C3%B3n-relevante.

general. Interestingly, the early emphasis on social justice has evolved into a stress on social inclusion in the Deepening Democracy through Community Mobilization type, which is present in PB in several North Atlantic cases, as described in Chapter 5.

Latin America is also home to the first Mandated PB processes, which emerged in the second wave, and focus on improving local policymaking as a technical tool, not social justice. Chapter 4 outlines how several participatory programs in Asia morphed into mandated PB in the Philippines, South Korea, and Indonesia. We also see some expansion of mandated PB into Poland. With the exception of South Korea and Indonesia, which are discussed more in Chapter 4, the results from this experiment have generally been disappointing. In Peru, local leaders are not always interested in upholding the national mandate and the processes often become empty and formulaic. Chapters 4 and 6 elaborate on the many of the disappointing results for mandated PB process.

Latin America also hosts the Social Development and Accountability type (El Salvador) and Deepening Democracy (Mexico). We do not have impact data from these nations but do know that the El Salvador case provides interesting data about the potential sustainability of the donor-led process; 60 percent of the programs continued even after funding from USAID was discontinued. This is an important finding for the newer cases of social development and accountability types of PB, which are the very common in Africa.

Conclusion

In Latin America, PB emerged as a radical democratic project meant to engage new actors in local decision-making and subsequently morphed into a popular public policy tool adopted by hundreds of governments across the region. From its birth in the late 1980s until today, PB has transformed in several ways. Most importantly, the original focus on redistribution and social justice is no longer a vital component of most PB programs. Many programs now emphasize social inclusion (see Noriega, Aburto, and Montecinos 2016, for example). This is a noteworthy goal, but these programs do not require that additional resources be allocated to low-income and poor communities. The evidence also suggests that governments have decreased the percentage of their budgets that they allocate to PB programs. The earliest and most successful cases of PB allocated upwards of 15 percent of their annual budget to the process. By 2020, it is far more likely that governments will allocate less than 2 percent of their annual budget through PB.

Given PB's longevity and breadth in the region, researchers studying Latin American PB programs have generated a large body of research and therefore developed a base for much of our understanding about the causal mechanisms that lead to individual and community-level changes. Case study and medium-N comparative studies demonstrate that PB changes participants' sense of personal efficacy as well as their own views about what it means to be a citizen. It also teaches average citizens about budget making and the tough decisions that go into investment spending (Wampler and Avritzer 2004; Baiocchi 2005; Wampler 2007, 2015; Montambeault 2016). A smaller set of studies document that government officials also learn more about their constituents' preferences and neighborhood needs during PB meetings (Wampler 2015; McNulty 2018).

PB's effect on civil society and state–society relations is also well documented in Latin American cases. PB can change civil society's density and alter the existing relationships between CSOs and the state (Baiocchi 2005; Van Cott 2008; Baiocchi, Heller, and Silva 2011; McNulty 2011, 2015; Touchton and Wampler 2014). McNulty (2013) finds that CSOs are strengthened in some cases by creating new alliances and providing new forms of technical assistance. Montambeault (2019) finds that PB can democratize cooperation between state and civil society actors in limited cases. Thus, the nature of civil society is an important conditioning factor for outcomes.

Research from Brazil has documented changes in citizens' ability to hold government officials accountable as well as government's ability to collect taxes (thereby holding citizens somewhat accountable as well). Changes in accountability can partly be understood through PB's oversight process, which is embedded in PB's core design. In most places, participants form an oversight committee to monitor the projects and spending commitments that emerge from the annual process. Even when relationships do not shift to a more collaborative nature, the oversight committee can ensure that officials are spending investment funds in a responsible and transparent way. Importantly, however, in many PB processes around the region, the oversight process is not strong. This means that improved accountability may not emerge in many contexts.

Finally, evidence from Brazil suggests that PB programs improve well-being. We note, however, that there are just a handful of articles that empirically establish these associations in one country (World Bank 2008; Gonçalves 2014; Touchton and Wampler 2014; Wampler and Touchton 2019), therefore there may something unique about Brazilian PB that generates these positive associations with well-being. It is theoretically possible that other PB programs around the world have similar positive associations with well-being, but no one has systematically identified empirical relationships between PB and well-being in other contexts. This is an urgent task that researchers and international organizations would be well advised to undertake.

Research from Latin America has also generated a clear consensus that several mitigating factors explain why PB generates positive outcomes in some places but not others. First, the nature of civil society before implementation is crucial as has been extensively analyzed in the Brazilian and Peruvian cases. The government can co-opt organizations through PB when civil society is not strong or organized (Van Cott 2008; McNulty 2011, 2015, 2019; Garrido and Montecinos 2018). Second, the support of public officials also determines the extent to which these outcomes emerge. And finally, as noted in the comparison between Brazil and Peru, the design of PB itself will also condition the outcomes. Research in other countries echoes these findings.

Thus, it is important to keep in mind that the impacts that we describe do not magically appear after PB is created and implemented. PB must be designed for particular contexts to effect positive changes like those described above. There is still much more to document about PB in Latin America, even with the robust body of literature that now exists. For starters, we need more cross-national research that systematically explores PB's impact. We must also continue to gather longitudinal data on these processes to generate hypotheses that can be tested in new environments.

Latin America provides an interesting place to compare the outcomes associated with design decisions and types of PB, as many of the PB types documented in Chapter 1 exist in the region. It is especially interesting to compare the original Empowered Democracy model, with its overall positive effects on communities and individuals, and the Mandated PB, such as those in Peru and the Dominican Republic. For example, in the Dominican Republic, where PB must take place in all municipalities by law, research shows that PB has not taken hold in the way that reformers had hoped due to the lack of commitment by both citizens and political leaders (Hernández-Medina 2007; Allegretti 2011; Gutiérrez-Barbarrusa 2011; Garrido and Montecinos 2018). PB has been implemented in varying degrees around the country and is not considered to have transformed municipal spending (de León 2005; Hernández-Medina 2007; Gutiérrez-Barbarrusa 2011; Reyes and González Molina 2011; González 2019). Thus, the results of both Peru and the Dominican Republic's nationally mandated PB processes have been disappointing; neither country's PB projects have led to the kinds of results that advocates originally hoped for. This suggests that the empowered PB type may generate more robust long-term results than its nationally mandated counterparts. Of course, more comprehensive research is needed to test this assertion.

Having documented the creation and initial diffusion of PB in Latin America, the following chapters analyze the ways that PB has been adopted and adapted in three additional regions of the world: Asia, the North Atlantic, and Africa. Chapter 4 documents PB's spread in Asia where, like Latin America, democratization processes led to innovations in cities. However, the early examples were not identified as "Participatory Budgeting." The programs developed rules based on similar principles and were eventually transformed into PB programs, following mimetic adaptations. Like Peru, the three countries (South Korea,

Indonesia, and the Philippines) analyzed in Chapter 4 now all have mandated PB programs. Like Brazil, reformers tried to keep the social justice aspects of the original PB model; however, they did so in new ways. Thus, Asia presents an interesting region in terms of better understanding the spread of this democratic policymaking tool.

4

Parallel Paths to Local Democracy
in Asia

Extensive experimentation with new democratic institutions took place in Asia across the 1980s and 1990s, but PB only formally arrived in Asia at the beginning of the twenty-first century. The transition to democracy in countries like the Philippines, Indonesia, and South Korea spurred the development of local democratic, participatory institutions during the late 1980s and early 1990s, allowing citizen mobilization in municipal-level policymaking processes. These participatory programs were not initially branded as "PB," but they shared similar principles and designs. The parallel creation of comparable institutions to PB took place in a broader context of extensive citizen mobilization that was pressing for national democratic reforms. Political movements to establish democracy in these three countries emphasized expanding the direct role of citizen participation in public life, using public resources and state authority to improve citizens' social and living conditions, ending the arbitrary abuse of state authority, and citizens and CSOs monitoring state activities (Lee 2005; Gibson and Woolcock 2008; Lah 2010; Melgar 2010; Olken 2010; No 2017). The spread of PB across Asia thus builds from democratic impulses to empower citizens in new democracies.

During the 2000s and 2010s, we see the direct transfer of PB programs and rules from Brazil to Asian governments, as part of PB's third wave of diffusion (see Chapter 1). Government officials and NGO activists developed relationships with Brazilian policymakers, party officials, NGO activists, and researchers as well as international organizations (the World Bank in particular), which helped pave the way for the adoption of PB (No 2017; Porto de Oliveira 2017a).

In this chapter, we focus on three countries—South Korea, the Philippines, Indonesia—to illuminate key trends in the region. We see a clear pattern. A small number of local governments initially adopted "PB-like" programs. Positive evaluations of these programs then spurred national governments to mandate PB to incorporate large segments of the population in public decision-making. These three countries are on the cutting edge of participatory reform among Asia's democratic regimes. In all three countries, political reformers and democracy activists looked for ways to activate existing democratic practices in the hopes of improving the quality of their governments. All three countries' elected governments, nationally and locally, faced intense demands on their limited resources and state capacity. Achieving the dual tasks of providing public services and improving

Participatory Budgeting in Global Perspective. Brian Wampler, Stephanie McNulty, and Michael Touchton,
Oxford University Press. © Brian Wampler, Stephanie McNulty, and Michael Touchton 2021.
DOI: 10.1093/oso/9780192897756.003.0005

the quality of democracy is often an immense challenge for elected governments. It is within this broader context that governments began experimenting with programs that would simultaneously enhance civil society, improve the quality of democracy, and make better use of public resources. At the same time, elected officials, civil servants, and civil society activists advocated for the adoption of democratic innovations in very different national contexts. An additional focus, toward the end of this chapter, is the expansion of PB to China. Although our book focuses on PB in democratic environments, we include a short section on China because it helps to illuminate how the malleability of PB's rules enables local governments to implement the program in authoritarian contexts; the use of PB by authoritarian governments is one of the most controversial issues facing PB today.

We find three types of PB programs in South Korea, the Philippines, and Indonesia. In each country, the early programs are best categorized as either Deepening Democracy through Community Mobilization (Philippines, South Kora, Indonesia cities) or Social Development and Accountability (Indonesian villages). In all three countries, the national government then mandated that local governments adopt PB. In all three countries, subnational decentralization was key; national governments then mandated that municipal governments adopt some form of direct citizen participation in budgeting exercises. Table 4.1 below provides an historical view of PB in the region, including its key variants and diffusion over time.

Table 4.1. PB in Indonesia, the Philippines, and South Korea

PB type	1989 to mid-1990s	Mid-1990s to mid-2000s	Mid-2000s to 2020
Empowered Democracy and Redistribution			
Deepening Democracy through Community Mobilization		1 city in the Philippines (Naga City, 1997) 3–4 Indonesian cities (early 2000s) 1 South Korean municipality (2002)	
Mandated by National Government		490 Indonesian cities (2004)	609 Philippine local governments (2011) 1,590 Philippine local governments (2015) 74,000 Indonesian villages (2014) 514 Indonesian cities (2004) 241 South Korean cities (2011)

PB type	1989 to mid-1990s	Mid-1990s to mid-2000s	Mid-2000s to 2020
Digital PB			
Social Development and Accountability	Several hundred Indonesian villages (across 1990s)	65,000 Indonesian villages (2007)	609 Philippines (2011) 74,000 Indonesian villages (2014)
Efficient Governance			

From Deepening Democracy through Community Mobilization to Mandated by National Government

The Philippines

In the Philippines, we find the parallel development of a "PB-like" program in the early 1990s, which transformed into formal PB across the country, especially in rural areas. This is due to the unique role of the national government running PB from a national-level ministry.

The original development of participatory programs took place during the 1990s, a period of democratic renewal. In 1986, a popular social uprising forced the Filipino dictator, Ferdinand Marcos, from power. His successor, Corazón Aquino, took office in 1986 and helped to stabilize democratic rule. President Corazón Aquino oversaw the drafting and adoption of a new national constitution, the establishment of a bicameral national legislature, and eventual democratic rule. She also fended off several coup attempts intended to reverse democratic progress. The Local Government Code of 1991 established the legal right for national and subnational governments to formally include citizens and NGOs in policy and budgetary processes (Magno 2013: 19). Thus, a window of opportunity for participatory innovations, similar to Brazil, developed in the Philippines in the 1980s and early 1990s.

What is now PB has its roots in the adoption of an innovative democratic program in Naga City, a mid-sized city located on the Philippines' main island (Melgar 2010). In Naga City, an elected mayor and a group of political reformers adopted a PB-like program to help alter the basic structures of local state–society relationships. Fölscher and Melgar both identify the Naga City case as having rule-structures and programs similar to Brazil's PB (Fölscher 2007; Melgar 2010). In this program, citizens and community groups were mobilized to attend government-sponsored meetings in which citizens had the opportunity to deliberate and then vote on the government's policy priorities. The program did not include a specific social justice requirement, which differentiates the Naga City PB process from the more radical PB experiences in Brazil.

The mayor who led the political coalition at the head of the reform movement in Naga City, Jesse Robredo, would become the national Interior and Local Government Secretary under President Benigno Aquino III (2010–16). According to one government official, Robredo used his time as national minister to promote the national expansion of participatory reforms. Although formal PB programs did not expand much beyond Naga City during the 1990s and 2000s, there were numerous participatory and transparency initiatives taking place at the local level. For example, Roadwatch is a well-known Filipino initiative in which citizens organized themselves to actively monitor road construction (Aceron 2019; Fox 2015: 9; Magno 2013). Broadly, the 1990s and 2000s featured significant institutional creativity, much of it centered around new forms of state–society interactions. But the more specific PB programs from Naga City did not spread across the rest of the country. The absence of an ideologically coherent, strong party, such as the Workers' Party in Brazil, meant that the Filipino left did not win many elections, and when they did, there were no clear mechanisms available to induce local governments to adopt more radical programs.

PB's fortunes changed significantly with Benigno Aquino's 2010 election to the presidency. Aquino campaigned as a political reformer, emphasizing transparency, participation, and accountability (Magno 2013). Once in office, Aquino's governance-related reforms centered on transparency, openness, and participation. In 2011, for example, the Philippines was a founding member of the Open Government Partnership (www.ogp.gov), indicating that the Aquino government was interested in promoting a broader social reform agenda. More pertinent for this book, Aquino's 2010 election ushered in the rapid expansion of PB in the Philippines.

The most important transformation in the adoption and spread of PB in the Philippines lay in the involvement of a national-level ministry, the Department of Budget and Management. The Philippines is the only country we know of where a national-level department actively implemented PB in thousands of different local government units, without national legislation (as in Peru) or a legislative mandate for participation in budgeting or planning (as in Indonesia). Rather, a newly elected government, led by President Aquino, implemented PB as part of their reformist policy agenda that emphasized greater participation and transparency.

This ministry-led PB process was initially branded as Bottom-up Budgeting (BuB); later, it would be referred to interchangeably as BuB and PB. There are several noteworthy institutional features that differentiate Filipino PB programs from those elsewhere, including: (a) the direct involvement of the National Department of Budget and Management; (b) financial incentives designed to induce villages and towns to invest in PB; (c) the creation of a new decision-making body that includes 50 percent citizens and 50 percent policy experts; and (d) a focus on both infrastructure and social programs.

The National Department of Budget and Management incentivized cities, towns, and villages to adopt BuB by offering them additional resources if these subnational governments directly incorporated citizens into a series of public meetings and ensured that these citizens could exercise a consultative (non-binding) vote on policy projects. Under BuB, local governments were required to hold open forums in which citizens deliberated and then voted to select public works projects that the local government would implement. The national government provided basic technical support, including a common template for how the meetings and the process were supposed to be administered. Thus, the Aquino government sought to support adoption by providing a toolkit that subnational governments could follow as they introduced PB. Importantly, project selection emphasized development efforts, such as roads to improve access to markets, the reform or expansion of health facilities and schools, and building small dams to capture water.

The obvious incentive for local governments to actively support BuB was the additional resources they would receive from the national government. According to a government official who helped to organize the program, the national government hoped that the adoption of BuB would also generate changes in local state–society relations (see also Lim 2017; Aceron 2019). Government officials thought that PB's deliberative process would empower citizens. Lim argues that "BuB created a parallel mechanism that provided a more meaningful space for participation. It provided effective incentives that encouraged civil society and local governments to engage each other in participatory planning and budgeting" (Lim 2017: 7).

PB's advocates and program designers first sought to alter who participated in decision-making processes by taking advantage of the country's relatively dense civil society. "The target audience for participation is organized citizens' groups at the city or municipal level. There is no restriction [on participation], except that relatives of local government officials/employees cannot represent organizations" (Lim 2017: 10). The BuB was also designed to encourage unaffiliated citizens to participate, unlike places like Peru and Indonesia where most participants were invited to attend PB meetings through CSOs. Some evidence suggests that PB is changing civil society in the Philippines. Lim writes that "BuB has expanded the number of CSOs that are engaged by local governments since local governments can no longer decide who they engage with. Some local governments have begun to appreciate engagement with CSOs and some relationships have improved because the process is repeated every year" (Lim 2017: 12).

In addition, government officials hoped that additional oversight would decrease corruption, and a broader range of local development projects would improve citizens' lives (Lim 2017). We would also expect PB to improve well-being over time due to its focus on economic and social programs and not just infrastructure projects. The BuB program thus encourages CSOs to participate, but also promotes the involvement of a wider range of CSOs in order to move beyond the mayor's allies.

BuB uses a two-stage process to select projects. Citizens in a general assembly prioritize projects in the first stage. The selected projects must conform to the level of available resources as well as the policy channels through which local budgets operate. However, the Local Poverty Reduction Action Team (LPRAT) makes final project decisions in a second stage. "[This team is] composed of 50% local government officials and 50% representatives of the CSO assembly. Decisions in the LPRAT are often made through negotiation and consensus between local government and civil society, although voting can occur" (Lim 2017: 12). The two-stage filtering process may limit "elite capture" because participants know that a combination of policy experts, civil servants, and CSO leaders will review their policy recommendations in a subsequent stage of the policy process. However, it is possible that local governments could also work with their CSO allies to ensure that projects selected through BuB align with the elected governments' interests. Thus, the two-stage decision-making process creates great opportunities to initiate social, political, and policy change, but we lack evidence of the extent to which the BuB actually results in sustained social, political, and policy improvements.

Philippines PB programs are distinct from many others in that they include both infrastructure projects and economic and social service programs. Common infrastructure projects include road paving and building or refurbishing public facilities such as schools, community centers, or health clinics. Economic and social service programs include training on small business development and increasing access to markets, which are both aimed at helping rural residents identify ways to generate income. In this case, BuB should empower citizens by expanding their economic opportunities. This program was part of larger effort to simultaneously allocate greater resources in rural villages, broaden the number of citizens involved in the policymaking process, and increase development opportunities. This is also the clearest example covered in this book of how a presidential administration brought new political and policymaking processes to subnational governments and incorporated citizens directly in decision-making.

Coordinating BuB's vertical integration has been a major challenge because the national government wanted to delegate decision-making authority to local governments while also monitoring their actions to ensure that national resources were used well (Aceron 2019). Between 2014 and 2016, the national government extended BuB to 1,300 municipalities, many of which were poor, small, and rural (Lim 2017). This delegation of authority created many new opportunities for mayors and citizens to work together in participatory forums, thus permitting an expansion of voice and vote in the public arena. However, municipal governments struggled to implement projects that citizens selected because local state capacity was low and the "release" of funds by the national government was cumbersome.

Although the BuB programs include a redistributive component from the national level to local levels, there were additional rules that required funding to be spent in poor and underserved communities. These programs were attentive to deep regional and urban–rural inequalities that mark the Philippines but BuB didn't require that resources were directed to the neediest citizens. The national government provided additional resources to poorer, rural municipalities through the BuB program. By using a poverty-based indicator, the national government generated a redistributive effect, implicitly attempting to promote social justice by getting more resources into the poorest places in the country.

Government-generated data demonstrate that the program allocated significant resources to BuB (USD494 million in 2016 according to http://openbub.gov.ph/data), reaching a large portion of the country. The national government first included roughly a third of Local Government Units (LGUs) in PB, but quickly expanded to cover most Filipino cities and municipalities. The level of resources allocated to PB more than doubled between 2013, the rollout year, and 2016. Although there was considerable investment, as Table 4.2 demonstrates, there is no systematic research to demonstrate if these changes in spending have had an impact on well-being, civil society, or accountability.

Like many PB processes in developing nations, a significant limitation of the BuB model is the difficulty of implementing selected projects due to the program's institutional design and the lack of state capacity (Lim 2017; Aceron 2019). Following project selection at the local level, a combination of national- and local-level administrative units developed the projects (e.g., drafting of technical plans, securing legal permission). Local governments, especially in smaller villages, did not have the technical expertise, such as civil engineers, to design infrastructure projects, which then slowed implementation. Local governments relied on national administrative bodies to provide technical expertise, but these national units also faced capacity issues as they were understaffed and overburdened (Lim 2017; Aceron 2019). Furthermore, the national government administrative units struggled to efficiently allocate money to the LGUs. Thus, even with correct planning documents, local governments faced difficulties in soliciting contracting bids and paying for projects. The national government-led BuB program created the opportunity to expand participatory programs to villages and towns across the country but the program was eventually hamstrung by the national government's inability to systematically implement projects. Additional research is needed to determine if the BuB had a systematic impact on well-being, civil society, or accountability. When the Duterte administration took over in 2016, they initially scaled back the PB program, but pressure from mayors led the administration to continue funding it. However, this support was short lived and the BuB program disappeared from the Philippines.

Table 4.2. Philippines: Bottom-up Budgeting 2013–16

Fiscal year	Number of target LGUs	Number of cities/ municipalities that had PB programs	Budget allocation (in 2013 USD)	Number of projects
2013	609	595 cities and municipalities*	US $200 million in 2013 dollars	5,898
2014	1,233	1,226 cities and municipalities*	US $448 million in 2013 dollars	19,506
2015	1,634	1,590*	US $451 million in 2013 dollars	16,269
2016	1,514** (excluding ARMM)	1,514	US $475 Million in 2013 dollars	14,324

Notes: *Some did not receive PB funding in 2013 and 2014 because they did not go through the required participatory process or did not submit a list of priority projects.

**The LGUs in the Autonomous Region in Muslim Mindanao were removed from BuB due to the reorganization of the regional government.

Source: Lim (2017: 15).

South Korea

In South Korea, the PB type, Deepening Democracy through Community Mobilization, transitioned into Mandated by National Government. We also find extensive use of online and digital technologies in the PB programs, however the continuing face-to-face participation in most Korean PB programs means these programs do not meet the criteria for Digital PB. South Korea's PB programs emerged in the broader sociopolitical context of democracy-building, as Korea transitioned to a democratic regime in 1987, as well as rapid state-led economic development (Kohli 2004). As a result, efforts to build Korean PB programs as a means to deepen democracy occurred in a context in which policy experts and state bureaucrats were widely credited with successfully managing the country's industrialization (Choi 2014).

South Korea's first PB was established fifteen years after the country's democratization in 1987. It began at the subnational level in 2002 when a leftist, union-oriented elected political party was elected to the municipal government in Gwangu, a city of 1.4 million. The leftist party elected in Gwangu was in contact with the Workers' Party in Brazil, which helps to explain why the government chose the specific format of PB (No 2017, 2018). Normative pressures (creating space for the working class inside the government) as well as mimetic pressures (PB as an internationally recognized democratic policymaking instrument) drove the adoption of PB in South Korea.

South Korea's PB did not incorporate the more radical forms of participatory democracy for several reasons. Most importantly, the sequencing of adoption, both domestically and internationally, pushed it toward a less radical form of PB because PB arrived in 2002, nearly fifteen years after the mass mobilizations. The mass mobilization of 1987, led by students and union members, led to a new democracy but direct citizen engagement in policymaking was not at the core of the new institutions (Lah 2010). Second, South Korea made some attempts to expand citizen participation during the 1990s, but these were complementary to representative democracy rather than being envisioned as a radical democratic renewal (Lah 2010; No 2017). Thus, PB was not initially created during the key democratization moment of the late 1980s and early 1990s, as in Brazil. Second, PB arrived in South Korea when democracy was already fifteen years old; PB became more of an incremental citizen participation innovation rather than a radical form of participatory democracy that strongly emphasized broad, popular mobilization. Third, by the 2000s, the internationalization of Brazil's PB (the Porto Alegre model) focused more on the rules that made it a successful, incremental democratic policymaking institution than a radical democratic innovation.

The Gwangu case marks the first clear example in which an elected government in South Korea adopted a program that promoted citizens' direct participation in policymaking (No 2017). Won No notes that "although it was the very first case in South Korea that named the program 'participatory budgeting,' the type of participation allowed in the first year was close to a public consultation rather than co-production or empowerment because the district head was in charge of constituting the PB committee and calling for meetings" (2017: 9).

Building on this initial case in Gwangu, PB began to spread across South Korea. In 2005, the national government passed legislation to "permit" municipal governments to design participatory programs that directly engaged citizens in budgetary processes (No 2017). This increased the rate of PB adoption across the country because municipal governments were more willing to institute the program once it became clear that it was legal for them to do so. The spread of PB following its first adoption was also spurred by the interest of President Roh, who advocated for "participatory democracy" (Lee and You 2013; Cho et al. 2020). Local governments gradually created PB programs over the next several years; by 2010, just over 40 percent had adopted PB (Song 2013, cited by No 2017).

In 2011, the national government passed legislation *mandating* that all local government units incorporate citizens in the budget process (No 2017). There were two distinct ways that this could be done: 1) "heads of local governments were required to establish procedures that allowed resident participation in local public budgeting processes, and 2) heads of local governments were required to enclose written statements that included residents' opinions of the budget proposal and submit them to the local council" (No 2017: 11). As a result, over 90 percent of South Korean municipalities adopted PB by 2012, suggesting that local governments were very interested in complying with the directives of the national government (Hwang and Song 2013). In a short period, by 2014, almost all Korean municipalities actively adopted PB programs (No 2017). This suggests a relatively high level of local government interest as the governments were actively involved in adopting PB as part of their policymaking process (No 2017).In this sense, the South Korean case is similar to the Peruvian case in that PB was first adopted at the subnational level, then expanded to all municipal governments through a national mandate. Yet, the South Korean PB experience is distinct because it appears that there was much more interest in program adoption among Korean mayors than among Peruvian ones. The reasons why South Korea's local governments were more likely to support PB include: (a) greater resources to implement projects; (b) greater levels of local administrative capacity; (c) a competitive two-party system with one leftist party strongly supporting increased citizen participation; and (d) a stronger, more energized civil society (Cho et al. 2020).

In Korea, technology has been used as a participant recruitment tool as well as for providing information about budgets (Kim 2016; Park et al. 2019). Local governments use different social media communication strategies, such as texting, websites, and Twitter, to galvanize support. Local governments also have good access to budget data, which they then publish online. However, South Korean PB programs have not emphasized online deliberation or voting features, which are more prevalent in Europe. The presence of high-quality budget data suggests that having a well-functioning, high-capacity state may be a key ingredient to producing a favorable environment for transparency and learning. We turn now to the case of Seoul to better explore how local governments adapted PB to meet their local needs.

PB in Seoul, the capital of South Korea with a population of over 10 million, adopted PB in 2011. Due to its large geographic size and massive population, the government created a decentralized governance system within PB that is similar to the Porto Alegre model. Namely, Seoul is divided into twenty-five districts where citizens make decisions, with additional decisions reserved for nine thematic areas (No 2017). Further, any Seoul resident is eligible to vote on the final proposal (No: 2017). This is a clear example of mimetic adoption as the program's institutional rules align with the Porto Alegre model. However, these rules also move beyond the Porto Alegre model in a few key ways.

Seoul's PB uses three stages of project selection at the district level. Citizens first propose projects. Government officials then review them to ensure compliance with legal and fiscal guidelines. Next, a voluntary citizens' committee evaluates the proposals, providing a score for the broader group of citizens who vote in the final stage. The city government then randomly selects committee members, working to ensure a balance along gender, age, and home neighborhood (No 2017). The committee then evaluates all proposals through eight criteria: 1) needs; 2) urgency; 3) publicness; 4) effectiveness; 5) accomplishment; 6) subject fit; 7) gender equality; and 8) project cost appropriateness (No 2017).

Seoul's public administrators manage the final round of deliberations but mainly rely on volunteer facilitators to guide the deliberations. This represents a key adaptation of the decision-making process in PB. Seoul draws facilitators from the citizens' evaluation committees, which means that these facilitators are volunteers who were randomly selected to be part of the committee. Won No found that Seoul's PB meetings are more "deliberative" under very specific conditions. She argues that the "meetings can be deliberative 1) when public managers are not dominating the discussion and the facilitators are not being authoritative, 2) when both the public managers and facilitators are not dominating the discussion, or 3) when there is a female facilitator and the public managers are not dominating the discussion" (No 2017: 105–6). This analysis demonstrates that governments are more likely to reshape the decision-making process when they invest in deliberative processes. Won No's work highlights the possibility that the decision-making process can be transformed to promote a robust and healthy debate, but it also demonstrates the strong and genuine commitment to deliberation by governments is necessary to achieve these outcomes.

The Seoul case affords the opportunity to assess how PB might generate changes across civil society, accountability, and well-being (Choi 2014; No 2017; No and Hsueh 2020). There is a wealth of data on Seoul and its PB programs, which has been utilized by researchers to investigate outcomes similar to those researched in this book. One of the most important findings is that the Seoul program is very attentive to social inclusion. Although no specific social justice rules *require* PB projects to be allocated to poor communities, the strong emphasis on social inclusion means that PB is more likely to invest in projects that address the needs of poorer communities. Looking ahead to Chapter 5, this is a relevant finding for PB in New York City, where the program strongly emphasizes social inclusion but also doesn't have specific rules mandating that resources are spent in low-income communities.

Won No's work finds this to be true, demonstrating that "poor districts got more resources even though they had no specific rules that promoted social justice" (No 2017: 51). No (2017) offers three explanations for why the program generated positive social justice outcomes. First, the institutional design and processes encouraged people to consider community needs as they made decisions. Citizens appear to have been influenced to make voting decisions that are equity-based by incorporating the idea of "need." In turn, they supported a greater number of projects in poorer, underserved communities. Second, districts that successfully incorporated a broader group of citizens into their processes are more likely to produce pro-poor outcomes. This suggests that the use of social inclusion rules will create a broader cross-section of participants, which contributes to improvements in well-being. Third, groups from poor neighborhoods secured additional resources when they formed alliances during the deliberation and voting phases. These citizens generated "bonds of solidarity" through which they advanced their shared interests (Alexander 2006). Finally, smaller groups that were unable to form similar alliances viewed these alliances as negative.

Hong and Cho's (2018) research also demonstrates that Seoul's PB program results in greater spending in poorer neighborhoods in comparison to middle-class and wealthy neighborhoods. Hong and Cho (2018) found that an increase in citizen participation from poorer communities was associated with greater spending in these communities. "The results of our study suggest that citizen participatory budgeting results in more redistributive policy outcomes than traditional bureaucratic budgeting" (Hong and Cho 2018: 494). Furthermore, they argue that the results of this study indicate that there was little trade-off between equity and effectiveness when budgeting decisions are made with input from citizens. "Our data show that gains in equity were much more pronounced than losses in effectiveness" (Hong and Cho 2018: 494). Overall, the evidence suggests that Seoul's PB program took initial steps towards allocating increased resources to poor communities. Combined, this research hints that PB is changing the nature of civil society and will probably improve well-being over time.

In sum, the research of Cho, No, and Park (2020), Hong and Cho (2018), No (2017) and No and Hsueh (2020) demonstrate that Seoul's PB program results in the redistribution of resources to poorer communities. This success stands in sharp contrast to mandated programs in Peru (Chapter 3), Poland (Chapter 5), and Indonesia (see below) where researchers have either found little to no positive redistribution effects. More broadly, the Korean case stands out from other examples of mandated programs because the available research indicates that its PB programs are working relatively well. The principal reasons why the Korean cases are working better than those in other countries include: (a) ample resources to implement projects by citizens, (b) capable, efficient local states, (c) strong local government support, and (d) an engaged civil society. However, we note that there is limited comparative analysis of Korean cases, so it is difficult to generalize from Seoul to a broader number of cases. However, we note that the high level of mayoral support in Seoul for PB suggests that the outcomes in Seoul are most likely better than in other cities.

Deepening Democracy and Social Development and Accountability to Mandated by National Government

Indonesia

During the 1990s, under the Suharto dictatorship, community-driven development programs, which share many principles with PB, spread across rural Indonesia. Local governments and civil society leaders developed new institutional venues to encourage deliberation and citizen-oriented decision-making.

Following the fall of the Suharto dictatorship in 1998, social movement activists travelled to the Philippines to gather information about how local governments developed new participatory mechanisms. By 2014, the national government mandated participatory planning and budgeting programs used by 490 Indonesian cities (Rifai 2019) as well as in 74,000 villages. However, the legislation that mandates PB utilizes a broad category, "participatory planning and budgeting," which means that subnational government units have extensive flexibility to adapt rules to best address local problems. Indonesian PB programs follow two distinct tracks: one situated in the cities and a second in the villages. The roots of the "cities" track are drawn from the Deepening Democracy through Community Mobilization type. The programs in the "villages" track are most similar to the Social Development and Accountability type; however, because of the large number, we do not know the extent to which Indonesia's villages have actually implemented programs that we would classify as PB. Further, PB is now mandated at both levels. We first address the PB in Indonesia cities.

Indonesian Cities

Adoption of PB at the city level quickly followed national democratization after General Suharto's removal from office in 1998. According to a civil society activist, in 2000 the Ford Foundation provided funding for NGO activists from three central Javanese cities to travel to the Philippines to learn about participatory planning processes. This activist identified that specific trip as the key factor behind the introduction of a pilot PB program in Surakarta, an industrial city in middle of Java. The proto-PB program in Surakarta included several notable features that would continue in PB processes that later spread to all cities. First, government officials invited participants to PB meetings, following a longstanding cultural and government tradition of officials inviting local elites to meetings. Civil society leaders who were not invited to PB meetings were not likely to know about the meetings because they were not widely advertised. If a civil society leader who hadn't been invited to the meeting happened to learn about it, there was a strong bias against them attending. Thus, while all citizens legally enjoy the right to attend and participate in these meetings, most participants were invited by government officials.

Second, government officials and local community leaders in Surakarta drew upon existing community organizations and structures in several ways to organize who they would invite to participate. For example, women's groups, which were a key part of social organizing under the Suharto dictatorship, became important sources of participation. Further, Javanese cultural tradition places a strong emphasis on allowing community leaders and elites to deliberate and hopefully reach consensus (Barron et al. 2011). Java's deliberative traditions thus dovetailed nicely with the principles of democratic deliberation associated with PB (Warren 2007; Rifai 2017). Finally, government officials embedded the PB process in administrative state structures that form Indonesia's government, inserting it into the two lowest levels of government (Ruken Tetangga and Ruken Warga): community and neighborhood levels that permit government officials to directly connect with community leaders and citizens. The benefit of this approach is that PB organizers could draw upon existing civil society engagement as well as state support, but the clear defect is that these existing state–society relations may not be conducive to promoting social change. Surakarta's model would soon spread across Indonesia.

In 2004—six years after the establishment of democracy, four years after NGO activists travelled to the Philippines, and three years after the Surakarta city government set up PB—the national government mandated that all 490 cities in Indonesia must use a participatory planning and budgeting process (Rifai et al. 2016: 12). The 2004 law requires a *Musrenbang* process, which is a combination of participatory planning and PB. Based on a series of interviews in Java in 2018, citizens and community organizers were highly enthusiastic about PB's prospects as they sought to build new institutions that would directly involve citizens in deliberative decision-making processes and improve the quality of democracy (see also Rifai et al. 2016: 13–15). Local governments didn't just adopt PB "as is," but they significantly transformed the rules to improve basic governance while simultaneously building local democracy.

PB's first transformation was a shift to both planning and budgets.[1] According to Rifai, Asterina, and Hidayani (2016):

> Though there is quite a clear demarcation between planning and budgeting, the laws also indicate that both the planning and budgeting processes are considered to be interrelated processes. *Musrenbang*, as mentioned in the Law of SPPN, is a communal form for constructing development planning, but can also be viewed as a space for participatory budgeting.   (15)

However, we should note that Indonesia's cities account for a very small percentage of the overall public budget—between 1 percent and 3 percent of the national budget. One consequence of this disparity between local and national funding is that the cities have limited resources to implement specific projects that citizens select. Within Indonesia cities, another adaptation was the creation of two parallel tracks for participants: Neighborhood PB and City-Wide PB.

---

[1] Broad guidelines permit cities to adopt very different sets of participatory processes. We therefore draw heavily from one research document, "Improving Transparency, Inclusivity and Impact of Participatory Budgeting in Indonesia Cities: Solo, Yogyakarta, Surabaya, Makassar, Bandung, Kebumen," which was written by three authors employed by the Kota Kita NGO. In addition, one of our researchers conducted a field research trip to two cities on the leading edge of PB adoption—Surakarta and Yogyakarta.

Neighborhood PB

Within Neighborhood PB, the city distributes a block grant to the lowest administrative unit, the Ruken Tetangga (RT). The resources from this grant support community organizing and, secondarily, are invested in small-scale infrastructure projects (e.g., drainage). The local government officials host meetings to which they invite community leaders to foster social solidarity and build community. Citizens participating in Neighborhood PB have autonomy to decide how to spend the resources in their own communities.

However, the very low levels of funding made available through the block grant system mean that many of the projects implemented through Neighborhood PB are quite small. For example, PB Neighborhood funds are used to increase drainage or to pave short sections of narrow roads. Several community leaders indicated that they needed to raise additional funds to expand the potential impact of these projects. One community leader requested donations from major businesses (e.g., hotels, formal restaurants) while two others sought funds from area residents. These strategies suggest that a neighborhood's location and makeup likely impact its ability to employ the block grant to achieve substantive local results. Those communities located near wealthier business centers or which include a larger middle class capture greater levels of resources from private companies and households. In addition, multiple interviewees indicated that they use a system of "self-help," whereby local residents contribute their labor to build an infrastructure project. We note that governments and international donors often view this practice positively because the willingness to provide additional resources suggests that local community members actively support the reform project. A common criticism, however, among community activists is that their "labor participation" is an additional form of taxation.

City-Wide PB

City-Wide PB is a consultative participatory process in which citizens vote on a series of projects that they want the municipal government to implement. Citizens and communities first deliberate over a list of potential projects. City officials then have discretion to decide which projects to implement. The municipal government is not required to implement any of the selected projects and may add or "pick and choose" from the list. City-Wide PB, then, is not a case of "strong democracy" in which citizens have real decision-making authority (Barber 1984). Rather, it is a consultative process in which citizens provide the city with a wish list. A common complaint among our interviewees is that the citizens' list does not correspond to what the city planning department will eventually implement. Although the City-Wide PB process marks a significant step forward in allowing citizens to express their voice in public, its core limitation is that the government has complete power to decide which projects will be implemented.

Rather than open calls for participation, the Indonesian PB model relies on government-issued invitations to community leaders to deliberate over projects to be recommended to the government for implementation. According to several community activists and CSO leaders interviewed in 2018, a cultural tradition within Javanese society creates a sense of obligation to attend meetings to which one is invited and, conversely, not to attend meetings to which one is not invited (see also Barron et al. 2011). Javanese culture is one among many in Indonesia, but the 140 million people on the island of Java represent the majority of the population. Although no one is legally denied permission to attend public meetings to which they are not invited, community activists stressed that only invited community leaders are likely to attend. We spoke with representatives from one NGO as well as one community organizer who stated that they had attended meetings without an explicit invitation; their tone was one of defiance and breaking of tradition. We recognize the courage of these community leaders to attend a PB meeting without an invitation, but we also believe that it highlights the limited nature of ordinary citizen participation. If it is a major step for community leaders to attend meetings uninvited, one can only imagine the difficulty facing poor, vulnerable residents to attend these meetings without a formal invitation.

Indonesian City-Wide PB processes use deliberative, consensus-based decision-making systems. A vote is only called as a last resort if participants are unable to reach consensus. According to several interviewees, PB is embedded in a deep cultural tradition of local elites discussing issues; one community leader claimed that they would sometimes deliberate all weekend to reach consensus. Unfortunately, we lack more in-depth analyses to understand if these deliberative processes are dominated by local elites. Theoretically, deliberative scholars from Mark Warren to James Bonham place a high premium on fairly equal social standing in deliberative bodies. It is possible that deliberations in Indonesia's PB programs are among individuals who are fairly equal, but this would be due to the restricted nature of participation, in which mainly invitees attend.

An important adaptation in City-Wide PB is the use of gender quotas to increase women's participation. Women must occupy 30 percent of all PB-related positions; for example, women must fill two of the positions on a six-person oversight committee. The inclusion of this rule was to promote greater social inclusion and expand the voice of women in these new spaces. There is mixed evidence regarding the ability of women to play a more active role in these deliberative bodies (Barron et al. 2011; Olken 2010).

There is a not a strong formal commitment to social justice considerations within the City-Wide PB programs. Nevertheless, there are two ways that PB in Indonesian cities addresses social justice concerns. First, the government uses four criteria that determine how much funding each neighborhood receives when it allocates Neighborhood PB block grants: population size, size of the territory, percentage of poor residents, and percentage of residents who pay their property taxes on time. Thus, the most funding would go to neighborhoods with larger populations, covering broader areas with more poor citizens who pay their taxes on time. The expansion of this rule to incorporate 25 percent of the resource distribution suggests that program designers are aware of participatory programs' bias in favor of wealthier groups. However, it is crucial to note that these PB programs are not required to distribute resources to the neighborhood's poorer areas.

Rifai, Asterina, and Hidayani compare the cities of Surakarta and Yogyakarta to tease out the different ways that Indonesian cities fund PB. The two principal ways include the block grant and development funds. In general terms, the evidence suggests that the cities allocate a relatively small percentage of their overall budget to PB (see Table 4.3 below).

Although the percentages are relatively low, at 3 percent to 5 percent of direct spending, these funding levels align roughly with PB-related spending in other middle- and upper-income developing countries. Thus, the funding data suggest that PB in Indonesian cities is likely to have a limited impact on well-being because the governments are not allocating enough resources. The use of the block grant permits neighborhoods to allocate resources to their high-demand projects while the broader use of development funds now means that all three cities can implement projects that citizens select.

A second way that PB in Indonesian cities advances social justice is through deliberative processes. Several community leaders assert that the process of deliberation that focuses on local issues allows for a better understanding of the needs of the poorer and more vulnerable parts of the population. Participants discussed how the allocation of resources could potentially affect different groups living within the community. These discussions focused on households' different needs, especially those living below the poverty line or in environmentally precarious positions.

Finally, the city of Surakarta stands out for remarkable advancements in their employment of technology to promote improved public services. Much of the credit goes to an NGO, Kota Kita, which initiated a neighborhood mapping exercise. Kota Kita's team first used Geographic Information Systems (GIS) to identify the type and location of existing infrastructure in each neighborhood. This

Table 4.3. Percentage of total budget allocated through PB in Indonesian cities

	Surakarta	Yogyakarta	Surabaya
Block grant: Neighborhood PB	2.56%	0.45%	N/A
Development: City-Wide PB	2.05%	2.91%	3.22%
Total	4.61%	3.35%	3.22%

Source: Adapted from Rifai et al. (2016).

information was vital to help residents understand the location of public goods such as health-care clinics, schools, drainage, sewage, and public toilets. In addition, Kota Kita collected household-level social and economic data. This data was then aggregated to the sub-neighborhood level, allowing residents to gain a better understanding of variation across their neighborhood. NGO professionals at Kota Kita argue that providing neighborhood mapping improves the quality of deliberations because citizens gain a better understanding of their communities' needs (Rifai et al. 2016). The Kota Kita map provides a solid base for citizens' policy deliberations. The mapping exercise is an excellent example of a well-designed and well-managed use of technology; the principal downside is that the PB program did not offer citizens sufficient resources to address many of the identified needs.

Grillos' (2017) work on Surakarta brings a significant note of caution to the argument that PB fosters a commitment to social inclusion and social justice. Grillos created a unique dataset based on information on project resources and distribution from Surakarta's city government and Kota Kita. Grillos (2017) found that fewer resources were allocated to the poorest communities and argues that the bias against the poorest neighborhoods begins at the earliest stages of the PB process: Projects that are sent to the city for possible implementation are primarily located in better-off neighborhoods (Grillos 2017). These findings highlight one potential downside to consultative PB processes: Poorer neighborhoods may receive fewer resources when governments "cherry-pick" the projects they want to implement (see also Font et al. 2018). Relatedly, Grillos' careful analysis of PB in Surakarta suggests that only half of PB infrastructure projects came from citizens. This finding can be interpreted in two very different ways: Concluding that, because roughly half of infrastructure projects come from citizen forums, Surakarta has made great advances in citizen participation, or that 50 percent of projects are added outside of the formal meetings, suggesting weak or marginal advancements in transparency.

Indonesian Villages

The path to PB's adoption across Indonesia's 74,000 villages was a bit more complicated, based in a 1990s-era social development project supported by the World Bank and Indonesia's national government. The Kecamatan Development Project (KDP) introduced a participatory system of village-level decision-making that allowed citizens to directly decide which small-scale development projects to implement (Barron et al. 2011; Gibson and Woolcock 2008). KDP is an excellent example of the creation of participatory institutions parallel to the PB programs being developed in southern Brazil. The program channeled resources directly into Indonesian villages and placed a series of institutional checks on spending to ensure that the resources would be used properly. The program also required multiple meetings to discuss proposals; facilitators worked with women's groups to provide information on how to use the new process, and villagers were elected to monitor local resource distribution and the implementation process.

In 2007, the Indonesian national government renamed KDP as Program Nasional Pemberdayaan Masyarakat Mandiri, or PNPM, and expanded it to roughly 65,000 villages. The principles of the PNPM were drawn from the KDP experience with relatively minor changes. In 2014, the national government rolled out the basic program design to all 74,000 villages. National legislation (Village Law 6 of 2014) mandates that all villages use participatory planning and budgeting (Musrenbang). Thus, KDP's principles (democratic decision-making, oversight, local control) and rules (three rounds of deliberation, oversight committees, etc.) spread from a small number of pilot cases to the adoption by most of Indonesia's 74,000 villages in twenty years (1998–2017).

There were three major adaptations, including the annual transfer of funds to villages from the national government, the hiring of local villagers to administer the process, and the use of facilitators to help community members deliberate. One important difference between the original KDP program and Indonesia's village PB is that the "PB Villages" program had specific sources of public revenues transferred from the national government. The Village Law (2014) is a funded mandate, as each village annually receives between USD100,000 and USD200,000 from the federal government. Seventy percent of the resources must be spent directly on development projects, while 30 percent can be allocated to personnel or community organizing. Thus, the Musrenbang/PB process includes specific parameters for community organizing and development projects. Having a funded mandate encourages local governments to be actively involved in the process. However, we see limited evidence that demonstrates how many of these villages have actually adopted this mandated program; it is vital for researchers to gain a better understanding of how these PB program may be working across Indonesia's 74,000 villages.

The election of a local leader and payment of a stipend to organize the process is another adaptation that circumvents the costly involvement of the national government. Instead, the elected official manages the PB process and reports back to the national government. In the village-level process, citizens prioritize projects that they would like to see the government implement. Given the deep structural poverty in many rural communities, citizens are often unable to contribute additional funds to expand the resources the federal government provides. However, rural communities are often strongly encouraged to contribute their labor and time through "self-help" projects. Based on multiple conversations, we know that the monthly wage paid to the elected official is slightly higher than the national median wage, which means that the position is attractive to most rural community members, but is not a means for leaders to become wealthy.[2]

---

[2] https://www.ceicdata.com/en/indicator/indonesia/monthly-earnings.

Another Indonesian adaptation at the village level is the use of facilitators in deliberative decision-making processes. The KDP process, introduced by the World Bank in 1998, relied heavily on the use of facilitators to guide discussions. As Barron et al. 2011. argue, well-run KDP programs in which facilitators can steer deliberative processes help communities to reach decisions that reflect the interests of different community groups. KDP can thus mitigate conflicts and promote better relationships among community members. However, Barron et al.'s book (2011) also illuminates how weak facilitators do little to lessen conflict among community members. Although the current Musrenbang/PB process is distinct from the original KDP or the subsequent PNPM, there remain enough similarities that we feel confident that core lessons from the KDP process are applicable to the Musrenbang/PB process as well.

Similar to Indonesian cities, villages use an invitation-based system to draw participants to meetings. Indonesian villages must also fill gender quotas to increase women's participation in PB. Thus, women must occupy 30 percent of all PB-related positions in villages as well. This explicit rule is designed to induce greater numbers of women to participate because it ensures that women will hold positions of authority within PB programs. Yet, direct participation does not necessarily mean that these women will exercise the authority that has been formally extended to them. There is some evidence from one of PB's predecessors, the PNPM, that including women in village-level meetings has not meaningfully altered women's roles in these meetings (Azarbaijani-Moghaddam 2014).

The village PB program involves a direct allocation of national funds to villages, which have higher poverty rates than cities, in an effort to bypass regional political elites and redistribute money to rural areas. The Musrenbang/PB process directly injects more than USD7 billion per year into these villages. However, there is not a specific set of rules that ensures that these resources are then spent to address inequalities within each village. Anecdotally, during our field research in rural villages on the island of Java, we heard multiple stories about how villagers were often willing to support projects that benefit more vulnerable parts of their communities (e.g., irrigation to a far-flung field or building a footbridge to help a small number of households). However, we have no evidence if these anecdotes are representative of broader trends.

In terms of social inclusion, the Musrenbang requirement that women hold at least 30 percent of all PB positions could, in theory, expand women's deliberative and decision-making opportunities. Based on evidence from the PNPM (2007–14), the precursor to the Musrenbang/PB (2015–present), there is some well-done analysis suggesting that many women incorporated into the PNPM process had limited voice and vote; they also performed traditional roles such as providing and serving food and drink to the other participants (Barron et al. 2011). The implication is that the formal, mandated structures of these participatory processes may not be able to overcome cultural attitudes that discourage women's active involvement in public decision-making processes.

We found no evidence that Indonesia's villages use technology as part of their PB processes. The primary reason is cost: Villages lack resources to develop meaningful software that could illuminate their core challenges. We did find, however, that the Indonesian national government created a national financial reporting system that is designed to produce efficiencies and increase transparency. Tens of thousands of municipalities now use this system. Technology is therefore used to link villages to the central state, but villages do not appear to have used technology in their PB processes.

Data about KDP allow us to assess the impact of PB on village-level outcomes. KDP was adopted in the late 1990s and would eventually spread across the archipelago to involve over 70,000 villages. "From the early days of the KDP, the World Bank emphasized rigorous baseline studies and impact evaluations to determine the effectiveness of the program. It financed several randomized, controlled trials, building on new applications of these methods to policy analysis" (Friedman 2014: 15). We recognize that KDP programs have several important differences relative to PB, but we believe that the similarities in principles and basic rules allows us to draw inferences from them (Olken 2010; Friedman 2014).

First, analyses of KDP highlight the programs' general success in promoting development and well-being outcomes. Barron, Diprose, and Woolcock argue that in "a strictly organizational sense, KDP has clearly been deemed successful by the entity that has a democratic mandate to allocate public resources as it sees fit, namely, the Indonesia government" (2011: 80). Their premise is that conflict is an inherent part of "development" in rural areas because the introduction of new resources will alter the existing balance of power. They find that "micro-conflicts related to KDP are common but that these rarely escalate and almost never turn violent" (Barron, Diprose, and Woolcock 2011: 139). The authors demonstrate that a well-run KDP program can ease tensions in a community. However, the authors caution that poorly performing KDP programs can have negative effects on communities, which suggests that the mere introduction of formal rules is insufficient to ensure positive outcomes for aspects of development and well-being.

Barron, Diprose, and Woolcock's (2011) work on KDP also argues:

> KDP appears to be effectively reengineering the relationship between citizens and the state at the local level. It brings a set of rules and norms concerning, among other things, who should participate in decision making, the criteria that should be used for resource allocation, and the checks and balances that should be in place to control local power. . . . The evidence shows that the program is helping to democratize village life. Marginalized groups, in particular, women, are far more likely to take part in KDP meetings than in other village

government meetings and increased participation in KDP also appears to be spilling over into other domains of village life.   (208)

This suggests that Indonesia's KDP programs led to an expansion of accountability. Although we do not yet know if the current version of PB will produce the same impacts as KDP, we can be reasonably optimistic that the similar institutional design and financial transfers to villages will help to produce these changes. Within Indonesian cities, the relatively small budgets dedicated to PB limit the programs' impact on accountability.

Finally, research shows spillover effects from KDP programs. Torrens (2005) identified KDP's "comparative advantage in village infrastructure development as compared to the government's long-established top-down approach" (Torrens 2005: 41). Torrens found that KDP projects were more cost-effective than working through a contractor, a benefit to using local building supplies and local labor, and that "officials now face high expectations from their communities for similar levels of transparency and openness in managing future village projects" (Torrens, 2005: 41). Thus, the KDP programs helped establish the foundations for generating improvements in civil society engagement, accountability, and development/well-being outcomes.

PB and Authoritarian China

As noted previously, municipalities and national leaders in authoritarian nations began to adopt PB as a means to improve budgetary efficiency and development outcomes. China is an excellent example of this trend, one that has just begun to take off. PB arrived in China in the mid-2000s, toward the end of the second wave and at the beginning of the third wave of PB's spread across the globe. Simultaneously, other participatory and deliberative programs, such as Deliberative Polling, were also introduced to the country as another way to gather information about citizens' interests and preferences (Fishkin et al. 2010; He 2011; Wu and Wang 2012; Cabannes and Ming 2014; Cabannes 2018). In a series of semi-structured conversations in 2005, one informant used the metaphor of a traffic light to explain how they worked with local governments, explaining that they had a "green light" from central authorities to work with local governments to adopt different citizen engagement and participatory institutions. They worked across China in order to introduce multiple PB programs over the course of the 2000s and 2010s, in the hopes that local governments would better engage citizens. National government officials oversaw their efforts, giving "yellow light" signals when they needed to slow-down innovation and "red light" signals when they needed to stop their work. Importantly, over a decade later, it is increasingly clear that the Chinese national government was dramatically reducing opportunities for local governments to implement PB.

Baogang He's work also demonstrates that local officials had considerable leeway to experiment with local policymaking programs. He argues that early PB program in China followed three distinct logics "based on administration, political reform, and citizen empowerment. Each logic denotes different conceptualisations and understandings of PB, constituting different frameworks in which PB programmes and activities operate" (He 2011: 122). He argues that when "the administrative logic dominates PB, the concept of citizenship is likely to be diluted and even lost other than in terms of the possibility for some public scrutiny of budgets" (2011: 122). This is most similar to the Efficient Governance type (similar to Germany and Poland described in Chapter 5), whereby governments adopt PB to improve their allocation of scarce resources. He also argues that the "political reform logic differs from the administrative logic in that some local officials, scholars, and NGOs have used PB to rejuvenate the local Peoples' Congresses in China to make them work more effectively and to make the deputies more powerful" (He 2011: 122–3). This observation is crucial because it suggests that local government officials sought to use PB to strengthen the role of the authoritarian Chinese Communist Party (CCP) that monopolizes political power. Thus, what is distinct in the Chinese case is that an authoritarian system can use PB to empower political elites at the local level, thus further entrenching the government's authority. Although political renewal also takes place in democratic countries with PB, a key difference is that democratic political parties must compete with other parties whereas PB can be a tool for reinforcing the local authority of the CCP.

Finally, He demonstrates that the logic of "citizen empowerment" may also motivate governments to adopt PB: "The citizen empowerment logic is characterised by activist citizens and NGOs who regard citizen participation in the budgeting process as a political right, and demand the power to decide the allocation of budgets in local communities. PB aims to cultivate and empower citizens and, in doing so, changes the relationship between the state and citizens in favour of the latter" (2011: 123). Although He identifies the possibility that this "citizen empowerment" approach may be present, he finds little evidence of this logic at play. Rather, "most PB projects are a top-down process with limited input from the bottom-up. This differs from the case of Brazil where participatory organisations have been set up by, and gained support from, the leftwing political party. Chinese PB takes place without a two-party system and electoral pressure. The CCP plays a central role in backing, approving and monitoring PB experiments. Often, local party organisations make the crucial decisions on PB projects" (2011: 125). The general thrust of He's argument is that most PB programs are used to either improve the efficiencies of local government spending practices or to try to politically revitalize local government officials. Although there is the possibility that PB may generate citizen empowerment, He finds that a weak civil society as well as single-party rule makes it very difficult.

In contrast, Cabannes and Ming are much more positive about the potential for PB to serve as a catalyst for democratic empowerment in China (2018). They focus on Chengdu, a large metropolitan region in China's south-west, and argue that PB developed with few international influences. This "home-grown" experiment thus allowing local leaders to focus on issues such as the urban–rural divide. In Chengdu, PB now takes place in over 2,600 rural areas and 1,400 urban areas. Over ten years, these programs allocated more than USD1.2 billion in public investments through PB (Cabannes 2018). The central claim of Cabannes and Ming's analysis is that PB is providing great opportunities for citizen empowerment and is thus helping to lay the foundations for accountability. Similar to African PB processes (described in Chapter 6), programs in Chengdu are designed to generate citizen engagement and to revitalize local governance systems. Thus, Cabannes and Ming's conclusion is that PB helps to generate important change that is altering basic state–society relationships. Interestingly, this is a very similar claim to what was made in other countries, such as Brazil, Peru, Kenya, and Indonesia, regarding the adoption of PB following the establishment of democracy at the national level. However, it is unclear if the adoption of PB in authoritarian contexts will lead to an expansion of citizen voice and accountability or if PB will help a single-party government (CCP, in this case) to further consolidate its control. We must seriously consider how to conceive of a program that moved from a radical democratic experiment in the early 1990s (Genro 1995; Avritzer 2002; Baiocchi 2005) to a technical tool (Baiocchi and Ganuza 2017) to a governance tool employed by authoritarian regimes to consolidate their support at the local level. This is a crucial theoretical and empirical puzzle that researchers need to address carefully.

Comparative Analysis

Across the three democratic cases highlighted in this chapter, a clear pattern emerges. In each case, local governments initiated some form of participatory democracy that was then transformed into PB, which was then mandated by the national government. In some ways, then, this region has similarities with the cases of Peru and the Dominican Republic in Latin America (see Chapter 3), Poland in Europe (see Chapter 5), and Uganda in Africa (see Chapter 6). The push from the central government to mandate participatory democracy is driven by the idea that the local level is the best place to make decisions about local needs and that citizens should be involved in policymaking processes. National governments, generally those with a reform-oriented government, seek to reconfigure state–society relations from afar. By mandating PB, national governments hope to inject more transparency and participation into state-sanctioned policy-making processes in far-flung places.

However, evidence about these cases build on findings about Peru and suggest that most mandated programs function poorly because they suffer from limited local government support, insufficient resources, and weak citizen engagement. The Indonesian villages experience illustrates this process quite well—when the KDP program was initially created, there was extensive technical, financial, and political support from the National Ministry of Finance and the World Bank. These organizations worked with local governments and community leaders to refine the rules, which would then be rolled out to the rest of the country. However, once PB was mandated, there was much lower technical and political support. Villages receive, on average, USD150,000 per year, but there is little over-sight from the national government regarding how the programs function in practice. The Indonesian experience is most reminiscent of Peru, where a reform-ist government sought to induce local governments to use PB in the hopes of better engaging citizens and promoting transparency. Unfortunately, the evidence does not indicate that mandated programs will work well.

We also note that there are some cases, such as Seoul, South Korea, where local mayors invested extensive resources into making PB a vibrant political and poli-cymaking process (No 2017; Cho et al. 2020; No and Hsueh 2020). In many ways, Seoul is quite similar to Porto Alegre or Belo Horizonte; leftist governments incorporated an already mobilized civil society in public venues to hold spirited debates to allocate resources. Thus, the vital roles of government will, state capac-ity, available public resources, and civil society are well situated in thirty years of research on PB: PB outcomes are strongly associated with the degree of support provided by the government and civil society's ability to mobilize itself. Thus, when PB programs are mandated, we should expect that some places will still produce high-quality programs because of their pre-existing support from local elites and community organizations. But many other governments will see PB as an unfunded mandate that provides few political and policy pay-offs. Similarly, many CSOs will be unprepared or uninterested in taking on the dual role of pol-icy implementer and community mobilizer.

We also see similarities between the adoption of PB in rural areas of Indonesia and El Salvador. The World Bank spearheaded Indonesia's adoption of PB, while the USAID led the effort in El Salvador. In both contexts, local PB programs were designed to build trust, limit violence, and advance development projects. Indonesia is a remarkable case because the country scaled up from a few hundred pilot PB programs in the 1990s to all 74,000 villages based on the perception that the programs produced successful outcomes. The Salvadoran programs were much more modest—USAID supported a few dozen villages and towns. The remarkable aspect of these PB cases is that USAID's withdrawal did not result in PB's disappearance. Rather, PB programs were continued (or resumed) by local reformers even without ongoing technical and financial support from USAID or the central Salvadoran government (Bland 2017).

Conclusion

The spread of PB across Asia was driven by windows of opportunity associated with transitions to democratic rule. South Korea, Indonesia, and the Philippines democratized during the 1980s and 1990s as mass mobilization brought national-level regime change. New democratic institutions emerged in subnational spaces with principles and rules similar to the pioneering cases of PB in Brazil. These initial democratic efforts later included a drive to align with prevailing international norms of the period: combining citizen empowerment practices with democratization in incremental policymaking venues. International organizations such as the Ford Foundation, the World Bank, and the Asian Development Bank provided bridges between these new democrats and the cutting-edge institutional designers that advocated for the expansion of citizen participation in decision-making. Thus, normative and mimetic impulses of adoption fueled creative adaptation in these contexts. Over time, there was a more explicit move from the normative adoption of democratic institutions to a mimetic adaptation based on the prevailing international standards.

There is no one PB type in Southeast and East Asia, as each has significantly different roots. But what stands out in the three countries covered in this chapter is that national governments in all three programs built upon municipal-level programs to mandate that subnational governments use PB. Interestingly, all three countries crafted different types of national mandates in response to their political and social context. Importantly, the early emphasis on democratic principles helped fuel the normative impulse that then led to a strong emphasis on change within civil society, accountability, and well-being. Here we briefly identify the most important trends in the region.

Creating a stronger civil society is a key goal for all four programs (BuB in the Philippines, PB in South Koreas, and PB Cities and PB Villages in Indonesia) and there is some evidence that this is taking place, albeit unevenly across the four cases. Government officials and their civil society allies believed that the direct inclusion of citizens in budgeting processes would give citizens access to information and expand their voice. Across the four programs covered in this chapter, the preliminary evidence suggests that the most significant potential advances in strengthening civil society may occur in the two programs that are most different from each other: Indonesia's village program and South Korea (Gibson and Woolcock 2008; Barron et al. 2011). The Indonesian village PB programs offer the greatest potential to strengthen civil society because these programs have greater local control over public resources, influence how local leaders are elected, and encourage extensive public deliberation regarding how specific resources are spent. Existing evidence from PB's forerunner programs (KDP and PNPM) suggests that the growth of civil society was strong, but we do not yet know how PB design has affected PB across the broader universe of 74,000 villages. In South Korean cities, government programs that support participation and implement projects selected by citizens have had an empowering effect on civil society as well (No 2017; Hong and Cho 2018). More research on this outcome is needed. In the Philippines, the different rules and processes put in place—inclusion of new CSOs, the creation of a split committee (half CSOs and half technical experts), and increased spending in rural districts—suggest that the government sought to strengthen civil society. However, Aceron's work suggests that the government was unable make much headway on revamping civil society or state–society relations (Aceron 2019).

Broadly, we lack evidence that allows us to know if and how these programs might have generated greater accountability. First, it is difficult to decipher the extent to which the Philippines' PB program strengthened accountability, given the limited research on the programs. We have small nuggets of information that suggest that the Philippines' programs share similarities with the better-studied programs in Brazil (Baiocchi et al. 2011; Wampler 2007) but we remain at the speculative stage of analyzing these programs' impact (Lim 2017; Aceron 2019). There is also very little work about PB programs' relationships with accountability in South Korea. But there are some important clues that suggest that these programs may strengthen accountability. For example, the normative adoption of PB in South Korea suggests that many elected governments sought to use PB to empower citizens and to alter basic state–society relations. Governments that are normatively committed to PB are more likely to promote accountability, whereas those governments using PB mandated by national legislation are less likely to provide the necessary support to strengthen PB programs and any subsequent impact on accountability.

Improving well-being is another key goal for these four programs, which all included efforts to improve service delivery and allocate more public services to underserved communities. However, we lack systematic data that might permit us to assess the extent to which these outcomes were achieved. Filipino and Indonesian village programs included an explicit attempt to distribute greater resources to small, poor municipalities and villages. The expectation was that the use of PB resources on basic development projects would have a positive effect on well-being. Although we lack direct evidence from Indonesia's more recent PB programs (under the Village Law), the precursor program, the KDP, has been extensively researched. Key findings demonstrate an important multiplier effect in these municipalities; by turning resources over to villages and through direct citizen engagement there was a greater local impact. The limited evidence from Indonesian cities indicates that resources allocated at the neighborhood level are insufficient to make meaningful differences in social well-being. Preliminary evidence from South Korea suggests that PB programs allocate increased resources to poor neighborhoods (Hong and Cho 2018; No and Hsueh 2020). Although we cannot conclusively assert that this greater level of resources results in changes in well-being, we believe that we can safely assert that additional resources would have a positive effect on more generalized sources of well-being.

The cases from Asia reviewed in this chapter offer the promise of social and political change. Given that subnational data are not systematically collected and published, we still lack enough information about these programs' specific impact. Based on the available data and analyses, however, our interpretation of these cases is mixed. The internal rules and institutional processes suggest that PB program design contributes to citizens' empowerment, allocates resources to poorer communities, and fosters better relationships between elected governments and citizens. But, as is well known, institutions often produce unintended consequences or do not function as designed, which means that we need to temper our analysis with the understanding that we continue to lack basic information to evaluate PB's impact across Asia.

Importantly, Asia is also the site of several prominent PB programs in non-democratic environments, namely China and Eastern Russia. The former is largely consultative, with a strong emphasis on a process in which citizens provide feedback to proposals prepared by government officials (He and Warren 2011; Cabannes 2018). The latter focuses on delivering development projects in an accountable way, which places it closer to PB programs in sub-Saharan Africa (Shulga and Sukhova 2019). The PB programs in Eastern Russia appear to be most similar to the Social Development and Social Accountability type and the PB programs in China seem to fall within the Efficient Governance type. The growing adoption of PB in authoritarian contexts is noteworthy because it suggests that PB may be evolving into a signaling body, designed to improve the quality of governance although not necessarily promoting the expansion of democracy. There are two distinct ways of interpreting the meaning and impacts of these programs. PB advocates believe the approach inculcates public learning around rights, citizenship, and government responsibility; in this sense, PB programs in non-democracies have the potential to act as radical bodies of change (Cabannes and Ming 2014; Fan 2018). However, PB programs are also understood to serve as technical programs that improve local governance. From this perspective, PB could help to legitimize authoritarian governments. We return to the topic of PB in authoritarian countries in the book's conclusion. At this point, we simply want to acknowledge the presence of the PB in non-democracies, primarily in Asia.

In Chapter 5, we turn our attention to the spread of PB across older, wealthier democracies in the North Atlantic region, Europe and two countries in North America (Canada and the United States). The rapid spread of PB in these wealthy and established democracies is an excellent example of the policy diffusion from the Global South to the Global North. This expansion is driven by activists' and politicians' desire to improve the quality of democracy in an age of citizen apathy and distrust. As it expands, we see evidence of a continued emphasis on social inclusion (like in Asia) and more extensive use of digital platforms. Chapter 5 tells a fascinating story of PB's use in a context very different from those discussed so far.

5

Re-engaging Citizens in Europe and North America

The spread of PB in the North Atlantic region (Europe, the United States, and Canada) is taking place as citizen apathy, declining trust, social exclusion, and growing inequalities spread in these wealthier democracies.[1] In fact, these North Atlantic democracies are generally considered to be the birthplace of modern representative democracy, as the forerunners of an industrialization process that built up wealth and institutions over time, the creation of which resulted in a strong working class, a larger middle class, and a robust social safety net. By the early twenty-first century, many of these democracies faced economic stagnation and also struggled to include citizens' voices in policymaking processes, leading to a related decline in social trust. Many scholars identify these trends as a sign of weakening support for democratic practices. In 2020, a general malaise around democratic practices and institutions marks political life in many well-established democracies in Europe and parts of North America.

The shortcomings of modern representative democracy inspired civil society groups and political reformers to advocate for the adoption of PB as a potential solution. By 2018, major cities such as New York City, Paris, Madrid, Barcelona, Lisbon, Chicago, Boston, Seattle, Toronto, and Seville adopted some form of PB. These adoptions took place at the tail end of the second wave of adoption (mid-1990s to mid-2000s) and across the third wave (mid-2000s to 2020). We see significant institutional innovation in these PB processes as PB's original rules have been reimagined to address different types of problems. Most notably, New York City and Chicago initiated their PB programs at sub-municipal levels (e.g., city council districts and wards) at the behest of city council members, thus significantly altering the scale at which it was implemented. Many places, like New York, Toronto, and Chicago, are focusing on social inclusion as a means to achieve social justice. Córdoba and Seville initiated PB programs in the early 2000s that were quite similar to the Porto Alegre model, although both programs changed the rules to incorporate people differently. By 2018, Paris, Madrid, and Barcelona

---

[1] Mexico, of course, is geographically part of North America. For the purposes of this book, we include Mexico in the Latin American analysis because its political, social, and cultural features share more in common with South American and Central American countries than with the United States and Canada.

Participatory Budgeting in Global Perspective. Brian Wampler, Stephanie McNulty, and Michael Touchton, Oxford University Press. © Brian Wampler, Stephanie McNulty, and Michael Touchton 2021.
DOI: 10.1093/oso/9780192897756.003.0006

had adapted their PB programs to strongly emphasize online participation, thus drastically limiting the face-to-face deliberation that was central to the pioneering Porto Alegre model. In addition, governments adopted PB in France and Germany as a technocratic strategy to improve policymaking processes to generate efficiencies (Sintomer et al. 2016).

In most of these North Atlantic countries, a combination of centrist and leftist governments and civil society leaders drove adoption of PB programs as they sought to revitalize democratic practices. PB traveled into these European and North American democracies through the networks and activities of "PB ambassadors," who brought the concept of PB from Brazil to the Global North (Porto de Oliveira 2017a). There are now hundreds of PB cases across the North Atlantic region, which makes it nearly impossible to provide a simple story of "PB in Europe" or "PB in North America." There is a greater diversity of PB programs in Europe, in comparison to North America, because of these countries' varied histories and political systems. In this chapter, we include cases that are most representative of the broader PB trends we see in the region. Importantly, there is a very limited number of empirical studies from the United States, Canada, and Europe that demonstrate the impact of PB on key outcome indicators such as attitudinal change, and improvements in communities' quality of life. The absence of clear, well-defined results means that many PB advocates' support for PB is based on evidence from Latin America (mainly Brazil) as well as political and ideological aspirations that PB will generate change. Table 5.1 below presents the history of PB in the two regions covered in this chapter, including their key variants and diffusion over time.

South-to-North Diffusion: PB Comes to the North Atlantic Region

The adoption of PB in Europe and North America represents a very interesting and relatively rare example of South-to-North policy diffusion (Allegretti and Herzberg 2004; Porto de Oliveira 2017a). PB adoption was initially stronger in Europe but rapidly spread across the United States during the 2010s. Giovanni Allegretti and Carsten Herzberg captured this South-North flow of ideas as the "return of the *caravelas*," an allusion to the Portuguese and Spanish colonizers who fanned out across the Americas in search of treasure (Allegretti and Herzberg 2004). The former colonies, most notably Brazil, were now in a position to provide European countries with new ideas concerning how they could encourage democratic innovations. The diffusion took place through organizations such as International Observatory on Participatory Democracy (OIPD), United Cities and Local Governments (UCLG), and European Union-sponsored Urban Program (URB-AL), all of which helped to develop networks across Latin America (e.g., Brazil-Ecuador) as well as bring these ideas back into Europe

Table 5.1. PB programs in Europe and North America

PB Type	1989 to mid-1990s	Mid-1990s to mid-2000s	Mid-2000s to 2020
Empowered Democracy and Redistribution			
Deepening Democracy through Community Mobilization		Toronto (2001) Córdoba, Spain (2001) Palmela, Portugal (2002) Saint-Denis, France (2005)	Chicago (2009) New York City (2011)
Mandated by National Government			1,500 Polish towns and villages (2011–18)
Digital PB			Madrid (2016) Barcelona (2015) Paris (2014)
Social Development and Accountability			
Efficient Governance		German Municipalities (2000–)	Soport, Poland (2011)

Source: Authors.

(Allegretti and Herzberg 2004; Porto de Oliveira 2017a). These organizations had strong ties with left-of-center parties, especially among the early adopters of PB in Spanish municipalities.

In Europe, many of the pioneering cases were in small towns and mid-sized cities (e.g., Córdoba, Spain) that had few participatory policymaking opportunities for citizens, making PB an appealing option. PB came later to North America. Across, the United States, Canada, and Europe, there were already multiple opportunities for citizens to participate in local governance. As a result, PB became an additional democratic policymaking venue in a somewhat crowded field. In the North American context, PB advocates creatively chose to introduce PB at "sub-municipal" levels, meaning city council districts (wards), public housing authorities, and schools because many mayors were unwilling to support the city-wide adoption of PB.

Four types of PB programs are present across Europe, the United States, and Canada: Deepening Democracy through Community Mobilization, Digital PB, Mandated by National Governments, and Efficient Governance. First, we find that the initial wave of PB programs are most closely categorized as Deepening Democracy through Community Mobilization. City officials and CSOs in Chicago,

New York City, Toronto, Seville, Córdoba, Tuscany, and smaller cities in France adopted PB as a means to rejuvenate stagnant democratic practices. A commonality among these programs is an emphasis on encouraging the participation of local residents to rebuild connections between citizens and governments. A second common type is Digital Participation, whereby local governments use innovative technologies and program design to engage citizens in online programs. These PB programs are innovative because they incorporate citizens in new ways, but we stress that they tend to focus on encouraging greater numbers of participants rather than promoting deliberation or increasing trust.

Mandated by National Government PB programs are also present in Europe, with Poland as the most prominent example while Portugal has now mandated PB programs for public schools. In these cases, national governments mandate that subnational units (e.g., villages or schools) implement PB programs. The national government provides technical assistance to support PB programming, although they do not necessarily provide additional funding to allow citizens to implement projects.

Finally, we also see the presence of Efficient Governance programs, which are the main PB type established in Germany. There is a strong emphasis on using PB to help modernize local policymaking processes as well as to generate governing and service delivery efficiencies. As a result, these programs de-emphasize the more radical democratic elements of PB and use PB to promote good governance.

Deepening Democracy through Community Mobilization

Efforts to deepen the quality of democracy strongly influence PB adoption in Europe, the United States, and Canada. The adoption of the earliest PB programs was led by leftist CSOs or leftist governments who sought to revitalize connections between citizens, communities, and government (Sintomer et al. 2016; Baiocchi and Ganuza 2017; Cabannes 2019). When we compare PB adoption across different regions of the world, the better-established democracies have the largest number of PB programs that were driven by governments' and CSOs' normative concerns for improving the quality of democracy, rebuilding trust, and strengthening civil society. In some ways, then, these European and North America programs best reflect PB's radical democratic roots in Brazil as they seek to empower citizens by providing opportunities for participants to engage each other in public forums.

We note that there are some crucial differences between the pioneering programs in Brazil and how they were adapted in the North Atlantic region. These programs did not adopt the explicit social justice rules to ensure that poorer, underserved neighborhoods would receive greater resources on a per capita basis than wealthier neighborhoods. Rather, the programs made a shift toward emphasizing social inclusion, whereby local PB programs sought to incorporate individuals and community organizations from marginalized communities. The language of social justice continued to be prevalent in PB programs, but programs lacked specific rules that require greater resource allocation to politically and socially marginalized communities. We begin by examining PB programs in Canada and the United States before turning our attention to Europe.

Toronto Housing Corporation

In 2001, the Toronto Community Housing Corporation (TCHC) adopted one of the earliest known PB programs in English-speaking North America.[2] The TCHC "houses over 164,000 tenants, six percent of the city's population, with a large number of refugees and new immigrants," giving it a substantial role in Toronto's social and political life (Foroughi 2017: 1). The initial impetus for PB came from TCHC leadership, which sought to increase participation among its residents. They developed contacts with activists and university researchers who were familiar with the famed PB program in Porto Alegre, Brazil, as they gathered information about available options, and decided to adopt PB (Foroughi 2017; Schugurensky 2020). Sergio Baierle, a key NGO leader from Porto Alegre, and Daniel Schugurensky were important "PB ambassadors" who provided information to government officials on how PB functioned in Porto Alegre (Lerner 2014; Foroughi 2017; Schugurensky 2020).

Toronto's PB program stressed the mobilization and inclusion of immigrants and poor residents living in public housing. The mayor and city legislators were uninterested in establishing city-wide or even ward-level PB processes, but TCHC was a viable option, allowing residents to deliberate over the allocation of small projects that could lead to improvements in the quality of life (Lerner 2014; Foroughi 2017). In 2001, PB participants allocated 9 million Canadian dollars (roughly 6 million US dollars at the time); this amount fluctuated between 5 and 9 million over the subsequent decade (Foroughi 2017: 2). Project selection focused on small-scale public works (e.g., landscaping, lighting, cleaning stairways) that would potentially improve individuals' quality of life. In 2015, housing authorities paused PB for a single year to allow the city to refine the rules as well as to finish implementing already selected projects; the program then resumed in 2016. Interestingly, three city council districts adopted PB in 2017 to incorporate citizens into sub-municipal policymaking processes. These districts were among

---

[2] The city of Guelph, a suburb of Toronto, created a participatory project in 1999 and renamed it "PB" in 2000 (see Goldfrank and Landes 2018). We focus on the TCHC because it remains in operation and the Guelph program was discontinued in 2012.

Toronto's poorest, which means that social inclusion in PB is a central part of a wider effort in Toronto to include marginalized communities.

Although there is not very much impact data, we know Toronto's public housing has significant diversity—it includes a mixture of individuals and families from multiple ethnic, racial, religious, linguistic, and national groups. Toronto is an immigrant-receiving city and Toronto's public housing has a higher percentage of non-Canadian born residents than the rest of the city. The Toronto PB program thus addresses a great need in the immigrant-receiving cities in the Global North: the inclusion of immigrants into democratic processes, thereby increasing connections and trust between government officials and area residents (Lerner 2014). We note, however, that including a diverse group of citizens is not necessarily an easy process. Foroughi (2017) argues that the PB process also created considerable tension between citizens and government officials. Participants in Toronto, as in many other places across the globe, placed a greater number of demands on government officials than the government was able to address.

In sum, Toronto's PB program was an important early anchor that contributed to PB's diffusion across Canada and the United States. The shift to a sub-municipal program had a cascading effect, as most programs in Canada and the United States would go on to follow this same approach (Peabody and Lerner 2019). A second important contribution was the shift to an emphasis on social inclusion and a move away from the more specific social justice rules that were central to early PB programs in Brazil. By adopting a PB program in a public housing project, Toronto's PB incorporated thousands of residents who were often marginalized from city-level politics.

Chicago and New York City

By 2020, there were dozens of PB programs in the United States, including in New York City, Chicago, Boston, Seattle, Phoenix (Public Agenda 2016; Russon Gilman 2016; Goldfrank and Landes 2018). Citizens selected over $300 million worth of projects across these programs by 2020 (PBP.org, accessed on January 22, 2020). The first case of PB, however, began in 2009, when Chicago Alderman Joe Moore put over $1 million of his council district's discretionary funds into this participatory process. After narrowly winning the Democratic primary in 2007 (the Democratic primary in his ward is the principal moment of political competition due to low voter support for Republican candidates), Alderman Moore sought to adopt new programs to better connect with his constituents. After learning about PB in Brazil and visiting Porto Alegre, in part thanks to outreach from the PBP, Alderman Moore delegated a portion of his discretionary funds to the PB process (Baez and Hernandez 2012; Lerner 2014; Russon Gilman 2016). Moore enlisted PBP to design a PB system that would help his constituents allocate nearly $1.3 million in public funds (Lerner 2014). In 2011, Moore won with 72 percent of the vote. "According to Moore, PB was the most common reason people gave for reelecting him" (Lerner 2014: 15). The alderman subsequently became an advocate for PB, speaking about it across the country, and received honors at the White House. PB spread from Moore's wards to cover roughly a third of Chicago's wards (http://www.pbchicago.org). Moore led efforts to show elected officials and CSOs beyond Chicago that PB was a viable venue to promote community mobilization, social inclusion, social justice, and public deliberation. Even more importantly, the Chicago program demonstrated that potential implementers could be creative as they thought about how to adapt local institutions. The lesson was that PB could be done in city council districts, in schools, and among the youth, depending on the interests of local social and political leaders.

The adoption of PB in New York City followed a similar process as Chicago but has become much larger over time. In 2011, four city council members adopted PB in their districts, turning over a portion of their discretionary budgets to citizens. The adoption was a combination of normative adoption, as progressive Democrats advocated for PB, and "mimetic" adoption, as city council members sought to align themselves with cutting-edge democratic reform. By 2018, PB had spread to over half of New York City's council districts; in each case, city council members initiated the process in their individual districts (Russon-Gilman and Wampler 2019). In November 2018, New York City voters approved a referendum to revise the city charter to expand PB to the entire city (65 percent of voters, nearly 700,000 individuals, supported the expansion of PB). Given the expansion, it is expected that PB in New York City will expand its resources to between $150 million and $200 million annually.

New York City's PB program places a greater emphasis on small-group deliberation than in the original Brazilian cases. The focus is on educating citizens, providing learning opportunities, and facilitating small-group discussions (see Russon Gilman 2016; Russon Gilman and Wampler 2019). There are several opportunities for deliberation within the program, which first occurs at the local neighborhood assembly meetings where residents identify neighborhood spending priorities. Neighborhood residents learn about their city's budget process and the PB process, and then break up into groups to brainstorm. Following the small group deliberations, participants generally vote for multiple projects, often through a show of hands or by using "dot voting," where people place a sticky dot next to the project they support. Thus, this process occupies a middle ground between the secret ballot (which often allows more vulnerable voters to express their preferences) and consensus-based voting (which is often more susceptible to elite domination).[3] In addition, during the neighborhood assemblies, participants

---

[3] In some of the more well-structured PB programs, there is a secret ballot at the end of the process, but the majority of districts did not rely on secret ballots to select programs.

volunteer to serve as budget delegates; they are not elected but instead choose to be part of the process, which means that the programs may experience "elite capture." Given the emphasis on deliberation, volunteering, and public voting, the New York City and Chicago PB experiences draw from existing US experiences of local democracy.

There are not specific social justice rules that determine the allocation of public resources to low-income communities in the Chicago and New York City PB programs. Rather, social justice considerations are part of the broader deliberation about how resources are distributed (Lerner and Secondo 2012; Pape and Lerner 2016; Goldfrank and Landes 2018). In both Chicago and New York City, program administrators and their civil society allies spent considerable time and effort to incorporate poor and politically marginalized groups (Lerner 2014; Goldfrank and Landes 2018). The active involvement of individuals from poor and politically marginalized groups greatly increases the likelihood that participants will raise policy concerns of central importance to these communities. Of course, incorporating voices from marginalized communities does not guarantee that these citizens' demands will be met. We need additional research to determine if social inclusion in project selection leads to changes in civil society or well-being, for example. Celina Su's (2017) initial evaluation of projects outcomes suggest that it may not, but Hagelskamp and her co-authors demonstrate that PB changes spending allocations in New York City, with greater spending on schools and in public housing projects and less spending on parks (Hagelskamp et al. 2020).

In addition, a focus on social inclusion helps to bring new civic voices into the process, but there is wide variation among PB programs regarding who participates. Some communities have successfully encouraged more diversity than others along various socio-economic indicators such as race, income, and education. Research on PB in the United States demonstrates that Black residents and White residents are generally overrepresented or represented proportionally to their community's general share of the local census tract, while Hispanic residents are often systematically underrepresented (Hagelskamp et al. 2016). With regard to education and income, there is a bit of bifurcation. Lower-income households are overrepresented or represented proportionally in most PB programs, thus meeting PB's goal of social inclusion. However, those with the highest education levels (undergraduate and graduate degrees) are overrepresented (Hagelskamp et al. 2016). This bifurcation suggests that PB programs are partially successful in attracting new political actors into the political system, most notably young, low-income residents. Yet, the programs still experience difficulties attracting Hispanics and those with lower education levels.

New York City's PB has been effective at ensuring that PB voters represent a larger percentage of marginalized residents than in traditional elections. In the period from 2014 to 2015, 51,000 residents voted. A majority of New York City PB voters—57 percent—identified as People of Color, compared to 47 percent of local election voters and 66 percent of the total population of the participating twenty-four districts (CDP and PBNYC 2015). The New York City process is thus successful at galvanizing traditionally marginalized communities, in part because of strong community anchors with deep ties to community members. The PBP, the lead technical nonprofit organizing PB in North America, is located in Brooklyn and Community Voices Heard (CVH), a multiracial membership organization that organizes low-income populations to influence policy change, is the grassroots organizing partner for the city's process. PBP and CVH have been advocates for PB adoption and leverage their networks to encourage citizen participation.

There is also evidence that links citizens' participation in PB with an increase in voting in regular elections. Johnson, Carlson, and Reynold created a unique database that links individual-level participation in PB with individuals' voting behaviors, finding that PB participation increased the probability of voting by 7.5 percent (n.d.: 15). There is an even greater increase among individuals from groups that historically vote at lower levels, including those who are younger, poorer, Black, and Latino. This suggests that PB generates a spillover effect where its emphasis on social inclusion helps to bring individuals from traditionally marginalized groups into formal participation spaces, which then leads these same individuals to turn out to vote.

PB in Chicago and New York City revolves around community organizing and allowing local politicians to connect with new constituencies. If the focus in Porto Alegre was an "inversion" of spending and policy priorities, PB in North America focuses much more on incremental change within existing budget processes (Goldfrank and Landes 2018). The decentralized PB process, with most programs at the sub-city level, necessarily has more limited funding. One key result is that budget allocations are relatively small compared to overall city budgets. Across forty-five PB projects in the United States and Canada during 2014–15, the average winning project cost was $195,506 (Hagelskamp et al. 2016). Looking across multiple PB programs in the 2014–15 cycle, parks and recreation projects were the most common ballot items overall, followed by school projects (Hagelskamp et al. 2016). Schools received the largest share of PB-allocated funds (33 percent). The least common types of projects on the ballot were public housing and public safety projects. Public housing projects rarely appear on ballots and also have a low chance of winning funding when they do appear because of their high cost.

Since the beginning of New York City's PB programs, researchers closely monitored the extent to which they generate changes in budget allocations. By 2020, researchers published several empirically rich analyses of New York City's PB, focusing on whether the presence of PB alters how city council members allocate their discretionary resources. Interestingly, there was significant variation in the authors' interpretations of the results. Calabrese, Williams, and Gupta (2020) find that PB is associated with an increase in the number of projects funded by the city council office. However, they find that each individual project is funded at lower absolute levels when compared to similar projects funded by city council offices not using PB as well as in comparison to how the same city council office previously funded projects prior to PB. Calabrese and his co-authors assert that PB permits elected officials to build more connections to greater numbers of local community associations, which, they argue, is evidence that these elected officials are establishing clientelistic relationships. This research fits within a longer tradition of scholars who are concerned that PB produces something closer to "participatory clientelism" rather than citizen empowerment (see Navarro 2003; Goldfrank 2011; Selee 2011; McNulty 2019; Montambeault 2019).

Shybalkina and Bifulco (2019) show that PB investments in New York City have a redistributive effect, demonstrating that PB increases funding to poorer areas of the city council district. Interestingly, the districts' poorest sub-district did not see an increase in spending but the second poorest sub-district did receive additional funding. This set of findings provides strong evidence that the presence of PB in New York City alters how the government allocates a portion of its resources, but also suggests that its redistributive power is not as strong as PB's advocates had hoped. The authors provide a preliminary explanation for why we see this effect, arguing that these spending patterns are the results of two main factors: 1) weak adherence to PB rules; and 2) the presence of greater numbers of poor citizens combined with the absence of the poorest segments of the population (2019: 64). Thus, Shybalkina and Bifulco's findings suggest that New York City's PB is making some strides towards social justice and that the majority of these gains accrue to poor, although not the poorest, communities.

Finally, Hagelskamp, Silliman, Godfrey, and Schleifer (2020) also find that PB produces a shift in spending patterns when city council districts adopt PB. The authors focus on the discretionary funding available to PB to demonstrate that PB adoption increases spending on schools, streets, traffic improvements, and public housing, and decreases spending on parks and recreation projects, housing preservation, and development projects. Hagelskamp et al. (2020) argue that most of the shifts in resources appear to be in support of poorer residents, which suggests that PB is addressing basic social justice issues.

Thus, a common finding across all three articles is that New York City PB is associated with changes in how city council members allocate scare resources. From a research perspective, these three articles mark an important advance in the field because they demonstrate how PB adoption leads to changes in government spending. However, there still is not sufficient evidence to determine if these budget changes translated to meaningful changes in peoples' well-being. The next stage of the research agenda will be for researchers to evaluate whether the new spending results in changes in well-being, accountability, and civil society.

In sum, the two earliest and most prominent North American PB programs share two crucial components. Both New York and Chicago adopted PB at the sub-municipal level. The obvious strategic advantage of this approach is that PB advocates bypassed the lack of interest among city-wide political officials. Because of the district-level focus, these PB programs were well-situated to promote community mobilization and social inclusion. However, we note that the small-scale effect of PB limits the programs' broader impact. The relatively low levels of public resources dedicated to PB limits its ability to have a large social policy or redistributive effect.

Córdoba, Spain

The early adoption of PB in Europe took place in Spanish municipalities in the southern region of Andalusia, which has a long tradition of civil society organizing and strong support for leftist organizations (Foweraker 2003). Political parties on the left in Spain turned to PB in the late 1990s as a means to renew the connections between political elites and citizens, to make the state more transparent, and to revitalize civil society (Baiocchi and Ganuza 2017; Francés et al. 2018). Government officials initiated PB in Córdoba in 2001 at the behest of a government composed by the post-communist United Left party (IU) and the Socialist Workers' Party (PSOE) (Nebot 2004). The earliest Spanish PB programs exemplify "normative adoption" as leftist political parties followed the lead of their Brazilian counterparts. Although there was some variation in institutional design, most Spanish municipalities adopting PB during this early phase maintained the basic Porto Alegre model.

In Córdoba, multiple interviews in 2007 showed that citizens initially participated in PB based on rules developed in Porto Alegre designed to promote the universality of participation and to encourage the participation of individuals not linked to existing CSOs. The government halted PB in 2004 because existing CSOs boycotted the process due to fear that individual-level representation did not sufficiently take into account their long history of organizing. According to a city council member responsible for PB, "the associations paralyzed the process in 2004 because they felt isolated from it." PB threatened the CSOs' privileged access to the government. After months of negotiations among PB participants, CSO leaders, and government officials, a new set of rules was adopted in 2004 that permitted PB to resume in 2005. The new rules included a mixed system of representation—citizens could attend meetings as individuals or as representatives of a specific CSO. One clear effect of the rule was to strengthen the role of formally organized groups within PB. The initial set of PB rules sought to encourage the growth of unaffiliated citizens as well as to foster the growth of new CSOs. The change in rules in Córdoba strengthened those groups who were already organized, thus expanding the role of the "usual suspects" rather than creating new actors.

Another important rule change in Córdoba was the remaking of the "PB council," where final budgetary decisions are made. Instead of an open vote, the new rules allocated most seats to existing, prominent CSOs. Out of a total of sixty-five seats, fifty-eight were directly appointed by CSOs, thus solidifying the control of the already organized groups. The remaining seven seats were allocated through the "PB thematic" process and could go to a non-affiliated CSO or be allocated to existing CSO leaders (Nebot 2004: 71). Therefore, a minimum of 89 percent of the seats on the PB council, the most important body for making decisions within PB, were held by appointed members of CSOs.

With regard to social justice, a defining feature of the Porto Alegre model, Córdoba's PB program did include a social justice component that could be considered by participants when distributing resources. However, participants were not required to utilize social justice in decision-making. Since social justice was not a significant factor that affects the allocation of resources, the incentives for low-income citizens to participate were not as great as in Porto Alegre. The lack of clear social justice criteria, in conjunction with rules that favored existing CSOs, meant that PB reproduced the distributional advantages and disadvantages associated with representative democracy. These changes in Córdoba are representative of the broader shifts across the country (Francés et al. 2018; Pineda Nebot et al. 2019).

In another example from Spain, a study by Font, Smith, Galais, and Alarcon (2018) used the methodological strategy adopted by the cherry-picking process to analyze the fate of 611 (and, in their 2018 study, 571) proposals from thirty-nine participatory processes in twenty-five Spanish municipalities in Andalucía, Catalonia, and Madrid from 2007 to 2011. The results indicate that one third of proposals were implemented fully with no changes and another third were partially implemented with some changes. According to the authors, such an impact depicts an achievement compared with the classic model of democratic governance. More broadly, we find that there is a general pattern across Europe of using consultative process that provide local governments with great leeway as they decide which projects to implement (see Pineda Nebot et al. 2019). What is not prevalent, however, is research documenting the impact that these and other changes are having.

The move toward online and digital PB programs is the most significant change in Spanish PB over the past two decades, between the initial phase of adoption (early 2000s) and 2020. Francés, Carratalá, and Ganuza's work demonstrates that over 90 percent of PB programs "incorporate some digital element within Participatory Budgeting. That said, these digital participation channels are used almost exclusively to provide further channels for input (providing proposals) and output of the final results (voting or prioritizing proposals). In other words, the internet is frequently used for submitting proposals and voting on them" (2018: 283–4).

Portugal

Portuguese municipalities were also early European adopters of PB programs (Júlio and Dias 2019). The deep connections between Portugal and Brazil partially account for why and how government officials learned about PB (Porto de Oliveira 2017a). Similar to Spain, leftist governments in Portugal initially experimented with PB, suggesting normative adoption as a driving force. In 2002, the small town of Palmela adopted PB, implementing a combination of the Porto Alegre model and a decentralized consultative approach similar to other European countries (Sintomer et al. 2016). Sintomer, Rocke, and Herzberg (2016) indicate that this small city then became the center of a network designed to support the adoption of PB across Portugal. Palmela's program is also relevant because it used a consultative process in which final project selection remained in the hands of the local city council and mayor; this marks a move away from "binding decisions" made by citizens in the Porto Alegre model and a shift to greater authority placed in the hands of elected officials. The process adopted by the Lisbon city government in 2008 stands out because they sought to use a combination of online and text messaging to recruit participants. The Federation of Portuguese Municipalities and Research Institutions, including the Centre for Social Studies at the University of Coimbra, played a crucial role of raising awareness about PB, which spread quickly across Portugal. By 2012, Portugal had the highest percentage of people living in cities with PB in Europe (Sintomer, Rocke, and Herzberg 2016).

In the 2018 book *Hope for Democracy*, Dias, Júlio, Martins, Sousa, and Biel evaluate the impact of PB in Portugal in comparison to the classic model of democratic governance. In a chapter based on several case studies, they characterize the impact of PB in Portugal as an experiment that provided an opportunity for citizens to determine a portion of municipal investments and also, in some cases, served as an instrument for municipalities to understand citizens' perceptions, thus influencing public policy (Dias et al. 2018: 271). Thus, it does appear that PB in Portugal is changing individuals' (both citizens' and government officials') attitudes and behaviors.

Importantly, the Portuguese national government created two new types of PB processes. First, they created a nationwide PB in a narrow number of policy areas, with the aim of incorporating the participation of older residents in small towns and villages. The program's budget was limited to 3 million euros per year (2017) so it is best to conceive of this project as a pilot test case (Dias et al. 2018; Falanga 2018). Second, the national government mandated that all high schools adopt PB in order to promote civic education (see Abrantes et al. 2018; Paz 2018). As Dias and his co-authors note, Portugal is the first country with PB at local, regional, and national levels (2018). Unfortunately, we continue to lack more systematic evaluations of impact that would permit us to better understand if these programs are generating social and political change.

France

In France, the adoption of PB programs by municipalities took place in the context of a broader national discussion on the perceived need to narrow the distance between citizens, CSOs, and a centralized state (Sintomer et al. 2016; Pradeau 2018). National legislation passed in 2002 allows for the establishment of neighborhood councils in all towns and cities with a population over 80,000 inhabitants (Sintomer et al. 2016: 79). PB programs in France were implemented at the behest of municipal governments and don't rely heavily on support from CSOs (Sintomer et al. 2016). This is an example of "mimetic adoption," whereby governments are seeking to improve efficiencies in democratic governance, rather than the normative adoption of governments motivated by the desire to promote social inclusion and social justice.

Early adopters include the town of Bobigny, a suburb of Paris that adopted PB in 2004 with a purpose of fostering active citizen participation in the decision-making process (Sintomer et al 2016). Saint-Denis, a suburb of Paris, followed suit in 2005, adopting a PB program that was largely informal and consultative, and importantly, retained a top-down approach (Sintomer et al. 2016; Porto de Oliveira 2017a). A notable exception is Poitou-Charentes, a regional PB program that is similar to the Porto Alegre model in two aspects: The government allots significant resources to the program and participants have decision-making powers through a vote that ranks projects (Sintomer et al. 2016).

Rather than using binding decision-making, most French PB programs are consultative processes in which citizens enter demands but government officials have complete discretion over which projects to implement, part of a broader trend that we increasingly see across the world. Sintomer and his coauthors argue that the French model is based on "cherry-picking" or "selective listening," which means elected representatives and civil servants possess the discretion to select which projects they will adopt at town-level meetings (Sintomer et al. 2016: 85; Font et al. 2018; Pradeau 2018). Many PB programs now permit citizens to be involved in voting for projects but the key decision-making authority regarding which projects will be debated and then implemented rests firmly in the hands of government officials. In sum, the French cases appear to occupy a grey area between the Empowering Democracy through Community Mobilization and the Efficient Governance types (see Sintomer et al. 2016; Pradeau 2018).

Unfortunately, there is limited academic literature that systematically evaluates the impact of PB in Europe. There is a wealth of single-case studies and process-oriented work, but we still have a limited understanding of PB's impact on accountability, civil society, and well-being in Europe (Enríquez 2019). However, one research team studied the impact from the social justice perspective. Sintomer, Rocke, and Herzberg analyzed the differences between first generation Latin American PB and the various European models in their book, *Participatory*

Budgeting in Europe: Democracy and Public Governance. Their first key observation is that European PB programs downplay the role of distributive justice and focus more on the process (2016: 185). As a result, there are limited social outcomes in the various European programs (Sintomer et al. 2016). According to these researchers, one way to understand the impact of these experiments is to evaluate the criteria with which policy design and implementation occurs. Rather than focus on social justice, these programs center on modernizing the administration, democratizing politics, promoting economic development, and building trust among social actors (Sintomer et al. 2016; Pradeau 2018). There is some research that found evidence for positive results surrounding administrative modernization and trust building, but less so for the delivery of social justice (Sintomer et al. 2016; Schneider and Busse 2019). This suggests an emphasis on oversight may help to generate changes in accountability, but is less likely to generate changes in civil society or well-being.

Sintomer et al. (2016) characterize the overall impact of the majority of European PB programs as being limited due to their emphasis on "consultative" processes (187). They argue, "if we consider European participatory budgeting as a whole, there have been some social outcomes, but apart from exceptions, they have been on a fairly small scale. They have usually involved affirmative action aimed at the most disadvantaged and occasionally allowing for specific groups, but the macro-social balance has remained unchanged" (Sintomer et al. 2016: 188). As mentioned in the beginning of this section, a majority of those PB programs fall into the categories of administrative modernization, trust building among actors, and similar criteria that are void of redistributive justice. Additionally, some of the most important measurements on which the European models show limited social impact are gender equality, local economic development, and sustainable growth (Sintomer et al. 2016; Pradeau 2018; Fouillet 2018). Nevertheless, there is some positive evidence that PB is associated with improvements in citizen well-being (Carcaba, Gonzalez, Ventura, and Arrondo 2017) as well as the promotion of greater community engagement (Font, Del Amo, and Smith 2016; Dias et al. 2018). Although there are a handful of research articles and reports that identify a series of positive impacts through PB, the overarching lesson is that researchers have not systematically demonstrated a wider range of positive impacts. Quite simply, we still lack sufficient empirical evidence to definitively assert that European PB programs generate extensive social and political change.

Digital PB

Another common program type in this region, Digital Participation, is an effort to include greater numbers of citizens in policymaking processes and represents a significant innovation regarding how citizens engage in PB. We find greater use of online participation to incorporate citizens in PB in Europe in comparison to the Global South. The obvious reason for the greater use of technology is the high levels of wealth in European countries, which lowers the relative cost for citizens and governments to implement these new programs. But we also see greater use of online technologies in Europe than in the United States or Canada. Although Madrid, Paris, and Barcelona are noteworthy examples of how governments are developing new technologies for PB, North American PB programs tend to emphasize small-group participation, deliberation, and public voting. The different emphasis is derived from a longer North American tradition of public deliberation among citizens in formal policymaking arenas as well as the NGOs/CSOs advocating change (Bryan 2003).

The cities of Paris, Madrid, and Barcelona are leading the way in promoting online PB participation and voting. We describe these programs below to better illuminate how online platforms are being used to incorporate citizens into participation. Because they are so new, there is very little data about the extent to which they are changing individuals and communities.

Paris

The PB program in Paris is noteworthy because of the high level of resources allocated to it and because half of participants only engage through an online process. In the first year of the program, the newly elected mayor began with a relatively small pilot project, committing USD15 million to the program. This quickly increased to USD125 million in 2015 and USD150 in following years (Arhip-Paterson and Fouillet n.d.; Fouillet 2018). This level of spending is far higher and much more extensive than in comparable cities such as Chicago and New York. Thus, there is a higher potential for generating changes through PB because there is a significant amount of resources being spent based on citizens' votes. We note, however, that we were unable to identify any research that demonstrates the impact of this spending on Parisians' quality of life.

Parisians can participate in two ways: They can choose to attend face-to-face meetings or they can do all of their participation online. In 2017 and 2018, about half of participants voted in person (generally at a weekend farmers' market) and about half participated online (Arhip-Paterson and Foulieet n.d.). According to a PB staff member in Paris, government officials designed their program to incorporate greater numbers of Paris residents as well as to incorporate younger residents. PB in Paris is primarily an online process, though citizens can also attend local meetings at the sub-municipal level. Paris introduced two significant changes to how citizens first propose and then select projects. Citizens can propose projects through an online portal, after which the government provides a cost estimate and carries out a feasibility study. The government then generates a list of proposals on which citizens may vote. Following the publication of this list, the government holds public meetings at the neighborhood level to give people the option of discussing projects prior to voting. But there is no requirement that citizens engage in either face-to-face or online deliberation. Citizens can either vote online or in ballot boxes that are distributed in public areas, such as Saturday markets. The majority of participants vote online.

The second Parisian innovation is a new way to finalize project selection. Citizens vote for specific projects, but these votes are not necessarily binding. The Parisian government places final decision-making in the hands of a committee comprising ten government officials and ten PB citizen-participants. The PB participants are randomly selected from among the individuals who submitted project proposals; this reflects the democratic idea of "the selectorate," in which random individuals are selected to form a governing body (Fouillet 2018; Peixoto et al. 2018). The purpose of this innovation is to overcome elite capture, whereby entrenched community leaders are more likely to dominate PB meetings. Thus, an interesting democratic advance associated with the Parisian model is that the program combines government expertise with a randomly selected group of participants.

The Parisian case has important drawbacks to accompany its innovations. First, the Parisian PB process does not promote extensive deliberation among citizens. This can be a "thin" version of participation whereby participants have limited information and vote online with little to no deliberation or knowledge accumulation (see Fouillet 2018). PB's role as a "school of democracy," through which citizens learn to engage each other, largely disappears in this context. In addition, the Parisian PB program does not specifically address social justice or social inclusion. As noted above, many programs in North America substituted social inclusion for specific social justice rules to better incorporate under-represented communities into the process. In Paris, our analysis suggests that the PB program is reinforcing access for wealthy and well-situated citizens rather than serving as an instrument to incorporate poor residents and immigrants (Nez 2016). The first way this occurs is through the program's strong emphasis on digital PB. Online processes tend to encourage the participation of middle-class sectors that have easier access to high-quality internet services. In addition, poverty in the Paris metropolitan region is concentrated in the areas *outside* of Paris' formal territorial boundaries. As a result, the PB program is being implemented in Paris, which largely comprises middle- and upper-income communities. The combination of online administration, a wealthier demographic base, and the lack of explicit rules to promote social justice means that the Parisian program is part of the worldwide trend of deemphasizing social justice in PB.

Madrid and Barcelona, Spain

Governments in Madrid and Barcelona adopted PB programs, but they deviated significantly from the Porto Alegre model. The principal innovation was that

Madrid and Barcelona's PB processes occur primarily online; they emphasize online proposal processes and voting to select projects. These decisions are relatively binding compared to those in Paris, but the programs also lack deliberative components. These two cities' platforms serve as the model for over thirty-five additional PB programs across Spain, Europe, and Latin America, suggesting that North-North and North-South diffusion of PB innovations is now occurring (https://consulproject.org/en/, accessed July 14, 2020). Greater access to technology in Europe and the timing of PB adoption account for why more technology is used in the North Atlantic region. Interestingly, the preexisting networks of exchange (which started through South-to-North transmissions) are now used in the North-South dissemination.

In Spain, there is also a broader trend that supports the incorporation of digital tools into existing PB programs. A study by Francés, Carratalá, and Ganuza (2018) underlines the impact of digital tools for PB, especially after 2015. They found that 91.7 percent of case studies use digital participation channels for proposal submissions and voting, while 61.7 percent of case studies use in-person meetings for participant deliberation (Francés et al., in Dias et al. 2018: 283–4). They also show that a majority of PB programs used a combination of online and in-person channels, though more populous municipalities use more digital tools in comparison to smaller cities. Such evidence is beneficial to evaluate the process or tools used in the PB process, but lacks an overall social outcome measurement, either of its success as a socially inclusive process or as an end goal itself.

Madrid and Barcelona promote their respective online platforms for other municipalities across Spain and around the world. In 2020, *Consul*, Madrid's open-source platform, is in use in thirty-three different countries (https://consulproject.org/en/, accessed July 14, 2020). *Decidim*, from Barcelona, is also open-source, but it is unknown how many municipalities use it. Each city holds parallel conferences for developers to discuss new features and write new code, with general technical assistance coming from the Madrid and Barcelona city governments. Madrid's PB program also has an in-person, deliberative component designed to incorporate the elderly, who tend to be some of Madrid's poorest residents, into the process. Holding in-person meetings and managing the online platform is costly in terms of time and resources. Government officials in Madrid thus face some of the classic trade-offs between Digital PB and traditional, in-person PB. Online processes are more cost-efficient ways to engage larger numbers of people populations. Participant numbers are very high in these programs (Paris had upwards of 7 percent of the population participate in 2016), but participation is thin, and deliberation is often non-existent (Arhip-Paterson and Fouillet n.d.) Participation is more intensive for in-person programs, but participants are fewer and meetings are costly to hold.

Efficient Governance

We find greater use of the Efficient Governance type in Europe than in the other world regions. In comparison to the Global South, this is likely because local governments in Europe already had high state capacity and high levels of human development. These European governments do a remarkable job of providing basic public services to their populations. However, these governments, especially in the context of Germany, face intense pressures to continue to provide services in a time of tightening budget constraints. In this PB type, PB moves from being a radical democratic project to a governance strategy designed to allow citizens to help government officials make difficult decisions.

Germany

An effort to combine administrative reforms and participation in pursuit of efficient governance is a noteworthy feature of many German PB programs; governments were less driven by normative concerns of "deepening" the quality of democracy and more interested in generating governance efficiencies. The first known PB program in Germany was in 1998 in the small municipality of Monchweiler (Sintomer et al. 2016: 115). By 2010, ninety-six municipalities adopted some form of PB into budgetary decision-making processes (Schneider and Busse 2019: 3). In most places, government officials designed PB to help address the lack of adequate resources to deliver programs, leading to innovative approaches that focused on improving the efficiency and effectiveness of the local administrations (Sintomer et al. 2016). Sintomer and his coauthors characterize German PB as an attempt to link participation and modernization in public administration based on the New Public Management reform, in which citizens are customers and public servants are managers of the public programs (2016: 126).

PB in Germany differs considerably from that of the Porto Alegre model. The Brazilian cases strongly emphasize co-governance whereas the German cases mainly emphasize consultative processes, with final decisions being made by the local legislature, as well as management efficiencies (Geissel 2012: 165; Franzke and Kleger 2010; Schneider and Busse 2019; Stolzenberg and Wampler 2018). Thus, scholars identify PB in Germany as a public management tool and not a democratic reform (Baiocchi and Ganuza 7; Sintomer et al. 2016: 125–7). The driving force behind adoption appears to be a desire to improve governance efficiencies in the budget and policymaking process; a secondary concern revolves around improving the quality of democratic governance.

Researchers are also very skeptical about PB's impact in Germany. Schneider and Busse argue that PB is popular among government officials, but they do question its legitimatacy among the broader population (2019: 11). Further, they don't find much evidence of any impact of PB on mobilizing marginalized groups and improvements in budget effectiveness and efficiency (Schneider and Busse, 2019: 11). Schneider and Busse note that a "general problem of PB in Germany (and elsewhere) is socially biased participation. Most participants are from 35 to 65 years old and well educated" (2019: 267). Furthermore, a comparative analysis carried out by Nuenecker indicated that there is limited evidence that PB alters the spending patterns in cities that adopt it (cited in Schneider and Busse 2019). Overall, Germany's programs seek to raise awareness of the difficult budget trade-offs faced by local government. The involved population are well-educated members of the middle classes, thus dampening the likely civic education impact that might be otherwise be extended had participants been drawn from immigrant, low-income, or other politically marginalized communities.

Mandated by National Government

We find several cases of mandated PB programs in Europe, most notably Poland, Portugal, and Scotland (but not the rest of the United Kingdom). National governments mandate programs in their efforts to "fix" some sort of governance deficit at the local level, trying to legislate social and political change from above. We turn our attention to Poland because it has the highest number of subnational governments that are required to adopt PB programs.

Poland

In Poland, PB emerged in 2011 in small towns and villages; by 2018 it had been adopted across nearly fifteen hundred towns and villages throughout the country. This process is thus analogous to Indonesia, South Korea, and Peru, where local PB experiences paved the way for national-level mandated programs. In 2018, the Polish national government required larger towns and some cities to use PB. The sheer number of PB cases in Poland now means that these programs represent the majority of PB cases in Europe. Like Indonesia, there are two parallel processes— one at the village level and a second among larger towns and cities.

In 2009, the Polish national government created the Solecki Fund to promote participation and empowerment at the lowest levels of governance (towns and, below them, villages) (Sześciło and Wilk 2018; Keblowski and Van Criekinger 2014). Each year, towns must formally declare their intentions to "earmark" specific funds for their villages. The levels of funding are relatively low. According to Bednarska-Olejniczak and Olejniczak, "in 2016, in as many as 417 municipalities the expenses from the Village fund exceeded the equivalent of 10 Euro per capita, while in 562 municipalities their share exceeded 1% of total expenditure" (2018: 343). After a town officially decides to delegate resources to some or all villages, residents then attend a public meeting and decide how to allocate those resources. The town then implements the selected projects provided that they are financially and legally viable. Following the implementation of the project, the town may apply to the national government to be reimbursed up to 40 percent of what they spent on this community participation program. Thus, similar to the Philippines, Polish PB serves as an effort to provide additional resources to local governments to support the citizen participation process. However, we note that villages and towns do not have a clear set of rules or institutional design to follow. Sześciło and Wilk argue that this village-level participatory process can work well if "it is accompanied with significant incentives and grants, as well as the extensive autonomy and flexibility of local communities" (2018: 179). For this approach to work well, it would require sustained and consistent support from the national government. However, we simply don't know if the national government is will-ing to invest in village-level participatory programs. Bednarska-Olejniczak and Olejniczak raise a significant concern, which is that the "total freedom of the local authorities in undertaking decisions on the conduct of consultations stems from the voluntary nature of these procedures" (2018: 2). Local governments at odds with the national government may choose to withhold their support from the local PB programs and the national government could choose to punish specific villages or regions by withholding funding; under both of these scenarios, the pro-gram wouldn't work well at the local level. This program, like other participatory programs across the world, therefore depends heavily on the political interests of the government as well as the configuration of civil society. Unfortunately, we lack any systematic research to account for how Poland's 1,450 PB programs function.

Parallel to the village-level PB process, a group of community activists in 2011 in the town of Sopot (thirty-eight thousand residents) convinced the local gov-ernment to formally adopt PB. The purpose was to open dialogue between the government and citizens: "Deliberation is not an objective here—citizens are sup-posed to merely express their support or disapproval regarding projects prepared beforehand by the local administration" (Keblowski, and Van Criekinger 2014: 373). Rather than being a project that emphasizes democratic renewal, the emphasis of this first program was on citizens voting on projects from a list selected by the local government. Unlike Spain or France, where the first cases of PB are best conceptualized as Deepening Democracy through Community Mobilization, the earliest cases in Poland are more similar to the Efficient Governance cases that dominate the German PB experience. Keblowski and Van Criekinger argue that Sopot is now the model that other PB programs would copy (2014: 370). Bednarska-Olejniczak and Olejniczak estimate that "in 2013 PB was implemented in more than 50 municipalities, in 2014 it was about 150 and now it is between 200 and 250 municipalities" (2018: 8).

Preliminary research on Sopot and other PB cases in Poland is not positive: "PB in Sopot—very much a symbolic, frontier-like case in Polish local politics—reflects few achievements and many flaws of PB in Poland. These flaws are fundamental, as PB Polish-style actually preserves the current, criticized system of urban management and power, [and] conserves the status quo" (Keblowski and Van Criekinger 2014: 377). Given the relatively recent adoption of the national legislation requiring that all towns include citizen participation as a part of the budgetary and policymaking process, there is insufficient evidence to know what type of impact Poland's PB processes will have. Like with many other mandated PB programs around the world, we do not see evidence that PB is strengthening civil society or contributing to improvements in local quality of life. There may be marginal improvements in accountability but even those are difficult to identify clearly.

Comparative Analysis

The early adoption of PB programs in Spain, Portugal, and France was driven by leftist political parties that sought to mobilize civil society, address high political apathy, and improve low levels of trust. Different from the Brazilian experiences (where PB was created simultaneously with the re-establishment of democracy), these European PB programs were largely efforts to deepen existing democracies and mobilize the community in a context of weak democratic practices rather than being co-founded with new democratic regimes. Thus, PB in Europe is an institution with much more of an emphasis on incremental, policy reform relative to the original radical democratic experiences. This helps to explain why researchers have found limited social and political change associated with European PB programs. Germany is the principal location of the Efficient Governance type. Interestingly, we don't see this type in many other places in the world although some programs may share characteristics with the German PB programs. We surmise that many German governments are actually already quite efficient, but that the adoption of PB is a way to leverage citizen participation to improve governance-related issues.

Digital PB, principally in Paris, Madrid, and Barcelona are excellent examples of governments innovating. In these cities, greater numbers of citizens participate at some point in the process and the level of resources dedicated to PB is much higher than elsewhere. However, this is rather "thin" participation, by which we mean that citizens can vote on projects, but there is little deliberation, expansion of accountability, or strengthening of civil society. Of course, there is also a trade-off between an increase in resources, greater numbers of participants, and more limited forms of engagement. Governments are willing to dedicate greater levels of resources to PB because they have more control over where the resources will be allocated; civil society is a much weaker partner in the process.

In Canada and the United States, the most significant change in PB relative to the early Brazilian programs was its adoption at the sub-municipal level. The obvious benefit of this approach was to initiate grassroots, participatory democracy, bypassing disinterested mayors and city administrators. PB was led by city council members who were really interested in connecting with community leaders and constituents. However, the problem with this model is that city council members have limited resources as well as weak control over the local state administrative apparatus. A first wave of research demonstrates that PB is changing how city council members allocated their limited resources. But, we must now wait for additional research to assess whether these budgetary changes result in shifts in accountability, civil society, and well-being.

In comparison to Asian PB programs, one noteworthy difference for PB in the United States is that it has not scaled to cities or the national level. Moreover, PB has only been systematically mandated in one European country, Poland. National governments in Indonesia, South Korea, and the Philippines mandated PB after the national government deemed pioneering programs successful. In contrast, there has been no national level take-up of PB in United States and there are very limited examples of robust city-wide uptake. We do see "city-wide" approaches in places like Seattle and Boston, but these PB programs focus on the youth and do not incorporate many citizens or allocate a lot of resources. Thus, the Asian programs studied in this book now have much greater breadth because they cover significant portions of their countries. The North American PB programs are smaller in scope, which could be advantageous because they are led by people committed to making them work well.

Conclusion

PB spread across Europe, the United States, and Canada, again, largely at the urging of center and left-of-center political parties, civil society activists, and NGOs. There was a strong normative push among these actors to deepen the quality of democracy and improve social inclusion. But a secondary push is also noteworthy, in which many adopting governments were more concerned with improving efficiencies of governance by incorporating citizens' voice through consultative practices. Thus, we see the twin impulses of normative and mimetic forces driving adoption across the North Atlantic region. Interestingly, we also see extensive experimentation involving the use of cutting-edge technology among these programs, thereby allowing governments to incorporate larger numbers of people into PB, albeit with less face-to-face deliberation and engagement. Many of Europe's PB programs are therefore thinner versions of the original Brazilian models.

There are some single-case and small-N comparative analyses that demonstrate PB's positive impact on civil society. In Europe, local governments and CSOs incorporate citizens into PB programs often as a means to counter the centralization of authority in Brussels as well as their national capitals. In North America, governments often seek to overcome citizen apathy by returning to previous periods in which citizens were more actively engaged in their governments. Governments that are more strongly driven by normative pressures of adoption are more likely to generate civil society engagement. Conversely, the evidence suggests that when governments are primarily interested in strengthening governance (PB as a tool), they are less likely to support activities that might strengthen civil society.

The expansion of accountability is greater in those places where governments allocate more resources to PB as well as when they hold more face-to-face meetings. When PB occupies a greater role in policymaking processes, there is also likely to be a greater expansion of accountability. One significant drawback to the European and North American cases is that the majority of PB programs across the region remain relatively small with few resources and relatively low numbers of participants (with the exception of Digital PB programs, which have significantly higher turn-out and greater resources). These programs also tend to lack transparency in some areas—implementing governments do not often publish participation numbers, demographics, or geographic information about participants. Although it is possible that some of these programs may have robust levels of citizen participation, our decades-long research in the area suggests that governments are willing to provide participation numbers when they are high, but tend not to when they are low. The general lack of readily available information on European PB programs suggests that the governments are not achieving their desired goals. This reduces the more expansive potential impacts that PB could generate.

We also identify a contradictory turn: Recent innovations in the use of online programs increase the funds dedicated to PB, which increases its potential impact. However, these programs also tend to be associated with a move to online project selection, which has the effect of limiting potential gains in accountability and social inclusion. Although there is interest among the different actors involved to use Digital PB to expand access to government officials and information, the relatively low numbers of participants in relationship to the general population and the limited connections to CSOs make it difficult to expand accountability.

Finally, limited evidence exists regarding how PB might enhance well-being across Europe and North America. We start with the obvious: Most European and North American countries already have relatively high standards of living and an expansive welfare state (much more so in Europe than in the United States), which means that local budgets with relatively low levels of resources are unlikely to alter general well-being. In comparison to the evidence from Brazil, it is thus less likely that we will see similarly significant improvements in well-being across North Atlantic countries, as it is much more difficult to improve upon relatively high levels of well-being than upon moderate or low levels. We would expect that public infrastructure projects implemented through PB would improve specific local conditions and quality of life on certain streets or in certain neighborhoods, but we lack any evidence that might highlight how such projects improve general quality of life. Moreover, many PB programs in Europe and North America more heavily emphasize the social inclusion of participants in the process rather than focusing on social justice outcomes.

At the broadest level, we can see that PB in Europe and North America is more heavily geared toward civic education and community empowerment than toward a radical inversion of spending priorities that might alter the quality of life among the more marginalized members of society. PB is an incremental democratic institution in these contexts that does retain some of the radical features of the first wave. Most importantly, most programs retain the radical idea that a wide variety of citizens, especially those from politically weaker and more marginalized groups, should be directly involved in decision-making.

These trends are very different from PB in sub-Saharan Africa, an area where there is a greater possibility of improvements in well-being, but with significant limitations on resources and weak state capacity. PB has spread in Africa largely at the behest of international organizations and actors. There have been some interesting transformations as well, all documented in Chapter 6.

6

South-to-South and Donor-driven Diffusion in Sub-Saharan Africa

Sub-Saharan Africa began its experience with PB in the early 2000s, which quickly grew to more than one hundred and fifty programs by 2012 then more than eight hundred programs in 2020. Subnational governments (cities, counties, villages) in diverse places such as Kenya, Senegal, Mozambique, Uganda, and South Africa adopted PB. Although there are a few cases of normative adoption of PB, most subnational governments adopting PB did so in close collaboration with international donors, such as the World Bank, DFID, USAID, and Germany's Gesellschaft für Technische Zusammenarbeit (GTZ), suggesting a combination of coercive and mimetic adoption. During the first two decades of the twenty-first century, these multilateral donors promoted citizen participation in policymaking alongside their support for development projects and efforts to improve govern-ance. The hope was that increasing participation through PB would generate transparency and therefore accountability. Of course, international donors and funders play a larger role in sub-Saharan Africa than in other global regions, which helps to explain why the international organizations and NGOs are strongly associated with the adoption of PB in the region (Hyden 2016; Awortwi and Aiyede 2017; Baessa 2017; Ceesay 2019).

PB's diffusion across sub-Saharan Africa has led to significant adaptations as governments, CSOs, and donors sought to fit PB to meet local needs and chal-lenges. Three key shifts stand out across sub-Saharan PB programs as well as in low-income contexts around the world where PB has recently been adopted. First, PB is now being adopted in villages and rural environments that often have fragile local states, high poverty, and very limited public resources. The scope of public works projects selected through these programs is thus much narrower than in middle- and upper-income countries due to limited funding and state capacity. PB is much more of a citizen empowerment program that is helping to initiate social accountability in these contexts, rather than a way to distribute meaningful portions of local budgets. In many ways, PB in sub-Saharan Africa resembles community-driven development programs (CDD), with the key difference being that PB designates *local* revenue for development rather than World Bank funds (Chase and Holmeno 2005; Wong 2012). This is somewhat similar to PB in Indonesia, Philippines, Guatemala, and Bolivia, with the exception that external donors are almost always the impetus behind PB adoption. However, the shifts

Participatory Budgeting in Global Perspective. Brian Wampler, Stephanie McNulty, and Michael Touchton,
Oxford University Press. © Brian Wampler, Stephanie McNulty, and Michael Touchton 2021.
DOI: 10.1093/oso/9780192897756.003.0007

described above are distinct from those evident in new PB programs in Europe and North America, in Asia, or in middle-income countries around the world.

Due to these different enabling conditions, the scope of potential impacts for new African PB programs will likely be different than in the earliest PB cases. In rural areas, we might expect the scope of potential change to be linked to capacity building and basic citizen empowerment as citizens gain information about how their governments operate. The focus on many different types of projects may undermine some of the projects' connections to well-being, but may still promote civil society growth, transparency, and accountability. However, because the programs are relatively new and data are scarce, it is not yet clear what actual impacts have emerged or will emerge.

A second shift in sub-Saharan Africa is that PB programs are more likely to use consensus-based decision-making models instead of a secret or even a public vote (e.g., a show of hands). Not surprisingly, there are different interpretations of this new model. Advocates argue that consensus-based decision-making helps to unite disparate communities, overcome differences, and create shared ownership of the program. However, critics worry that a consensus-based model is more susceptible to elite capture, whereby traditional local powerbrokers will dominate the process and exclude marginalized groups.

Finally, sub-Saharan African PB programs are far less likely to use specific rules that promote social justice and mandate the distribution of greater resources to underserved communities. This is due in part to the absence of this rule within the broader World Bank framework (Shah 2007; Goldfrank 2012). It is an important omission because the need to serve poor communities is very high in most cities that adopt PB. Nevertheless, introducing PB to rural villages in sub-Saharan Africa redistributes resources to very poor communities and thus promotes social justice. Whether this general trend results in redistribution that corresponds to village needs may depend on whether PB is imposed on the village or whether local demands drives adoption.

Case Selection and Typologies

Several countries across sub-Saharan Africa have adopted and used PB, including Angola, Benin, Burkina Faso, Cameroon, the Republic of Congo, the Democratic Republic of the Congo, Ethiopia, Kenya, Madagascar, Mali, Mauritania, Mozambique, Niger, Senegal, South Africa, Tanzania, Togo, Uganda, Zambia, and Zimbabwe (Dias et al. 2019). These countries cover a range of experiences with PB, from active use and expansion (Kenya, Senegal, Mozambique) to limited use in a few cities (Democratic Republic of the Congo), transformation and co-optation (Uganda), and limited experimentation and abandonment (South Africa).

African PB programs overwhelmingly align with the Social Development and Accountability program type. Like elsewhere in the Global South, PB programs across sub-Saharan Africa exist in sociopolitical environments plagued by poverty with limited accountability, democracy, state capacity, and civil society engagement. As a result, these PB programs emphasize investing in development-related projects as they also build the foundations for accountability.

We focus on PB in Kenya, Madagascar, Mozambique, Senegal, South Africa, and Uganda. These countries were early adopters of PB in sub-Saharan Africa and feature some of the most widespread implementation of PB programs. These programs showcase different aspects of the Social Development and Accountability program type, from the rationale for their adoption to their potential impact. Importantly, we also include South Africa, a country where PB was attempted and then abandoned. Interestingly, city officials initiated South Africa's lone PB program, in Durban, without top-down pressure from either national government or international organizations, or bottom-up pressure from civil society groups. We address these programs by type, beginning with Social Development and Accountability and then continuing with Uganda, where PB is Mandated by National Government. Table 6.1 below summarizes the development of PB in the region, including its key variants and diffusion over time.

Table 6.1. PB programs in sub-Saharan Africa

PB type	1989 to mid-1990s	Mid-1990s to mid-2000s	Mid-2000s to 2020
Empowered Democracy and Redistribution			
Deepening Democracy through Community Mobilization			
Mandated by National Government		134 Ugandan districts (2001)	
Digital PB			
Social Development and Accountability		1 Malagasy municipality (2005) 2 Senegalese municipalities (2003) 1 South African municipality (2002)	7 Kenyan counties (2013) 269 Malagasy municipalities (161 by 2011, 261 by 2014) 53 Mozambican municipalities (1 in 2008, 53 in 2019) 121 Senegalese municipalities (2015)
Efficient Governance			

Source: Authors.

Social Development and Accountability

Governments in sub-Saharan Africa tend to adopt PB through external, donor-based channels (Shah 2007; Nylen 2014; Peixoto and Sifry 2017; Baessa 2017; Wampler et al. 2018; Touchton and Wampler 2020). Donor-driven PB is more of a technical policymaking tool to improve governance and achieve social accountability than as the radical democratic project of its Brazilian origins. In this sense, PB as a technocratic policy tool carries support from a wide variety of actors far beyond those on the political left (Baiocchi and Ganuza 2017). Reformers seeking efficient local government through decentralization, international donors seeking to empower citizens, and politicians seeking legitimacy and votes in newly competitive electoral environments all support PB.

International donors provide the primary impulse to adopt PB across sub-Saharan Africa, which makes a powerful new actor with the broader PB landscape. This dramatically shifts accountability relationships to *external* accountability from local, social accountability. By external accountability, we mean the relationship of local governments to international actors, such as the World Bank. External accountability is closer to vertical accountability than to social accountability, with the key difference being that local governments are situated between international organizations and citizens. Since the impulse for PB comes from international donors in many cases, it is plausible that local governments may be more focused on generating positive outcomes for these donors than for their citizens.

Senegal, Mozambique, and South Africa began experimenting with PB in the 2000s, but PB in sub-Saharan Africa also includes continued expansion of PB in the Democratic Republic of the Congo, Madagascar, and Kenya in the 2010s. International donor interest combined with decentralization policies facilitated PB's expansion across sub-Saharan Africa. Constitutional reforms occurred in all countries whose PB programs we evaluate in this chapter, with Senegal's reform processes beginning as early as the 1970s. As in most countries using PB, decentralization creates local governments with at least some resources and authority over budgets—two prerequisites for meaningful PB. Decentralization has deepened as countries have more thoroughly implemented constitutional reforms and local governments have expanded their revenue and capacity to implement policy. However, local budgets in sub-Saharan Africa are often very small relative to those in other decentralized contexts around the world. PB programs and local governments in general may therefore generate limited local impacts simply because they do not have sufficient resources to create meaningful change.

Domestic government officials support PB as part of their efforts to pursue technocratic reforms in conjunction with citizen participation. World Bank-led programs are the best example of efforts that merge the interests of international technocrats and domestic reformers. Whether the domestic partners are strongly committed to PB or whether they are simply capturing available resources is unknown. In addition, international NGOs, such as the Ford Foundation and the Open Society Foundation, support PB projects in a diverse range of countries, including Uganda.

Government officials also often support PB as part of their electoral strategy in sub-Saharan Africa. PB tends to be popular, especially among poor voters, and elected officials may promote PB as one way to expand their political base (Baessa 2017). Elected officials are often critical in the adoption of PB but are not always involved in the daily aspects of administering a PB program. In general, local bureaucrats in budget and planning offices administer PB programs on a day-to-day basis. Citizens often play a secondary role to government officials when PB acts as a discrete, self-contained policymaking venue. These officials work with CSOs and citizen delegates to recruit participants, solicit proposals, hold meetings, and select and implement projects in the course of the PB cycle.

Civil society has a powerful role in PB adoption, implementation, and monitoring in many countries; however, we do not find this to be the case in most PB programs adopted in sub-Saharan Africa. Civil society is often underdeveloped compared to other regions where PB has recently spread (Carbone 2005; Lorch 2017). Thus, expectations that CSOs will mobilize their fellow citizens, engage in contentious politics, and deliberate broadly are not borne out in countries in sub-Saharan Africa that now practice PB. In many cases, this is because CSO density and capacity are very low in the rural, low-income areas where PB programs now operate. CSOs may not exist to mobilize or inform citizens and those that do exist may be stretched too thin to participate effectively in PB.

PB now occurs in heterogeneous institutional contexts across the continent. Contexts range from rural, low-resource environments to urban contexts with somewhat greater budgets and administrative capacity; the thread that links these adopting governments is the presence of local reformers and international support. This means that PB in rural Kenya is quite different from PB in urban Maputo, Mozambique, or Dakar, Senegal—even with the same general program type. Moreover, PB is associated with different political projects in different contexts. It seems that principles of accountability for public spending, citizen participation, and transparency have overtaken the radical democratic ideal of PB's origins in Porto Alegre in Brazil.

Kenya

National legislation approved in 2011 requires Kenyan counties to include some form of public participation in budgeting processes, but not necessarily PB. This coincided with constitutional reforms decentralizing Kenya's system of government. These reforms created forty-seven counties as the primary subnational administrative unit and the one responsible for determining how to comply with the constitutional mandate for participation in budgeting processes. As of 2017, seven of the forty-seven counties had adopted PB to meet the constitutional requirement, with at least four additional counties considering PB adoption (World Bank 2017). Thus, PB is one option among many for Kenyan counties to fulfill constitutional requirements, but is not mandated by the national government. The World Bank provided key technical assistance to support county governments as they sought to implement PB.

Participation in PB includes discussions and deliberations of projects at multiple levels. Project proposals and discussions typically begin at the village level and extend upward through several layers of administrative units (e.g., village-cluster, sub-ward, ward, sub-county, county). Delegates from lower levels discuss local needs and potential uses of PB funds in meetings at higher levels. Participants deliberate over their priorities but these decisions are consultative rather than binding. This process culminates in project selection in each county's wards, a sub-county administrative unit of roughly a dozen villages, and subsequent ratification in countywide forums.

PB programs in Kenya tend to use a consensus-based model of decision-making. Many of the PB programs are in rural areas, which means that project selection has focused on small-scale projects (e.g., digging wells) that are of importance to local farmers and herders. Kenya's counties operate PB programs, which translates to PB meetings in thousands of villages in some counties, and hundreds of sub-wards and wards across the others. Kenya's PB programs allocate a relatively large share of county funds. The percentage of local budgets used in PB varies across the counties, but at least 30 percent of the total county budget goes to development projects. Roughly half of this total development budget is allocated through PB, which means that 15 percent of the total county budget theoretically goes to PB projects. However, the percentage of the total budget ultimately allocated to PB projects varies from year to year and from county to county. For example, in Makueni County, in the financial year 2016–17, PB projects comprised 12 percent of the total county budget (Touchton and Wampler 2020). Distributing 10–15 percent of total spending through PB is very similar to the highest level of spending for Porto Alegre's PB program and two or three times greater than in most Brazilian cities with PB (Wampler 2007).

Currently, in most counties, each ward receives an equal share of development funds regardless of its population or residents' income. Makueni County passed a development bill in 2016 to promote equity in distribution of development resources across the county's wards. Each ward now receives equal development funds, regardless of economic conditions or political connections. This rule could effectively add a social justice component to the PB programs, to the extent that poorer wards now receive the same resources as other wards. When PB works well in Kenya, we see results like those we witnessed in 2018. Prior to the adoption of PB, the presence of a convent spurred the Kenyan government to drill a well to bring the nuns water. This occurred, in part, because a brother of one of the nuns occupied a key position in the national government. But, the surrounding villages and schools did not have access to a water supply. In 2016, villagers organized themselves within the PB process to advance their demand that PB furnish the resources to pipe water from the well to a nearby village and school. The most important change was that the decision to invest development funds went from being based on personal relationships to one in which local villagers expressed their policy preferences to their fellow citizens and to government officials.

Citizens propose projects at the village level in some counties, but primarily select them in ward-level meetings across the country. Kenyan PB programs mainly select projects or have citizens voice their preferences by consensus, not voting. They only call a formal vote on a project when consensus cannot be reached. There are notable limitations to consensus-based decision-making in Kenya. In much of our experience men, especially older men, tend to dominate these deliberations (Baessa 2017; Cele 2017; Meriabe 2017). In 2018 the authors visited Kenyan villages where PB meetings took place across three counties. In several instances, local officials introduced us as observers and asked the women to sing a traditional welcoming song and dance. The meetings then proceeded without women saying a word. That is, until county government officials insisted they do so "to show the visitors that women participate in the budget, too."

This dominance limits the role of women, youths, and other marginalized groups in PB. As a result, consensus-based processes may reinforce social power dynamics within a community rather than confront them. These types of PB proceedings may then lend themselves more readily to elite capture as the most powerful social and political actors already dominate the process.

Project-selection mechanisms represent an unresolved issue and we do not have research that evaluates the potential trade-offs between the different voting methods. Kenyan county officials themselves told us that inclusivity, representation, and voice for marginalized populations is a key challenge for their PB programs. Women and youth participants are in scarce supply in many rural areas and traditionally powerful segments of society (e.g., older men, those with more education, those with local authority) dominate many PB processes. Access to information is difficult for much of Kenya's population and budget forums are often inaccessible for the very poor due to high direct transportation costs and indirect opportunity costs to attend meetings.

The authors repeatedly heard arguments from local CSOs that consensus-based decisions really reflected the will of elders, the village chief, or local government officials. For example, Makueni County officials regularly spoke to us about how they needed to educate villagers and ward residents to select projects that went beyond individual community needs in favor of broader projects reflecting county priorities. Consensus-based decisions are easier for county officials to reach in conjunction with community leaders, but these decisions may or may not reflect individual citizens' preferences, much less the spirit of PB.

More than half a million citizens now attend at least one PB meeting a year in Kenya (World Bank 2017). It is not clear how often these citizens participate, but the total number of attendees represents over 10 percent of the population in the counties that use PB. There is some evidence that the total number of participants has grown in the short time that PB has been in place and, in particular, that some counties' efforts to recruit women participants and members of other marginalized groups is succeeding. Citizens have selected hundreds of projects through PB but most of these projects have yet to be implemented, due at least in part to the relatively short time that PB programs have been in place. Similarly, the portion of the county development budget allocated through PB is growing in Kenyan counties. Makueni, Elgeyo-Marakwet, and Baringo counties all began their PB programs with roughly 30 percent of the development budget allocated through PB in fiscal years 2015 and 2016, yet all three counties allocated 50 percent of the development budget through PB in 2017 and 2018, with goals to expand up to 70 percent in the future (Karanja 2018; Maratim 2018).

Kenya's PB programs do not use specific mechanisms to ensure that poor or traditionally marginalized groups receive a greater proportion of projects or funding than other citizens. However, some Kenyan counties, such as Makueni, devote additional energy to monitoring implementation by creating a project management committee composed of community members to give the county government regular progress reports. Some counties also require an even distribution of PB resources across wards, regardless of the wards' economic conditions or political influence. This requirement may have a redistributive effect that promotes social justice in the county even if ward-level spending decisions do not expressly include a social justice component (similar to PB in the Philippines).

We have more evidence for impact on participants in Kenya than for other countries in the region. We draw from our own (Touchton and Wampler) large survey of PB participants, a control group of non-participants, our own participant observation, and over forty interviews with key stakeholders. Our evidence points to several encouraging developments regarding citizens' attitudes and their behaviors. The survey results show that PB participants generally believe that their participation is worthwhile, that PB is working well, and that it is creating opportunities for citizens' engagement in policymaking (Touchton and Wampler 2020). We also found that PB participants were very vocal in many meetings, especially surrounding the implementation status of projects selected in previous years. In Makueni County, much of the discussion in PB meetings surrounded stalled development projects, which citizens had already selected, but the government had not yet completed. Many of these projects were selected in 2016 and 2017, but had yet to be contracted out in 2019, much less begun in earnest. Others had been partially completed, but were stalled for various reasons. Citizens in meetings asked county officials about these specific projects and questioned the officials as to why delays persisted. The officials offered new information on stalled projects and promised that all 2016 projects would be completed by the end of 2019. In this context, PB participants pursued *retrospective* accountability whereby they consistently pressured county government officials in the executive branch to explain why specific projects had not been implemented or completed. We do not ultimately know if all of these stalled projects were completed, but similar PB meetings in Kenya's other counties suggest that, at a minimum, PB promotes some accountability for development projects in a context where publicly questioning government officials' actions would have been very uncommon before PB.

Our results also highlight several key challenges for PB in Kenya. First, we infer from the survey that citizens do not have a solid base of information about the budget and therefore acquiesce to county government officials' spending priorities. PB programs exist in counties with relatively homogeneous politics; participants and non-participants alike are strong supporters of Kenyan county governments. We argue that this broad support may lead to general public enthusiasm about PB programs but result in few incentives to use the programs to contest traditional authority or shift distribution of development projects toward community needs. Second, the survey evidence suggests that PB respondents are uneasy and uncertain about the informal authority that traditional powerholders—local chiefs—play in their villages. Third, the organizational structure that integrates citizens into the process from the village, to the village-cluster, to the sub-ward, to the ward, and, finally, to the county level appears to have stretched the county government's administrative units thin. Finally, our qualitative interviews suggest that some community groups feel excluded from the process. Several community leaders felt that the county government deliberately excluded them from the meeting by not providing timely information on the venues and meeting schedule as well as canceling meetings without sufficient notice in some cases. In Baringo and Makueni Counties, some CSO leaders reported being barred from meetings or having meetings adjourned immediately upon their arrival. These leaders alleged that only CSOs who were already collaborating with county governments in other areas, such as churches or teachers' organizations, were invited to PB meetings; in other words, Kenyan PB functions as more of an invited space than a "claimed" space in many cases.

Madagascar

The World Bank introduced and funded Madagascar's first PB programs in nine municipalities in the 2000s. These programs expanded a limited PB pilot in Ambalavao, one small, rural municipality that began a PB experiment in 2005 at the suggestion of the Swiss Agency for Development and Cooperation (World Bank 2010a). PB advocates designed the expanded programs to improve decentralized governance, which the World Bank promoted throughout the 2000s (World Bank 2013). The World Bank and the national government also intend PB programs to build capacity and increase legitimacy in these contexts. The nine original municipalities were diverse with locations in rural and urban areas as well as in mining and non-mining regions (Cabannes 2014). PB spread to at least 160 municipalities by 2011, with many local governments adopting PB with support from the national government, but without direct World Bank support (Dias 2014; Kanouté and Som 2018). Further, the national government expanded the program to an additional 100 municipalities by 2014. Antananarivo, the capital city and the largest in the country, allocated 20 percent of its budget through PB in 2016 (Randriarilala and Melly 2017).

The World Bank was instrumental in initially bringing PB to Madagascar but PB has expanded throughout the country with the national government's assistance. PB is not mandated, but the national government promotes the program and assists municipalities with the technical challenges of implementing programs (similar to the Philippines). Local support has also increased over time and most municipalities now fund PB through an increasing percentage of their own budgets (Ravelomanantsoa 2016; Fenomezantsoa 2019). This is distinct from many other contexts across sub-Saharan Africa, such as Kenya, where World Bank funding and technical support are critical for PB's impetus and sustenance.

The World Bank, the national government, and local governments all promote PB as a way to improve decentralized governance, build capacity, and increase legitimacy. PB is thought to bring transparency and reduce corruption among newly created local governments. The World Bank also promoted PB as a tool for improving efficiency in allocation of local budgets and to increase local revenue through tax compliance (World Bank 2013; Kanouté and Som 2018). Specifically, PB advocates supported the program as a way to give citizens in mining regions a voice in debates on the distribution of mining royalties (World Bank 2015).

PB's rapid expansion across Madagascar continues to face serious challenges for bringing accountability to local governments. Local corruption is still very high, though PB has increased transparency in some areas. Most notably, citizens in mining regions are now more aware of how much their governments receive in mining royalties and how those funds are spent. Early evaluations showed that participation was relatively high in municipalities across the country, with about 3 percent of the population attending large, consultative meetings where deliberations set investment priorities. Further, locally generated tax revenues increased in municipalities with PB. Consultative PB processes may not empower citizens to directly allocate resources in their communities, however, large groups of citizens participate in Madagascar's PB programs and signs of improving tax compliance are encouraging. We do not have data on other outcomes but

Madagascar's PB experience shows considerable promise relative to others in the region.

Madagascar's PB programs tend to focus on small projects covering immediate needs. This emphasis generates a two-fold benefit: PB rewards citizens for their participation, which then helps to generate citizen support. In turn, citizen support leads to government support for PB to please citizen-participants. PB programs often focus on immediate, localized issues because citizens typically have greater information and knowledge on local issues than they would have on more macro or national issues. In addition, local governments implementing PB have control over resources that can fund smaller-scale projects.

However, a significant drawback to the focus on small, "immediate needs" projects is that they might not produce the types of improvements that citizens and governments originally desired. For example, a new well improves citizens' health and reduces the time spent collecting water but will not radically transform local economic conditions. Thus, government officials and PB advocates need to temper their expectations regarding the range of social and political change that PB programs will generate. Although the emphasis on small, immediate needs is understandable, it severely limits PB's potential relative to early PB programs that "inverted" priorities.

The municipally driven expansion of many of Madagascar's PB programs is another indicator of potential impact. Many of Madagascar's rural PB programs are not directly supported by international donors but are driven by local politicians and CSOs (Porto de Oliveira 2017b). This implies a program that is gaining popularity across the country. Madagascar also has tens of thousands of annual participants in its PB programs—up to 3 percent of the population in the hundreds of municipalities with PB (World Bank 2015). As in Kenya, the money that Madagascan municipalities distribute through PB is an additional way to gauge PB's potential impact. Several million dollars a year are allocated through PB across Madagascar, with a relative concentration in a few large programs (World Bank 2015). This funding carries the potential for serious impact in the poor country, even though most of the projects funded are small, village-level efforts designed to address specific development challenges. In very poor areas, hundreds of projects and tens of thousands of participants across the island could work to improve residents' lives in many ways.

Mozambique

The capital city of Maputo first adopted PB in 2008, with the World Bank providing training and technical assistance in the years prior to adoption. Like in Kenya, PB in Mozambique emerged following 2004 constitutional reforms that decentralized political authority and established municipal governments. Unlike Kenya, however, Mozambique's national government is a competitive authoritarian regime, which strikes advocates for participatory democracy as unusual (Nylen 2014). Maputo's government initially struggled to fully implement PB and contracted with an independent technical assistance organization, IN LOCO, to improve implementation. PB is now spreading across the country, with a wider range of independent NGOs involved in implementing PB at the local level. By 2014, two additional municipalities (Nampula and Quelimane) had adopted PB along the Maputo model (Allegretti and Copello 2018). The UK DFID/UKAID municipal governance program, DIALOGO (2012–17), supported these programs and relied on technical assistance from IN LOCO. In 2016, PB expanded to the municipality of Matola with the European Union providing financial support and the municipality of Maputo contributing technical assistance.

International donors' role has been instrumental for the adoption, diffusion, and adaptation of PB programs across Mozambique. The chances of PB surviving in the few municipalities that already use PB would be low without international donors' support because PB adoption requires financial and human resources as well as consistent technical assistance that most municipalities cannot provide (Baessa 2017). In the case of Maputo, Nampula, and Quelimane, the presence of the NGO, IN LOCO, was fundamental for PB's early survival. In contrast, the lack of a comprehensive donor support network for the provision of specialized technical assistance undermined PB adoption and implementation in Matola (Baessa 2017; Matendjua 2019).

Mayors, international donors, and advocacy groups promote PB as a pathway to popular legitimacy in a political context perceived as deeply corrupt and poorly performing in terms of service delivery. In practice, PB in Mozambique frequently becomes an arena for political competition and party development. Mozambique's two major political parties use PB as a recruitment tool as well as to demonstrate their democratic bona fides and/or to claim credit for delivering public goods (Baessa 2017). Broad political support for PB is sparse and partisanship often dominates debates over PB adoption (Baessa 2017; Matendjua 2019). PB programs are difficult to institutionalize and risk being abandoned in competitive electoral contexts, with turnover among mayors' parties. However, multiparty political competition is growing in Mozambique and mayors in the country's larger cities face electoral challenges requiring them to reinvent themselves to gain voters' confidence—in this case, through PB as a social accountability tool.

Accountability through PB may be difficult to achieve in Mozambique for two central reasons. First, Mozambique's PB programs primarily use a consensus-based decision-making model. Project selection, then, may reflect the preferences of traditionally powerful actors over those of marginalized populations. As a result, PB programs, government spending, and government officials may not become accountable to the broad public but instead to narrow, traditionally dominant interests. However, we should also bear in mind that a consensus-based decision-making process may be most appropriate for post-conflict environments like Mozambique, where previous consequences of partisan disagreement have been fatal. Baessa (2017) argues that the use of a consensus-based system was preferable to a direct vote for a number of reasons. Supporters of consensus-based decision-making assert that secret-ballot project selection can lead to conflict in some circumstances, particularly if votes occur along ethnic, religious, or other social cleavages. Instead, advocates seek consensus in PB decisions as a way to build community solidarity in multi-ethnic, multi-religious countries with a history of ethnic or religious violence and to mitigate the risk of future conflicts. Furthermore, consensus-based decision-making may allow citizens to forge bonds of solidarity and create a greater stake in the process. It is entirely possible that both deference to traditional authority and building bonds of solidarity occur in the same PB programs. Such a result might limit accountability but also help to prevent violent conflict.

Accountability through PB may also be difficult to achieve because PB is highly politicized in Mozambique. Certain partisan voices are likely to gain representation in PB processes at the expense of other participants who are unaligned or affiliated with opposition parties. The potential danger of a politicized PB process is that PB can become exclusionary and drift toward participatory clientelism. A positive spin on this information is that PB helps socialize parties into democratic behavior with PB serving as the venue for public competition over scarce resources. In this case, PB serves as a lower-stakes democratic incubator in a younger, less-consolidated democracy, playing a similar role to that of innovation in older, more consolidated democracies. PB's influence may be conditional on its adoption by the country's largest party (FRELIMO) or by the opposition. Yet, intra-party competition and the need for mayors to expand their political network and support bases still provide an incentive for adopting and sustaining PB, as in Maputo (Nylen 2014). Moreover, smaller parties govern other municipalities and may adopt PB to demonstrate their claim to incorporate citizens into policy-making and seek democratic legitimacy while larger parties may use it as a way to retain power while making a public claim to redistribute resources.

An early measure of PB's likelihood of survival in Mozambique, and thus its potential for future impact, is PB's expansion beyond specific political parties or cities associated with the ruling party. For example, Mozambique's PB programs began with a party-driven program in the national capital, Maputo. PB now exists in more than fifty additional cities, including many not governed by the national ruling party. Furthermore, the total number of participants in Mozambique is in the tens of thousands annually. Maputo's PB program alone implemented over a hundred projects between 2012 and 2016 (Baessa 2017).

As in the other cases in sub-Saharan Africa, the money distributed through PB in Mozambique is another way to gauge the programs' potential impact.

Like Kenya and Madagascar, Mozambique allocates several million US dollars a year through PB with a relative concentration in a few large programs (World Bank 2015). Most projects in Mozambique are small and designed to address specific development challenges at the village level. We have no other evidence of impact, but relatively high levels of funding have a high potential for impact in a very poor country; millions of dollars a year funds hundreds of small projects.

Senegal

Senegal has been a leader in PB adoption across sub-Saharan Africa. More than ninety municipalities used PB by 2017, many of them in rural areas. Senegal is also one of the leading countries using PB in Francophone Africa (including Cameroon, Madagascar, and the Democratic Republic of the Congo), which also have PB programs (ENDA-ECOPOP 2006). Senegalese PB programs are consultative, as citizens have limited decision-making authority (Porto de Oliveira 2017b). International donors have primarily led the spread of PB in Senegal, although at least two cities adopted PB-like programs prior to the involvement of international technical advisors.

Senegal's early PB adoption incorporated several distinct experiences, including participation on public spending that emerged through parallel development in rural communities such as Fissel in 2002. The Fissel program featured limited citizen participation but incorporated community leaders into budgeting processes as delegates. This practice then expanded to urban contexts, such as Rufisque-Est and Dakar, the country's capital, by 2006. Senegal's national government did not promote or require PB; however, the Ministry of Planning and Local Authorities supported a law for "Local Authorities and Participatory Budgeting" which provided the legal basis for subnational governments to adopt innovative forms of citizen engagement as the country decentralized (Kanouté 2014, cited in Porto de Oliveira 2017b).

Decentralization began in the early 1970s with Fissel (thirty-four thousand inhabitants distributed in twenty-eight villages) and Ndiaganiao (forty-five thousand inhabitants, distributed in thirty-seven villages) among the first rural communities created as distinct administrative units. This process facilitated the adoption of different mechanisms designed to strengthen local government and empower citizens to participate actively in public affairs (Gaye 2008). The national government's 1996 decentralization law states explicitly that citizens can participate in local planning and may request information on public administration including budgeting expenses (UN-Habitat, ENDA-ECOPOP 2008). PB also emerged following decentralization as a way to enhance citizen control over public policymaking in rural contexts such as Fissel and Ndiaganiao in 2003.

As in Indonesian villages, PB in Senegal relied on facilitators to help run meetings and discuss community needs.

After these initial experiences, however, international and domestic NGOs also drove the implementation of Senegal's early PB adoptions. Specifically, the Institut International pour l'Environnement et le Développement (IEED), with funding from the United Kingdom, was instrumental in promoting PB. Similarly, ENDA-ECOPOP is a nationally active NGO based in Dakar (Espaces Co production et d'Offres Populaires pour l'Environnement et le Développement en Afrique, Co-Production Spaces and Public Opportunities for the Environment and Development in Africa). This organization facilitated adoption and provided technical assistance for PB programs throughout Senegal (Porto de Oliveira 2017b). Senegal's Ministry of Planning and Local Authorities also promoted PB's institutionalization in Senegalese municipalities through its 2010 Program for Local Development in partnership with ENDA-ECOPOP. This program fostered training and workshops surrounding PB for 133 collectives in different munici-palities around the country by 2015. No specific political party is associated with PB in Senegal but municipalities with mayors from left-wing parties tended to adopt PB (*socialistes*, *ecologistes*, and social democrats).

PB in Senegal faces several challenges. Electing PB delegates that represent common citizens' interests can be complicated due to religious leaders' and village chiefs' informal authority. Gender equity in participation is difficult to achieve—decisions on project funding often do not take women's input into account and women are rarely elected as delegates in PB processes (Porto de Oliveira 2017b). Men tend to dominate PB processes in smaller, rural areas (Baessa 2017; Porto de Oliveira 2017b; Meriabe 2017). Including women in PB processes is a key issue in rural communities as well as in places where women have a limited role in politics and policy discussions. Women play a greater role in urban areas, especially in entry-level participatory opportunities and in municipal-level processes.

A lack of infrastructure and local administrative capacity hinders institutional-ization of PB processes and project implementation in many contexts. Low edu-cation among local populations and few local champions also undermine PB's efficacy in Senegal, particularly in rural areas. However, there is some potential for local impact. PB programs in Senegal tend not to have explicit, pro-poor requirements for voting or project selection. Yet, these programs are located in the context of extreme poverty and focus almost exclusively on attending to citizens' very basic needs. For example, health projects (building, equipping, upgrading, and renovating health facilities), water projects (digging wells, building earthen dams, providing infrastructure to deliver water), education projects (building and equipping schools and early-childhood education centers), and agriculture projects (building cattle dips, slaughter houses, and irrigation networks) represent the bulk of projects that citizens select.

The number of PB programs in a country is a rough and preliminary indicator, but it is potentially telling for PB's potential for impact in sub-Saharan Africa. Like Madagascar and Mozambique, Senegal now has dozens of PB programs in rural areas. Similarly, the creation of local observatories for participatory democracy improve prospects for transparency and accountability (Cisse 2019). International donors did not drive the adoption of these programs. Instead, local politicians and CSOs sought a governance model that promoted development and helped to create and sustain the institutions (Porto de Oliveira 2017b; Kanouté and Som 2018). The potential thus exists for PB programs to produce outcomes beyond the Social Development and Accountability PB type. We do not have enough information about these rural Senegalese programs to classify them, much less to draw inferences about their potential impact.

South Africa

South Africa created a version of PB with Social Accountability and Development characteristics, but it never gained a foothold in the country. The city of Durban is the only South African municipality to experiment with PB, which it adopted and abandoned during the 2000s. Exploring cases where PB was adopted, but later abandoned, helps us to understand what factors might sustain PB as it spreads across the continent. In South Africa's case, the governing African National Congress Party (ANC) never supported the widespread diffusion of PB and invested little energy to delegate decision-making authority to citizens (Heller 2001). Durban's government officials discontinued the program after two cycles. However, South Africa may prove to be fertile ground for renewed PB adoption and adaptation because of opposition parties' recent electoral victories and President Zuma's departure from office.

South Africa's 1998 decentralization provided the constitutional and legal provisions that encourage participation in many aspects of governance, including budgeting. None of these provisions, however, provided specifically for PB. Nevertheless, the White Paper on Local Government (1998) promoted governments "committed to working with citizens, groups and communities to create sustainable human settlements which provide for a decent quality of life and meet the social, economic and material needs of communities in a holistic way" (12). Additionally, the Municipal Systems Act (2000) formally introduced the concept of community participation. The Act requires municipalities to "encourage and create conditions for the local community to participate in the affairs of the municipality, including in . . . the preparation, implementation and review of its integrated development plan . . . and the preparation of its budget" (15).

South Africa implemented its new system for local governments during the mid-1990s through 2000. Yet, only eThekwini, which encompasses the greater

Durban Metropolitan Municipality, adopted PB in its 2002/3 and 2003/4 budget processes. Neither civil society groups nor international donors drove the adoption of PB in Durban. In contrast, eThekwini's metropolitan administrators, the majority of whom were members of the ANC, promoted PB. Yet, the national ANC leaders remained disinterested in PB and did not provide support to scale the program out across the rest of the Durban Metropolitan Municipality, much less across the country. The scale of PB adoption, then, and the networks to support it, matter for PB's performance. A single, standalone case of PB may be less likely to survive than programs where a network of governments adopt PB and compare experiences with one another for improved implementation and performance.

Mandated by National Government

Uganda

Uganda's 1995 constitution and Local Government Act (1997) decentralized governance and served as the foundation for PB.[1] The constitution also requires local governments to incorporate citizens into formulating and implementing development plans and programs that affect them. Additionally, the Local Government Act explicitly includes popular participation in, and control of, decision-making as a policy objective. The Act also requires district councils to prepare comprehensive and integrated development plans that incorporate lower-level local governments' needs when they submit these plans to the National Planning Authority (NPA). The Budget Act (2001) also provides for participation of citizens and their representatives in the budget process.

Different actors had different roles in introducing and promoting PB in Uganda. International agencies like the World Bank promoted New Public Management (NPM) reforms that brought decentralization and later PB. These organizations worked with UN agencies to fund PB activities and develop training modules and guidelines. The Ministry of Finance Planning and Economic Development provided for PB in its budget calendars under the Budget Act (2001) and, more recently, in the Public Finance and Management Act (2015). The Ministry of Local Government was also instrumental in the adoption of PB by issuing official guidelines as well as training officials on how to implement and operate PB programs. Finally, local CSOs were also important for monitoring and facilitating PB.

[1] Angola mandated PB in 2019. We selected Uganda as our case study for this chapter because of PB's longer duration.

Kasozi-Mulindwa (2013) asserts that PB in Uganda did not emerge on its own merit but was imposed by the state. He argues that the National Resistance Movement government adopted decentralization and PB as a way to attain political legitimacy and as a response to pressure from donors who were proponents of NPM (Baiocchi and Ganuza 2017). In turn, PB became required of municipalities and is theoretically used universally among them; thus Uganda is a mandated case of PB within the region.

PB shifted in two important ways as Ugandan governments implemented top-down directives for participation. First, participation is no longer open to any interested citizens; rather, government officials invite individual citizens to participate (Makaaru 2017). This is a significant transformation, especially in a one-party state and is similar to Indonesia, where governments extend invitations to participate based on social groups created under the Suharto regime. In Uganda, a single-party government uses invitations to reward supporters and potentially co-opt opponents. Second, citizen-participants no longer introduce policy proposals or vote on the projects that government officials introduce. Instead, Uganda's PB programs are now much more consultative and reflect the limitations of invited, consultative spaces versus deliberative venues emphasizing co-governance.

Ugandan PB programs face several additional challenges beyond these shifts. Similar to other countries described in this chapter, unfunded mandates for decentralization make it difficult for low-capacity states and municipalities to operate as local governments, much less to implement projects from PB. Moreover, local civil servants and politicians may not be interested in supporting PB or participation in general, which reflects a central problem with top-down policy adoption as described in Peru and elsewhere in Latin America (see Chapter 3; McNulty 2019). Finally, incorporating marginalized groups, such as women, youths, the poor, and ethnic minorities has been limited in Uganda as well (Kasozi-Mulindwa 2013). Thus, it strikes us that Uganda has the weakest commitment to the five founding principles associated with PB (see Chapter 1) of all the cases included in this book that operate under the "PB" label. As a result, the potential for change through PB is also lowest in Uganda.

Digital PB in Africa

Technology is not widely incorporated into PB processes in sub-Saharan Africa, especially not compared to programs in Europe, North America, or East Asia. However, there are several interesting examples of different governments using innovative technology that are worth noting. The Democratic Republic of the Congo (DRC) provides an example of how technology can be incorporated into PB programs in sub-Saharan Africa. Local governments in South Kivu province invite residents to meetings via SMS messages with all mobile phone users in range of a particular cellular tower automatically receiving the date, place, and time of PB meetings (Estefan and Weber 2012). Residents also vote on project priorities using SMS messages. Governments respond by aggregating in-person and mobile votes before they announce project winners—also through automated SMS messaging. Finally, residents can provide feedback on project implementation and maintenance through SMS messages (Estefan and Weber 2012).

Some Kenyan PB programs use Geographic Information Systems (GIS) to help inform policy deliberations. For example, a local NGO in Nairobi, Kenya, built a platform, Map Kibera, which maps community needs and tailors projects to meet those needs, promotes transparency in budgeting for projects, and improves project monitoring. Map Kibera did not directly design this program to support PB, but Nairobi County administrators now use it with their PB program. In this context, the county would solicit residents' input on needs and reports on project implementation. Map Kibera would then relay this information to Nairobi's PB program and present information at program meetings. There are several additional opportunities to add civic technology to PB based on other African countries' experience. Peixoto and Sifry (2017) highlight MajiVoice in Kenya which facilitates mobile citizen monitoring and reporting of problems with water services. A similar initiative could connect mobile citizen monitoring to PB projects.

Recommendations for how to best use technology are currently underdeveloped but are emerging rapidly. The World Bank's PB publications include some discussions of technology but evidence on program design and user testing is limited—especially for the developing world. One exception is the World Bank's Digital Engagement Evaluation Team, which assessed some technological innovations surrounding PB in the DRC, such as using mobile phones to recruit participants, vote on PB projects, announce project winners, and provide feedback on project implementation (Estefan and Weber 2012). Another is a recent set of expectations drawing on global evidence surrounding participation and civic technology (Peixoto and Steinberg 2019). However, results of these evaluations are mixed and have not yet led to consensus surrounding technology and PB.

Comparative Analysis

The Social Development and Accountability type is dominant across sub-Saharan Africa. This represents a distinct PB track compared to other global regions, where considerable variation across PB types is much more common. We do not have evidence of governments adopting the Efficient Governance type, as we frequently see in Europe, the Empowered Democracy or Deepening Democracy type, from many Latin American contexts or North America, and only two cases of Mandated PB, as in some Latin American and Asian countries. Digital PB is almost entirely absent from consideration across sub-Saharan Africa.

It is not likely that the adoption of new Social Development and Accountability PB programs will produce similar results to the pioneering cases in Brazil. From the outset, subnational governments in sub-Saharan Africa lack resources, state capacity, and organized civil society. Furthermore, causal processes for PB in sub-Saharan Africa operate through theoretically distinct channels from the Porto Alegre model because of their different program designs and operational rules. Extending a vote to citizens on the use of public resources was a key PB innovation. Citizens were not only able to deliberate on budget priorities through PB (exercising voice), but their decisions would then determine how governments spent public resources. Voting systems based on the Porto Alegre model include (a) ranked voting where citizens have multiple votes, and (b) a first-past-the-post system, where citizens each have one vote and select a small number of total projects. Oversight committees monitor vote counting and project implementation to ensure that citizens' voices are respected in this model. A radical feature among early PB programs was that citizens' votes would direct the actions of government officials. This was a noteworthy shift because citizens in Brazil and across Latin America had little experience directing government officials' actions.

In contrast, external donors and national governments drive PB processes in Africa and civil society is largely absent. The Social Accountability and Development PB type that is far and away the most common across sub-Saharan Africa may lead to more development projects in more marginalized communities than for previous arrangements. However, this PB type is unlikely to promote much social accountability as it is currently implemented within the region. Coercive adoption creates external accountability rather than local accountability, which may still produce positive change in Africa. But the processes leading to change and the potential long-term impact on society will be very different than with the social accountability ideal. It is also safe to assert that the types of changes that might emerge in Africa will be different than those in Latin America. For example, it is possible that consensus-based PB models will produce greater social bonds than secret ballots and individual voting. But it is also possible that consensus-based decision-making models will lead to elite capture. This uncertainty and lack of evidence suggests that governments, citizens, and donors involved in the promotion and adoption of PB must be aware that there is a high degree of uncertainty regarding the types of outcomes that PB will produce.

Conclusion

PB is spreading rapidly across sub-Saharan Africa. In almost all cases, international development agencies and donors drive adoption in the region, which most clearly aligns with the Social Development and Accountability program type. PB's transformation as it spreads to different African contexts has moved it away from its roots in Brazil and makes it more of a technocratic, policymaking tool than a radical democratic project. Yet, PB programs in sub-Saharan Africa are varied and contribute some evidence from diverse areas to our conceptual model of change. Specifically, the data suggests some *potential* for positive change through PB for accountability, civil society, and well-being.

Accountability and expansion of civil society theoretically come from PB programs, not from specific projects per se. For example, creating co-governance spaces for project proposals, deliberation, selection, monitoring, and evaluation may embolden citizens and CSOs to hold government officials accountable for delivering these projects and expand beyond PB to broader accountability surrounding general governance. Similarly, PB offers spaces for civil society to work with governments, expand their reach, and incorporate more citizens into their networks. Improving well-being through PB is a little different: expanding access to health care or education comes from specific projects, such as health clinics and schools. Thus, PB can potentially improve accountability, expand civil society, and promote well-being, albeit through different mechanisms. It is important to note, however, that we only have direct evidence on PB's impact in sub-Saharan Africa in a few cases.

Most consistently, international agency-driven and donor-driven program adoptions shift accountability relationships from local and social to external, due to a reliance on international (or national government) actors and donors. Relying on donors, international agencies, and higher-level governments for funding and technical assistance strengthens external connections and makes public officials accountable to these external entities rather than to local publics. This means that external organizations can influence local governments much more than local populations. Stated a bit differently, government officials may administer PB programs with a greater concern for how they are evaluated by international organizations than for their transformative effects on local accountability, civil society, and well-being.

Importantly, consensus-based project selection in most programs is the norm because program organizers want to promote collaboration and understanding among competing ethnic groups as well as government legitimacy. Consensus-based project selection may also be easier for governments to implement and, concerningly, to control. This operational norm also shifts accountability away from local individuals. Avoiding ethnic conflict and seeking legitimacy are laudable goals, but their pursuit may also exclude voices from marginalized groups such as women, youths, and ethnic minorities in an abundance of caution to avoid confrontations. Again, donors support consensus-based decision-making to arguably create perceived ownership and local buy-in, which they suspect externally imposed programs would not generate. In many instances, it is not clear that the World Bank, USAID, or other advocacy groups even know how individual PB programs select projects until programs have been up and running for a few years. The result is that local accountability is difficult to generate when PB programs reinforce traditional power relations at the local level. Yet, the shift to smaller-scale PB across sub-Saharan Africa theoretically increases inclusion from a geographic standpoint, where villagers may have been excluded from municipal processes.

It is also not yet clear if PB in sub-Saharan African contexts will strengthen civil society. These countries tend to lack well-established domestic CSOs to work with local governments and populations to co-govern through PB. Thus far, PB has generated a large amount of citizen participation in the policymaking process but not the creation of CSOs or the broad expansion of existing groups. However, there is little research on PB in sub-Saharan Africa that might demonstrate these programs' impact. Quite simply, we just do not know the extent to which social and political change is occurring through PB, especially in terms of developing civil society or increasing transparency. Nevertheless, we have some clues that help us to assess whether PB contributes to positive social change in the region.

Most PB projects in sub-Saharan Africa purport to improve well-being, which suggests that impacts in this area may emerge over time. For example, Kenyan PB projects emphasize access to health care, water, education, agricultural infrastructure, and roads. These types of projects are very common among other countries' PB programs as well. Impact on well-being in across sub-Saharan Africa for any of these areas is therefore possible over the medium and long terms. However, to date we do not have evidence to determine if this is happening. Moreover, it is generally too early to expect a lot of measurable long-term impacts in terms of well-being, such as in health or educational performance, to emerge from PB programs in sub-Saharan Africa.

Unfortunately, PB in sub-Saharan Africa suffers from low state capacity at the local level. Many subnational governments are new and the quality of local administrations is much lower than at the national level in most countries in the region. Implementing PB processes and overseeing project implementation in a village represents a tall order—particularly in poor, vast, rural areas. Similarly, CSO partners are in short supply across the continent. As a result, technical assistance for PB facilitation and project implementation is difficult for CSOs to provide and CSO oversight is difficult to achieve. Citizens, for their part, often do not have sufficient education or information to participate effectively in PB processes.

Theoretically, adopting PB also serves to empower citizens who have been historically excluded from the political process, especially in sub-Saharan Africa. PB has some potential to reform traditional power dynamics and engage women, youths, the elderly, and members of ethnic minority groups. However, citizens in rural areas face difficulties attending deliberative forums and providing input on project selection. Many programs are not successful in incorporating women and other marginalized populations. Although technology has been used as an important way to mobilize participants, it is still not very widespread and is not central to PB programs in sub-Saharan Africa.

Finally, one-off investments are not likely to produce sustainable change but rather encourage CSOs and government officials to chase external funding or allow the quality of the process to decline. Medium-term investment and external support are vital for PB programs, which presents a challenge: What happens after donors leave or shift interests? Several of the conditions necessary for successful, independent program implementation do not always exist in sub-Saharan Africa. As a result, governments may abandon PB programs if donors decrease their support.

Conclusion: The Frontiers of PB

PB means distinctive things to a diverse range of activists, citizens, and government officials. For some, PB is a radical democratic experiment that offers the possibility of social transformation. For others, PB represents an opportunity to improve basic policymaking and implementation practices, thus leading to improvements in basic service delivery. At another extreme, others see PB programs as empty shells, whereby citizens are incorporated into the process with the promise of having real power, but are given little actual authority. The wide variation in PB's meaning around the world is best illuminated in the literature through the contrast between Gianpaolo Baiocchi and Ernesto Ganuza's assertion that PB has morphed into a "technical tool," and Nelson Dias' work, which portrays PB as a "hope for democracy" (Dias 2014; Baiocchi and Ganuza 2017; Dias et al. 2018). Given the diversity of program design as well as widely different interpretations of what PB programs should be and do, it is no surprise that it is somewhat difficult to create a clear, coherent image of how (or if) PB may produce change.

In this book, we make six broad contributions to academic and policymaking debates. First, we cover a wide range of cases in four empirical chapters, which demonstrate that PB is not a static institution. Rather, governments, their civil society allies and international organizations modified PB's design to better meet local needs. PB's flexible nature helps its spread across the globe; local governments and their supporters (i.e., citizens, political parties, international funding agencies) take advantage of the flexible design to pick and choose different parts of the original institution to create new forms of PB.

Second, we identify different motivations for why governments adopt PB. For some governments, there is a normative commitment to strengthening civil society, accountability, and well-being. Other governments are more moderate reformers, following international trends in the hopes that this "best practice" would improve local governance. We also find that many governments were required to adopt PB by their national government or they were strongly encouraged to do so by international organizations. These underlying motivations are crucial because they shape governments' commitments to PB, including issues such as rules being redesigned, the level of resources and administrative support provided to PB, and the use of oversight mechanisms. There is strong consensus in the literature that the degree of government support for PB is a vital component for its impact, which means that researchers and policymakers must pay particular attention to the institutional and political incentives that shape governments' support.

Third, PB programs adhere, with varying degrees, to five core principles—voice, vote, social justice, social inclusion, and oversight. We find it more useful to

Participatory Budgeting in Global Perspective. Brian Wampler, Stephanie McNulty, and Michael Touchton,
Oxford University Press. © Brian Wampler, Stephanie McNulty, and Michael Touchton 2021.
DOI: 10.1093/oso/9780192897756.003.0008

conceptualize PB as a set of principles rather than a set of specific rules guiding program design. Adherence to these principles distinguishes PB from other participatory programs. At the same time, we find that local officials attach varying degrees of importance to each principle. The wide variation in the motivations to adopt PB, willingness to adapt the rules to local circumstances, and adherence to the core principles has now produced a very wide selection of PB programs.

Fourth, based on the variation in motivations and differing adherence to the core principles, we developed a typology that helps us to classify specific PB programs. We identify six PB types in Chapter 1, based on the degree of adherence to the core principles as well as the motivation behind adoption (normative, mimetic, or coercive). We note that it is reasonable to expect that other PB types will emerge over time as governments and their CSO allies create new institutional variations. We also expect that some programs will transition from one type to another depending on changing motivations, shifting priorities, and the development of new rules. This typology helps us to better identify the parameters of likely change that may be produced by different programs.

There is a profound unevenness to what we know about PB programs. From Brazil, we know that the presence of PB programs is associated with a host of positive social and political changes. But the levels of evidence on positive change quickly drop off as we move beyond Brazil. As we document in this book, there is good evidence from a small number of cases, which we can then pair with the typology to understand the likely parameters of change, discussed below. By this, we mean that PB programs situated within a specific type are likely to produce outcomes that are similar to other cases within the same type.

Our fifth contribution is to present a "theory of change," described in Chapter 2 and in the next section of this chapter, that links individual-level change within PB programs to broader social and political changes. We are thus able to move from the micro (individual) to the meso (community) level. These causal mechanisms are similar but also distinct across the six types of PB programs. As far as we know, this "theory of change" is the most explicit attempt to illustrate the causal process that links individual-level change to broader change. This approach also includes macro- and meso-level factors that condition the likelihood that a specific PB program will produce change.

Our final contribution in this book is to provide ample documentation to demonstrate wide variation in the capacity of PB programs to generate significant outcomes across three areas: civil society, accountability, and well-being. The four case-study chapters include rich sources of data about different PB processes as well as the outcomes these programs generate. Although these chapters do not include a complete overview of all existing PB cases, they do provide the most comprehensive set of case studies analyzed within a unified theoretical framework. Our aim in this concluding chapter is to illuminate how the type of PB adoption conditions the range of impacts that may be generated. The closer to a radical democratic experiment, the more likely that social inclusion, social justice, and citizen empowerment flourish. The closer to a technical policymaking tool, the greater the emphasis on consultative deliberations and oversight, which will have a greater impact of producing accountability. We begin by returning to our theory of change as introduced in Chapter 2, to better identify the contours of social change associated with actual, existing PB programs.

Theory of Change

A key contribution of this book is the development of a theory of change that captures how and why PB can lead to social and political transformation, especially in the areas of strengthening civil society, expanding accountability, and enhancing well-being. As described in Chapter 2, a combination of macro- and meso-level factors mark the parameters of possible change. When PB programs function well, changes in attitudes and behaviors occur among citizens, elected officials and civil servants; these individual changes can then be aggregated to the broader community. This involves individuals acting as "thought-leaders" surrounding new ways of doing politics as well as influencing others to act in different environments, in an example of spillover effects. In addition, change is also produced through the types of public projects implemented through the programs; people who never attend PB meetings still use or benefit from the PB projects. Thus, our theoretical contribution is to identify the causal mechanisms within and around PB that produce variations in outcomes.

The theory of change is based on evidence from a broad set of cases, albeit from relatively few countries. Most of this evidence comes from Brazil and Latin America, but there is a recent increase in outcome-related research coming from the United States, South Korea, and Europe. At the same time, the absence of outcome-related data from the vast majority of PB programs around the world means that we do not fully understand if and how PB produces social change. It is feasible that some of these programs will function well, but it is also equally feasible that many PB programs will produce limited results.

In terms of social change, the most thorough findings on PB come from Latin America, mostly Brazil, where PB first emerged and where we have the most data. We see a broad mix of outcomes across the three areas we analyze: civil society, accountability, and well-being. These outcomes range from positive advances, to limited impacts, and, in some cases, negative impacts. There is evidence that PB changes participants' attitudes and behaviors in a wide variety of settings, most prominently Brazil (Abers 2000; Baiocchi 2005; Wampler and Avritzer 2004; Wampler 2007, 2015; Goldfrank 2011; Montambeault 2016). This can then lead to PB expanding civil society and altering relationships between CSOs and the state by establishing and practicing co-governance (Baiocchi 2005; Lüchmann 2008; Van Cott 2008; Baiocchi, Heller, and Silva 2011; McNulty 2011, 2015; Romão 2011; Touchton and Wampler 2014). In other words, PB can change both the density of civil society and new repertoires of action. PB also improves accountability in some cases (Baiocchi et al. 2011). Evidence from Brazil shows that horizontal accountability expands when governments follow PB programs' rules (Wampler 2007). Vertical accountability also improves when both civil society and government work together. Although we know very little about PB's effect on well-being around the world, Brazilian municipalities using PB reduce infant mortality over time and increase spending on health and sanitation (Gonçalves 2014; Touchton and Wampler 2014; Wampler and Touchton 2019).

PB has spread far beyond Brazil, to different sociopolitical settings, different types of adoption, and different program designs. The results vary across these contexts as well. In Latin America, many PB programs in other countries have not produced the positive results evident in Brazil. PB in Peru has not improved sanitation, for example, which suggests that nationally mandated PB processes may be less impactful than those that arise more organically from the bottom up (Jaramillo and Alcázar 2013; Jaramillo and Wright 2015). Top-down PB processes have generated disappointing results in Peru and the Dominican Republic; early evaluations suggest that PB processes are not taking hold in the way that reformers had hoped (de León 2005; Hernández-Medina 2007; Goldfrank 2011, 2021; Gutiérrez-Barbarrusa 2011; McNulty 2011; Reyes and González Molina 2011).

Latin American PB experiences help us to understand how and why several mitigating factors drive positive outcomes in some places, but not in others. The extent to which civil society is developed prior to PB adoption and whether public officials support the program are two critical factors influencing PB's subsequent performance. Additionally, research on PB in Latin America shows us how the program design and operational rules also condition outcomes associated with PB. Thus, it is important to keep in mind that several positive impacts are associated with PB in some Latin American contexts, but that simply implementing PB programs on their own is not enough to generate these outcomes, especially when national governments mandate program adoption.

What we do not know about PB programs dwarfs what we know, once we examine programs outside of Latin America. PB experiences in Asia, Africa, and the North Atlantic region offer the promise of social and political change. However, subnational data is rare in the Asian and African cases reviewed in this book. More data exists for municipalities in the North Atlantic region, but we lack solid information about these programs' particular impacts due to the small number of cases and the programs' relatively recent adoption.

Nevertheless, we do have some information about programs. For example, our interpretation of evidence surrounding East and Southeast Asian PB cases is decidedly mixed. PB's internal rules and institutional processes in these regions suggest that some of these programs contribute to citizens' empowerment, allocate resources to poorer communities, and foster better relationships between elected governments and citizens. Robust findings surrounding PB's impact on well-being come from studies on Seoul, South Korea, where several researchers found "pro-poor" or "social justice" impacts (Choi 2014; Hong and Cho 2018; No and Hsueh 2020). However, it is also clear that other programs within the region do not function as designed. We therefore must be cautious regarding our claims in Asia because we continue to lack basic information to evaluate PB's impact across the region.

In Africa, the data we collected suggests the potential for positive change through PB for accountability, civil society, and well-being. However, we lack direct evidence on PB's impact in sub-Saharan Africa as well. Most consistently, we uncover evidence that international agencies and donors drive PB adoption in the vast majority of cases. These externally driven programs shift away from emphasizing local and social accountability relationships to external accountability relationships due to a reliance on external funding and resources. A reliance on donors, international agencies, and national governments for resources strengthens external connections and makes local public officials accountable to these external entities, rather than to local publics or civil society. Additionally, consensus-based project selection has become the norm in most programs as PB programs spread across Africa. This norm also shifts accountability away from local publics and may also exclude voices from marginalized groups, such as women, youths, and ethnic minorities.

We do not have the evidence to know whether PB in sub-Saharan Africa will strengthen civil society. Countries in this region tend not to have well-established CSOs to work with local governments and populations to co-govern through PB. PB programs have generated considerable citizen participation in policymaking processes, but we have no evidence that they have also expanded civil society's density. Finally, sub-Saharan Africa's PB programs focus most of their attention on citizens' very basic needs in health, sanitation, water, agriculture, and education. Yet, we do not have any research to show us the extent to which social and political change is occurring through PB in sub-Saharan Africa.

We know more about PB programs in the North Atlantic region than we do about PB in Asia or Africa. PB in Europe and North America tends to be oriented toward civic education and community empowerment rather than toward a radical inversion of spending priorities. PB is thus an incremental policymaking institution in these contexts, but it does retain some of the radical democratic features of PB's first wave. Most importantly, most North Atlantic PB programs retain the goal that a wide variety of citizens from marginalized, vulnerable groups should be directly involved in decision-making (Lerner 2014; Public Agenda 2016; Su 2016, 2017). PB programs in Europe and North America take very different forms than those in Asia and Africa, but these also tend to be distinct from the

Porto Alegre model. Governments that support PB's normative ideals tend to work with CSOs to incorporate citizens into PB programs. However, governments that adopt PB to enhance governance through a new policymaking tool tend not to emphasize civil society or focus on expanding it through PB programs.

PB programs in Europe, the United States, and Canada take many different forms and these forms influence the extent to which PB makes governments more accountable. Governments expand accountability most when they devote greater resources to PB programs and hold face-to-face meetings. There is a growing body of research that demonstrates that New York City's PB programs allocate resources differently than previous budget-making processes (Shybalkina and Bifulco 2019; Hagelskamp et al. 2020). Many PB programs across the region remain relatively small, devote limited resources to projects, and have relatively few participants. All of these factors limit PB's potential to effect change in North Atlantic countries. Recent trends show rapid growth in online programs and the funds distributed through these programs. This theoretically expands PB's potential impacts in some areas, but decreases them in others as online programs limit potential gains in accountability.

Finally, there is limited evidence regarding how PB might enhance the quality of life in Europe, the United States, and Canada. It is much more difficult to improve well-being when it is already relatively high, as in this region, than to improve well-being when it is at moderate or low levels, as in Latin America, Asia, or Africa. In fact, the goals of PB in this region are often less about improving indicators of well-being and more about expanding democratic participation, improving governments' efficiency, and increasing quality of life. Still, some of the budgets allocated through PB are quite large in Europe, in particular, and these funds have the potential to improve residents' standard of living among other impacts. Unfortunately, we lack any evidence that might highlight how such projects improve general quality of life, much like in Asia and Africa. Future research in Europe and North America would do well to focus on developing quality of life indicators that are appropriate to major urban centers, such as increasing access to public spaces, public security/safety, accommodations for people with disabilities, inclusion of immigrants in the local community.

The "theory of change" developed in this book is based on the authors' extensive engagement with PB in all the world's regions. We have some empirical evidence that illustrates the theory of change, but this book also draws attention to our incomplete understanding of whether individual, specific PB programs are producing change. This area requires much better data before governments and CSO activists can know if they should invest their scarce time and resources into PB programs. Yet, in general, our review of the existing data demonstrates that there is a strong connection between the type of PB program and its likely outcomes. We explore these connections in the following section.

Typology of PB Programs

As this book makes clear, PB is not a static institution; rather, it has evolved over time as local activists and governments rewrote key design rules to better fit PB to the local context. Chapter 1 presents six types of PB programs developed across the globe. Given that there are now thousands of PB cases around the world, we see the general consolidation of PB into six types as reflective of a process of mimetic adoption, confirming DiMaggio and Powell's (1983) work.

The use of the PB typology permits us to identify the roots of the wide variation in the range of outcomes associated with PB. This book is the first cross-national, cross-regional analysis of PB programs that employs a single framework to assess the likely parameters of change generated by PB. We drew upon the excellent edited volumes, *Hope for Democracy* (Dias 2014 and 2018) as well as the *Participatory Budgeting World Atlas* (Dias et al. Júlio 2019) for their broad coverage of PB, but we move beyond these books by employing a unified analytical approach to account for process and outcomes. An important caveat remains, however: Much of the academic and policy-oriented research on PB focuses on describing PB processes because local researchers seek to explain how these new programs work. These studies are valuable, but we lack many comparative, medium-N, or large-N analyses that would permit researchers to make broad claims about PB. In this section, we synthesize the preliminary, incomplete data.

At the broadest level, we see governments moving away from programs that emphasize social justice through redistribution and toward programs focusing on social inclusion, especially in Asia and the North Atlantic region. The shift to social inclusion includes an emphasis on recruiting individuals and groups from politically marginalized communities (e.g., racial and ethnic minorities, the poor, immigrant groups) as well as those with limited public voice (e.g., women, people with disabilities, groups identifying as LGBTQ+); it also entails a move away from using specific rules to allocate more resources to these communities. This shift is evidenced by the near disappearance of the original PB type: Empowered Democracy and Redistribution. This PB type was largely situated in Brazil, especially among the early PB adopters, who were often radical democrats affiliated with the Workers' Party or social movement activists. The strongest body of empirical work on PB has been done in the Brazil, largely based on this program type. We now recognize that the most positive PB results found in Brazil may therefore not be transferable to other contexts, because many Brazilian PB programs used social justice rules to allocate greater resources to poor communities. Thus, we believe that is much less likely that newer PB programs will generate significant changes in well-being because most PB programs no longer use social justice rules, and because many governments have decreased the level of resources allocated to PB (Wampler and Touchton 2019). Thus, we expect that the six PB types developed out of the original PB program will have very different impacts than in the pioneering programs in Brazil.

We expect the Deepening Democracy through Community Mobilization to have the most robust effects in the area of civil society, in terms of increased CSO activity as well as changes in citizens' attitudes and behaviors. Most of these programs are located in wealthier countries with a stronger tradition of civil society engagement. Most of these programs also count on the strong engagement of local CSOs, which are often committed to greater social inclusion and public deliberation. Attitudinal shifts, in issues like trust, or behavioral changes, in issues like voter turn-out, are areas where we are likely to see change. We are less likely to see dramatic shifts in well-being through these programs because the level of resources allocated to PB is not enough to dramatically move the needle on well-being indicators, especially in wealthy countries where levels of well-being are already high, and services costly. We do expect to see improvements in residents' quality of life through these programs, but we expect these changes to be relatively narrow in scope because most programs operate with limited resources and have no social justice requirement. Thus, a major paradox of this program type is that community mobilizers often "oversell" the potential for change to successfully mobilize participants, but the programs are most likely to produce small-scale improvements in quality of life.

The fastest growing and most widely adopted PB type is the Social Development and Accountability type. We find that this type is most prevalent in the Global South and/or in rural areas (e.g., the Polish countryside; Russia's Far East; villages in Kenya and Indonesia). We expect moderate to low impacts through these programs because of their focus on modest and very low-cost infrastructure projects. These small-scale projects create the possibility that specific communities and individuals will benefit from new public works selected through PB. But it is difficult for us to evaluate whether these programs improve well-being more broadly because most Social Development and Accountability programs exist in data-poor environments. However, our worry is that the limited levels of resources devoted to PB will constrain the likelihood of a broader societal impact, even if budget percentages allocated through PB are high.

Most of the Social Development and Accountability PB programs emphasize transparency and participation. We argue that these programs have the potential to generate positive impacts on accountability because of the investment in empowering citizens and a focus on changing basic state–society relationships. Yet, the reality is that the evidence supporting any firm conclusions on these programs is very thin. Based on the existing evidence, we believe that it is less likely that Social Development and Accountability programs will generate significant changes in civil society because governments and donors drive most of the PB programs in this type; CSOs typically respond to government officials' policy initiatives rather than serving as co-equal partners in building new PB programs.

CSOs are unlikely to change when they are not equal partners in the process. Finally, we find that there are more opportunities within the Social Accountability and Development type to expand accountability than for strengthening civil society. Moreover, this will be contingent on the extent to which there is strong local government support for PB in these contexts. PB is more likely to generate changes in accountability when governments are willing partners; local governments are less likely to provide the systematic change needed to generate greater accountability when they are coerced into adopting PB.

We have better evidence from the Mandated by National Governments programs, which are similar to the Social Development and Accountability programs in the sense that an external actor (the national government) drives the adoption of these programs at subnational levels. The existing body of research suggests that Mandated by National Governments programs are not performing well. Within this type, some specific subnational governments produce more robust program outcomes, but these programs are the exception rather than the rule. Unfortunately, it appears that local governments interpret most PB programs in this type as "unfunded mandates," in which PB is another policymaking requirement that the national government places on the local government. However, we note that within Mandated programs, there are clearly examples where PB is working well. For example, Seoul, South Korea, is an excellent example of how some governments generate successful programs. In Seoul, the institutional mandate created an opportunity that a local government seized to enhance accountability, strengthen civil society, and improve well-being.

The variation within the Mandated cases highlights the importance of identifying the incentives for governments and civil society activists to support these PB programs. There are few political incentives for subnational governments to invest their limited resources when governments are required to use PB. There are opportunities, however, for some governments to use the new mandates to initiate a cycle of change. We expect that reform-oriented governments with stronger ties to CSOs will be more likely to take advantage of PB to produce change. Some Mandated and Social Development and Accountability programs will function quite well. However, the majority will not have a lasting impact because governments are not likely to invest their scarce time, resources, and political will into a program required from above. Thus, as outlined in Chapter 2, the macro- and meso-level conditions surrounding implementation will unfortunately limit these programs' effects.

The Digital PB and Efficient Governance types are based on consultative processes, which limit their ability to strengthen civil society and accountability because there are no specific empowerment mechanisms embedded in program rules. One clear benefit of the Digital PB type is that larger numbers of participants vote on how to spend relatively large levels of public resources. And yet, participation in these programs is quite thin: citizens have relatively weak *voice* and *vote* and there is limited emphasis on social justice or social inclusion. It is thus unlikely that we will see significant improvements in civil society activity or accountability through these programs because they do not empower citizen-participants or their organizations. Finally, the consultative processes associated with the Efficient Governance type are also unlikely to produce significant change in civil society or well-being. But this program's emphasis on oversight creates opportunities to enhance accountability, which is the most likely outcome associated with this program type. Of course, these programs may have additional goals, which means that they need to evaluated, in part, on the basis of how local designers adjusted the rules to meet local needs.

In sum, local governments across the globe creatively adapted PB's original design to better align with local needs and the local context. In doing so, they obviously altered the participation process but, perhaps even more importantly, they altered the outcomes that PB programs are likely to generate. Thus, researchers and policymakers are encouraged to be cognizant that the form of change produced in one country will be difficult to replicate in another. We now turn to a brief analysis of the key transformations beyond program type, which are also essential for understanding where PB is now and where it is going around the world.

Key Design Adaptations

Over the course of this book we carefully traced a series of context-specific adaptations that have led to significant transformation of PB's basic contours. Given the vast number of adaptations across the globe, it would be impossible to meaningfully capture every single change that has occurred and how it contributed to PB's transformation. Instead, we highlight additional examples that we believe are representative of meaningful trends within each region in Chapters 3, 4, 5, and 6. Drawing from representative cases now allows us to illustrate PB's transformations over time from an overarching perspective, which subsumes considerations for distinctive program types.

Scale: From Municipal Governments to Villages, City Sub-districts, and Nations

One clear transformation is the move from municipal-level PB to multiple levels of governments and agencies. The earliest PB experiences took place at the municipal level in Porto Alegre; today, PB programs exist in rural villages, towns, small cities, sub-municipal districts, large cities, states, and entire countries. The most common transformations in PB's scale, however, are: (a) sub-municipal/city districts, whereby PB is only implemented in certain parts of the city; and (b) village-level adoption. Sub-municipal processes have been particularly important in the United States as city council members who sought to alter how they engaged with the public drove early adoption (e.g., in Chicago and New York City). This takes the slogan, "Think Globally, Act Locally," to a new extreme because these PB programs induce people to focus on very localized problems. Of course, part of the reason that these programs are successful is because people are interested in solving problems close to home. One potential drawback of the devolution of authority to this sub-municipal level is that the amount of resources and the types of policy decisions that individuals may make are too limited to generate significant change.

The village-level adoption of PB programs is driven by the spread of PB into countries and regions with large village-based population. In many cases, villages have limited formal authority and resources, so PB represents an effort to establish greater local control over policymaking. Theoretically, the expansion of PB to the village level offers opportunities to expand citizen influence over how scarce resources are spent. However, we do not have enough research to determine how PB programs are functioning at the village level. We have some basic hints about how these processes might work, but we really cannot know. The best evidence comes from Indonesia where a PB-like program was implemented in the 1990s, with the support of the Ministry of Finance and the World Bank. The earliest cases of PB-like programs at the village level, from the 1990s, suggest that these participatory programs have positive impacts on civil society, decrease project costs, manage conflict, and provide strong economic multiplier effects. In the most optimistic reading, we can extrapolate from these early programs to assert that seventy-four thousand village PB programs in Indonesia, which allocate USD7–10 billion annually, generate positive change. However, we do not know if these initial programs were successful because they received greater technical and policy support from the national government.

The implications of the shift to village-level PB are not well understood. In theory, we may see less deliberation as PB transforms into a highly localized process, because rural areas that lack a relatively well-structured civil society may face extra difficulties in exercising their role in any accountability relationship. Another challenge in rural areas is the high financial cost and time required to participate because citizens have to travel much longer distances to attend PB meetings (McNulty 2011). In turn, it becomes more likely that government officials will dominate PB processes if civil society is very weak or does not participate. Finally, in many countries in the Global South, rural governments have low capacity, meaning they often are under-resourced and have limited staff, therefore it is hard to organize inclusive meetings and execute the approved infrastructure projects.

Voting Rules: From Majoritarian Secret Ballot
to Consensus-based Decision-making

A second major transformation in PB programs, mostly in sub-Saharan Africa and Southeast Asia, is the introduction of consensus-based processes to make decisions and select projects. The original PB model is based on a two-stage process—public deliberation followed by a vote. Voting now takes different forms: Some places use a secret ballot, while other places ask participants for a show of hands. Voters have just one vote and PB programs fund the top projects in some places, while voters in other places have multiple votes, allowing them to select multiple projects or programs to fund. In either case, direct votes represent an important innovation in budget processes because they allow citizens to deliver precise instructions to their governments on how to allocate resources following deliberation.

In contrast, many of the new PB programs in the countries we examine use some type of a consensus-based decision-making; votes are only held if consensus cannot be reached. Examples include Indonesia, Kenya, Uganda, and El Salvador. Deliberation is at the heart of consensus-based programs because citizens, theoretically, use public reason to decide how to spend public resources. Advocates of consensus-based decision-making argue that this generates greater support for the overall PB process among all participants, not just the "winners," because all participating citizens agree to the selected projects. All participants theoretically also retain voice in how resources are spent. In addition, these advocates argue that consensus-based decision-making helps communities move beyond racial, ethnic, religious, class, or other social cleavages through public deliberation processes that foster the recognition of mutual interests.

Some equally powerful theoretical arguments contend that consensus-based decision-making is prone to elite capture. In many cultures, this would entail older, wealthier-than-average men, who both speak and are listened to disproportionately (Mansbridge 1983; Bardhan and Mookherjee 2000; Agrawal and Gupta 2005; Shah 2007; Lund and Saito-Jensen 2013; Sheely 2015). For example, studies of deliberative institutional contexts demonstrate that speech patterns are highly gendered, and speaking in a meeting is a sign of power (Bryan 2004; Karpowitz, Mendelberg, and Shaker 2012; McNulty 2018). If this happens, the decisions made with consensus-based programs will potentially reflect the interests of more elite participants and imperil the goals of empowering marginalized populations and improving their lives.

Social Justice: From Redistribution to Social Inclusion

A third significant transformation among many new PB programs is the limited use of rules that are explicitly designed to promote social justice. By PB-related social justice rules, we simply mean rules that require public resources allocated through PB to be spent at greater rates on programs and in neighborhoods historically underserved by government public works. For example, Brazilian PB programs commonly used a "Quality of Life" index, which allocated additional money on a per capita basis to underserved communities. This index is also based on a critique of representative democracy's relationship with individual equality. The argument here is that representative democracy does not recognize the power dynamics in the broader sociopolitical realm, which often means that middle- and upper-class communities receive more public goods than low-income communities (Schattschneider 1960; Ross 2006). In addition to countering the elite bias of representative democracy, using a quality of life index provides poor residents with a strong incentive to be involved in PB.

As PB spreads around the world, fewer programs are adopting social justice rules. Most programs implicitly embrace some sort of social justice outcome, which explains why there is so much enthusiasm for PB around the world; however, this is not always made explicit. When not explicit, PB runs the risk of becoming an empty promise. The absence of a social justice component in new PB programs removes one of the strongest incentives for poor citizens to participate. The lack of a social justice requirement also theoretically increases the likelihood of elite capture because it renders PB similar to other policymaking venues. We expect to see a decreased likelihood of redistributing resources to low-income neighborhoods through PB in the absence of explicitly pro-poor rules. Our finding that there is an absence of a social justice emphasis in many African and Asian PB programs helps confirm Baiocchi and Ganuza's (2017) argument that PB is becoming a technical policymaking tool. PB's radical roots drove an effort to allocate more resources to poor, underserved communities. However, this effort is being replaced by a more general effort to use PB to better incorporate citizens in incremental policymaking decisions.

Although social justice rules are being diluted over time, more and more governments running PB programs seek to employ them as a means for social inclusion, meaning to incorporate individuals from historically marginalized groups. Many new PB programs do not require that project selection be directly linked to a community's relative or absolute level of poverty (as was with many early PB programs in Brazil), but they continue to make a strong effort to incorporate individuals and groups from politically vulnerable and marginalized communities. Efforts to include different groups require the direct, ongoing involvement of the government that administers PB, and often their civil society partners, to recruit participants. The active recruitment of individuals and groups from politically marginalized communities appears to be a necessary condition to promote social inclusion in more programs today than thirty years ago. In other words, governments and CSOs that want to make PB an inclusive program must actively and continually reach out to minority and politically marginalized communities.

We are more likely to see empowerment of minority communities and their continued engagement in PB programs when governments successfully recruit from and invest in these communities. For example, evidence from New York City suggests a 7 percent increase in voter turnout for regular elections among PB participants, which indicates both empowerment and spillover effects (Johnson et al. n.d.). In addition, evidence from both Chicago and New York City suggests that they were able to successfully incorporate individuals from a diverse set of communities, including immigrants, non-native English speakers, Latinos, and African Americans (Russon Gilman 2016).

In some cases, we also see evidence that the emphasis on social inclusion can have redistributive effects. This is the case in Seoul for example, where program administrators emphasized social inclusion, which then led citizens to select projects that were more beneficial for poor communities (Hong and Cho 2018; No and Hsueh 2020). Thus, although Seoul lacked an official rule that required participants to allocate additional resources to the poor, participants chose projects that most directly helped underserved communities because the program included the goals of social justice and social inclusion. In New York City, participants allocated more resources to public housing projects than had been allocated under more traditional policymaking processes (Hagelskamp et al. 2020). There is a greater likelihood that participants will select projects that benefit poor, underserved communities when low-income participants are mobilized to participate and when governments emphasize social inclusion.

However, we also identify a broad trend that involves reducing funding for PB programs. The original PB programs in Brazil had upwards of 15 percent of the annual budget (this, too, declined over time). Today, many PB programs allow citizens to negotiate over less than 1 percent of the annual budget. Importantly, PB programs now seek to incorporate a broader and more diverse group of citizens, but there are few available resources to implement projects addressed by these communities. The spread of the programs may thus raise expectations, which are then dashed by poorly preforming processes. The worry, then, is that PB becomes yet another empowerment program that doesn't empower citizens but absorbs the time and energy of people from politically marginalized communities.

Technology: From Ballots in Meetings to Online PB

For obvious reasons, the first PB experiences in the early 1990s did not utilize the kinds of technology that are commonly available today. As technologies advance, PB programs have incorporated them in interesting ways (Piexoto and Steinberg 2019). Budget information and project descriptions are now often available online, especially at the municipal level in middle-income and wealthier countries and cities. Programs also frequently use technology to advertise meetings and recruit participants. Some programs, particularly those in middle-income cities and countries, stream PB meetings online and use internet voting to supplement in-person voting, or, occasionally, as a substitute (almost exclusively in wealthy democracies). Some PB programs use text-messaging systems to advertise meetings, recruit participants, and vote on projects. Digital PB allows citizens to vote online in cities like Madrid, Barcelona, and Lima. Online voting greatly reduces participation costs, but issues pertaining to the digital divide are still relevant because middle-class sectors are more likely than poorer citizens to participate online (Spada 2016; Spada et al 2016). Moreover, internet access is still very limited in poor and rural areas of most developing countries and, some residents, especially older residents, may be technologically illiterate. European cities, like Paris, Madrid, and Barcelona, are at the forefront of efforts to use online platforms to implement PB. Online voting greatly reduces participation costs and many online PB programs incorporate hundreds of thousands of people into the project proposal and selection process. The result is a large group of pioneering PB programs that operate online, but that are dramatically different from the Porto Alegre model.

Looking Ahead: Exploring PB's Unresolved Issues

Despite the enormous literature on PB, many issues remain unresolved. Here, we focus on five unresolved issues. First, it is not clear how PB's purpose and impact will shift as it gains popularity in authoritarian contexts (He and Warren 2011; Wu and Wang 2011, 2012). This book largely focused on PB in democratic settings, because PB emerged as an extremely popular institution as democracy and democratization processes were gaining strength around the world. In more recent years, as authoritarianism increases around the world, PB has not receded as part of the "democratic decline." Rather, PB continues to gain support in hybrid and authoritarian settings.

Less is known about PB in authoritarian contexts. We do believe, however, that embedding PB in democracies increases the likelihood of positive outcomes because democratic officials have clearer motivations to promote PB's core principles; voice, vote, social justice, social inclusion, and oversight are squarely situated within the democratic cannon. We also believe that citizens and community leaders are more likely to promote their own interests through PB venues in democracies because they do not fear reprisals from government officials. We further note that most research on PB is in democratic environments, with a small, recent expansion in countries like China and Russia.

Will the spread of PB into countries like Russia and China introduce new ideas that produce unintended consequences, such as the demand for greater political participation by citizens? Or will it placate citizens' wishes to participate in decision-making and ultimately further assimilate them into the authoritarian system? In other words, will these PB experiences become an example of "partici-washing," where governments pursue legitimacy by placing a participatory veneer over traditional, authoritarian practices? By "partici-washing," we refer to use of participatory programs by governments that seek to gain policy and political benefits from the adoption of the participatory program, but without distributing any real authority or resources to citizens. Thus, the term is applicable to PB programs where government officials make a purposeful effort to create and maintain a PB program that increases perceptions of legitimacy but does not necessarily empower citizens or increase accountability. PB programs in Russia and China do not appear designed to address political and social issues such as strengthening civil society or empowering citizens to better position them to hold governments accountable. Instead, these governments appear to be establishing thin programs that reinforce business as usual, with limited efforts to promote social and political change. The prospect of partici-washing extends beyond authoritarian regimes. Mandated PB in democratic or hybrid contexts often reflects an unfunded mandate, and programs which local governments do not support. Local governments therefore implement mandated programs in a pro-forma way, with very thin participation, if any. Such mandated programs might allow national governments to take credit for incorporating the public into policy-making, without having actual commitments at the local level (McNulty 2011, 2019).

Of course, some PB and other citizen engagement programs were intertwined with the spread of national-level democracy, in some places even preceding it (Brazil, Indonesia). We therefore acknowledge the possibility that the presence of PB in some authoritarian environments could establish the foundations for democratic transition. However, we note that democratic movements seeking to dramatically recast state–society relations led the drive to adopt PB and PB-like programs in authoritarian regimes in the 1980s and 1990s. In contrast, the use of PB in currently authoritarian environments, such as China and Russia, is associated with government officials seeking to improve governance and legitimacy rather than transforming state–society relations.

To be sure, ineffective participatory programs and poor outcomes might be the result of poor program design, lack of capacity to run a program, limited state capacity to implement projects or lack of political support through coercive adoption. Yet, poor outcomes are not the governments' intent in these contexts, nor is it the intent of external actors (e.g., World Bank) driving many programs in low-income countries. In contrast, partici-washing seems especially likely in authoritarian contexts, like in Russia, where PB adoption was not a normatively inspired radical democracy project. Rather, Russian programs are excellent examples of mimetic adoption in which subnational governments adopt the programs to better align themselves with prevailing international norms (Cabannes 2018). It is unclear if these programs are intended to serve to legitimize authoritarian governance or if they are beginning to spread democratic practices and values among participants. A significant concern is that these programs aren't intended to empower citizens and transform governance but are tools that allow governments to capture citizens' policy preferences to inform top-down decision-making. Thus, PB may strengthen authoritarian rule rather than promote democratic values.

In China, the ruling CCP opened up the possibility for PB as part of its effort to make local government more accountable and reduce the rural–urban divide, especially in light of budgetary disparities among local governments (Wu and Wang 2011, 2012; Cabannes and Ming 2014; Cabannes 2018). In this case, PB has become a policymaking process that directs citizens' voice into specific venues. This allows an authoritarian regime to better identify citizens' preferences and potentially provide better services *while also* maintaining political control. In this context, policy entrepreneurs are adopting the principles of PB to improve governance, but not necessarily promoting democratic values associated with the more radical versions of PB. PB is thus adapted to serve the interests of a political party in power rather than being an emancipatory democratic project designed to improve citizens' well-being. Importantly, the basic principles of transparency, participation, and accountability are being discussed, albeit in the context of one-party, authoritarian rule. He's (2011) work demonstrates that citizens are indeed being incorporated in public venues as well, where they provide feedback and support to government actors. In Chengdu, China, for example, PB takes place in over 2,600 rural areas and 1,400 urban areas, and over ten years, decisions were made about more than USD1.2 billion in public investments (Cabannes 2018). Unfortunately, we simply do not have enough information to evaluate the extent to which new PB programs in authoritarian contexts may be expanding accountability, promoting civil society, or improving well-being.

PB is also emerging in hybrid, semi-authoritarian regimes, such as Kenya and Mozambique (Nylen 2014). For example, in 2018, seven of Kenya's forty-seven counties used PB to allocate their development budget. Hundreds of thousands of people participated in annual budget deliberations in these counties, but there is contradictory evidence. Some survey evidence suggests that individuals are very satisfied with their participation but other evidence suggests that little to no authority has been extended to citizens (Touchton and Wampler 2020). Importantly, Kenya has a multi-party system, but the two dominant parties win 90 percent or more of the vote in their strongholds. Thus, PB can be used as a governance tool, whereby government officials improve the quality of public services, but it can also be used to maintain or even strengthen local one-party rule. Obviously, these adaptations move PB substantially away from its roots as a radical democratic project. These experiences are notable due to their sheer size, and most are at least partially driven by the international donor community (China is the exception). And, they are used explicitly as a governance tool, and not as a radical democratic project. Their long-term impact on individuals and communities is still not well understood.

The adoption of PB in authoritarian and semi-democratic environments raises the issue of the extent to which these programs are examples of "partici-washing." When there is one-party rule, there is a greater likelihood of lackluster implementation because public officials have few incentives to expand power and authority to citizens. When entrenched parties adopt PB, there is a greater likelihood that PB serves as a tool to reinforce existing powerholders than serving as the means to promote a realignment of political power.

A third set of unresolved questions that looms large are those surrounding mandated PB processes, such as those in Peru, the Dominican Republic, Poland, and Indonesia, which are a subset of the coercive diffusion pressures discussed in Chapter 1. We estimate that more than half of recently adopted PB programs are nationally mandated or driven by external donors. Can national governments mandate robust, inclusive, and transparent PB in subnational governments? Can external donors provide subnational governments with offers they can't refuse and still create incentives for government buy-in? Under what conditions will these programs create positive change and under what conditions do they merely lead to increased disenchantment and distrust in government officials? If mandating PB is not effective, how can processes effectively scale up in sustainable ways? Mandating PB by national governments became slightly more prevalent when advocates realized that PB processes were not very sustainable in the absence of national governments' support. Instead, PB programs would emerge under particular leadership and could easily end when that leadership group leaves office.

Preliminary evidence from Latin America suggests PB is not very effective in creating the kinds of changes that are captured in our "theory of change" model when mandated by national governments. For example, McNulty's (2011, 2018, 2019) work in Peru demonstrates that many subnational government officials undertake PB in the most superficial way: simply calling meetings and accepting proposals, and then making decisions about project spending with their own technical teams. There is very little actual deliberation or oversight. In the rare case that it is more robust, it is usually because of the presence of local officials who are committed to the philosophy of participatory democracy and a relatively vibrant civil society sector that attends meetings and participates. More research is needed to explore the effectiveness of national mandates and PB and consider alternate models that may make PB sustainable. What happens if national governments rescind their mandate or when external donors leave? Will these PB programs carry on with local government support or will they disappear as fast as they were adopted?

A fourth unresolved issue concerns the role of external actors promoting PB in the developing world as part of the third wave of diffusion. Will PB become a legitimate tool for making policy decisions when promoted by international organizations and donors? Much of PB's diffusion across Africa and Asia is linked to international actors. Will these experiences end up as lackluster as many of those that are mandated by national governments in Latin America? There is a different dynamic at play in these new contexts—international organizations seek out local "champions" as partners in much of Africa, for example. This increases the likelihood that the programs will have greater local government support than in the mandated cases. We lack information concerning the intensity of this local support—do these local governments support PB because they really believe in its goals and processes? Or are they supporting it as an opportunity to secure additional resources from donors and multi-lateral organizations?

A fifth unresolved issue is PB's change of scale, specifically the expansion from mostly municipal-level processes into rural places, notably in Kenya, Indonesia, and China. As we note repeatedly in the book, PB was born in and first spread to municipal governments. In addition to scaling up to national mandates and national budgets, PB now takes place at the village level in many countries. In Indonesia, for example, PB is theoretically part of all village-level discussions. In many of these environments, state capacity is very low. Ideally, PB would represent a new moment in state-building—combining local knowledge and oversight with technical expertise—but we just do not know if PB can flourish in an environment in which governments are still in the process of building basic state capacity. Again, these processes are relatively new and it is not yet clear if they will effectively improve citizens' well-being, expand civil society, promote accountability, or improve other aspects of their communities; it will be very important to document these experiences as they unfold to determine their potential.

Researchers and advocates are not yet able to determine if PB's more positive impacts will be leveraged to larger, national-level changes in democracy or governance. Nor are we capable of determining if PB's positive impact, with its unique characteristic of direct citizen engagement in the policy cycle, would have occurred if another type of Social Accountability Institution (SAI) had been widely adopted instead. In other words, the mobilization of citizens, CSOs, and government officials might have generated similar results if governments had adopted a similar social accountability institution. In some areas, such as rural Ecuador or Kenya, it is feasible that the combination of technical assistance and governmental assistance, in any area, is sufficient to initiate social change. These are important topics that merit further analysis.

Finally, perhaps the most important unresolved issue facing people who are intrigued by PB is whether it is ultimately a "good" or "bad" way to give ordinary citizens decision-making power in government policy. There is an active debate surrounding this question. On the one hand, PB skeptics tend to come from the academy and civil society, where many scholars and practitioners note the ways programs have shifted away from PB's radical democratic roots and the lack of broad, systematic, consistent evidence on PB's impact. Skeptics point out that PB's democratizing potential is diluted as it spreads and the meetings become weak examples of participatory practices. PB's more consultative nature in many places, such as Africa and Asia, reduces citizens' power over the decisions that are made. PB is also ultimately very restricted in scope in most places, putting a small amount of resources in the hands of citizens. Critics also note that PB can be used as a tool to refinance the neoliberal shrinking of the state, placing the burden of governance decisions on ordinary citizens who are already overwhelmed with pursuing basic needs, much less able to shoulder increased pressures on their time through PB.

On the other hand, PB advocates from civil society emerged from across a wide variety of local contexts. Civil society activists see immediate benefits from some PB programs and are inspired to advocate for PB's expansion. These proponents believe in PB's democratizing potential and the way that it empowers ordinary citizens to learn about governance and make decisions that directly affect their well-being. They view PB as a way to "democratize democracy" by giving citizens power to make real decisions that affect their everyday lives. Yet, PB's proponents tend to agree that PB is not a panacea. Rather, it is one of many tools that we can use to strengthen democracy in an age of discontent with representative democratic institutions.

We do not seek to resolve this debate or take a normative position about PB. Instead, we document and analyze PB's complexities and contradictions in all of its forms and functions as it spreads around the world. We see the potential for change through PB, but we also see several pitfalls associated with using the program. We offer theoretical insights about PB's spread and conceptualize the mechanisms that drive its potential impact. By providing this documentation and evidence, we educate readers as they then determine their own positions in this extremely important discussion.

To resolve these debates and grapple with new ones, there continues to be a vital role for "PB ambassadors," a term coined by Osmany Porto de Oliveira, to capture the crucial importance of individuals and CSOs in the dissemination of information regarding PB. But, we see a more pressing need that involves undertaking research that better documents if and how PB is generating change. Many governments and activists continue to adopt PB based on the hope that the programs will produce change. Yet research does not provide the necessary evidence and analysis to support these claims. Researchers would thus do well to focus on comparative, longitudinal, and large-N analyses that would allow international organizations, government officials, NGOs, CSOs, and citizens to make informed decisions about which type of PB program they should develop, *if any*. Several efforts to do this currently exist, such as the recent development of a Global PB Research Board with the mandate to build collaborative projects with PB researchers around the world.

Key Lessons for Policymakers and Civil Society Activists

Given these unresolved issues, what can those who are interested in PB do now to ensure a more robust and participatory process? Research suggests that several policies can enhance PB processes. First, we know that certain sociopolitical conditions facilitate the adoption of PB: PB must take place within a decentralized state structure. Without effective decentralization—fiscal and administrative—it is hard to imagine how PB can generate meaningful impacts. Furthermore, PB theoretically works best in places where legal guarantees for freedom of speech and association allow participants to question their elected officials and publicly hold them accountable as well as when elected officials face electoral competition. PB requires an environment with at least some rule of law to be effective. This ensures that the budget is not fictitious and that PB is not simply a new venue for clientelism and corruption, which is common in PB processes in Latin America.

Second, we find that specific types of rules and designs can enhance PB's effectiveness, including:

- *The "social justice" requirement.* The earliest PB experiments in Brazil included a "social justice" clause, which requires governments to increase spending in geographic areas that are underserved and under-resourced (Wampler and Touchton 2019). Although many would argue that this is an implicit goal of PB beyond Brazil, most PB programs today emphasize social inclusion rather than social justice. If the goal is to ensure that poor communities get greater access to public goods, then it appears that having an explicit rule will help achieve this result.
- *Simplified proposal process.* To improve access to the process, it is important to create a simple proposal process to engage participants who do not have specialized knowledge about public works projects. For example, Grillos (2017) finds that participants from poorer districts in Solo, Indonesia, are less likely to submit proposals to their government than are residents from more affluent areas, because the technical requirements for submitting proposals are too complicated. As a result, PB projects did not tend to benefit the poor.
- *Binding decision-making rules.* It is important to ensure that there are incentives and even mandates that the government fund the projects that participants select in prioritization workshops. This increases the likelihood that participants will emerge from the process with a sense of personal efficacy and that projects will ultimately benefit communities.

- *Policies that incentivize widespread and inclusive participation.* Different PB design choices can open processes to historically marginalized populations. Examples include quotas for leadership positions and waiving a citizenship requirement for participation and voting, which allows all residents to propose and select projects.
- *Open vs. closed meetings.* Some operational rules engage individual citizens (open meetings), while others encourage or even mandate CSOs' participation, but exclude the public (closed meetings). Anecdotally, it seems that those programs that incorporate citizens directly, such as in the Porto Alegre PB model, will engage more people overall than those in places like Peru that restrict participation to CSOs.

The adoption of these rules would steer many PB programs back to the original type, Deepening Democracy through Redistribution, or to a second type, Community Mobilization. Among PB types, we have the strongest evidence that these two types are the most likely to produce robust, positive results.

Third, the local government must have sufficient administrative capacity to organize PB processes and execute the projects. Research has documented that participants in many PB processes already tend to prioritize "pro-poor" projects, such as those that target the community's most disadvantaged areas. However, this does not always translate to executed public works projects. One factor that can help ensure that PB projects are funded is the government's capacity to execute the projects. For example, subnational governments in some Latin American and Asian countries have a hard time spending their budgets because of weak internal financial systems. The implementing government needs training and resources to establish the different steps of the process in contexts where PB is new or mandated by national governments. An educated civil service sector trained about the goals, processes, and potential outcomes will also be able to develop and oversee a more participatory form of PB. This condition is also important when governments contract with organizations to execute PB projects during the implementation stage. For instance, the PB process has become a formality in most places in Indonesia precisely because these two key factors—advocacy champions and strong local governments—do not exist. District officials are not willing to share information with the public and the councils are too weak to implement the proposals (Sutiyo 2017).

Fourth, sufficient funding for outreach, training, and infrastructure projects is also important. PB programs were initially designed to promote the "inversion of priorities," which meant public spending would be allocated differently. However, the amount of money that is debated in PB meetings is generally quite small relative to the overall subnational (and national) government budget. This can mean that citizens eventually decide that PB is not worth their time, which has happened in Peru and Poland (McNulty 2011; Džinić et al. 2016). National budgetary requirements can also impede the effectiveness of the process in places where subnational governments rely on national budget transfer processes. For example, Peruvian local government officials often report that the national government's budget process makes it very hard to undertake PB annually. The national investment project database is clunky and hard to use and the national government will not fund infrastructure projects after PB approval until several costly feasibility studies (often absent from the original budget) are complete. Further, annual budget projections often do not align with final budget transfers. These complications have led many citizens to lose faith in the government's ability to respond to their demands in Peru.

Conclusion

PB began as a radical democratic innovation designed to address many of the social justice and participation deficiencies found in representative democracy. Early programs operated on a small scale and sought to bring services to marginalized communities, engage excluded groups, and make governments accountable. PB has spread around the world since its emergence in Porto Alegre and is expanding at an accelerating pace. This expansion has brought major shifts in program adoption, adaptation, and the political, social, and economic context in which PB operates. New programs are frequently online (mainly in wealthy democracies), driven by external donors, often consultative in low-income contexts, and nationally mandated across all subnational governments in other settings. More than half of PB cases are mandated or driven by external actors.

We see the potential for a variety of outcomes to match the mix of forms, functions, and contexts in which PB now takes place. PB carries the promise of positive change in some areas, but we are skeptical of the prospects for dramatic improvements in others. We do not have enough information to assess all of these outcomes, or even most of them yet. However, we know that PB is not a panacea for all of government's ills. Moreover, it might not deepen democracy, promote accountability, strengthen civil society, or improve well-being in many contexts. PB can be co-opted and many of the contexts where PB now operates face fundamental challenges of low education, low resources, and low capacity. Nevertheless, advocates find the ideas behind PB appealing enough to implement it all over the world—a trend we do not expect to see slowing in the near future.

It will be critical to keep the goals, design, and context in mind as PB continues its global expansion. This book takes an important step forward toward a better understanding of the theory behind PB, its spread, and its changes. Systematic evaluation of PB programs is crucial and has thus far been lacking. These efforts will be critical for matching program rules and structures to appropriate contexts if PB is to achieve its transformative potential and improve peoples' lives.

The most important aspect of PB is that it represents an effort to empower average citizens in decisions that matter for their quality of life. Keeping this larger goal in mind is of utmost importance, given the large body of knowledge about the institution and the many gaps in the research. In the absence of this larger perspective, PB runs the risks of becoming yet another democratic institution that fails to grant actual power to "the people," and simply reinforces the status quo.

References

Abers, R. (1998). 'From Clientelism to Cooperation: Local Government, Participatory Policy, and Civic Organizing in Porto Alegre, Brazil', *Politics and Society*, 26(4), pp. 511–53.

Abers, R. (2000). *Inventing Local Democracy: Grassroots Politics in Brazil*. Boulder, Colorado: Lynne Rienner Publishers.

Abrantes, P., Lopes, A., and Baptista, J. (2018). 'The Schools Participatory Budgeting (SPB) in Portugal' in N. Dias (ed.) *Hope for Democracy: 30 Years of Participatory Budgeting Worldwide*. Faro, Portugal: Epopeia Records and Oficina, pp. 469–76.

Aceron, J. (2019). *Pitfalls of Aiming to Empower the Bottom from the Top: The Case of Philippine Participatory Budgeting*. Washington, DC: G-Watch and Accountability Research Center.

Agrawal, A., and Gupta, K. (2005). 'Decentralization and Participation: The Governance of Common Pool Resources in Nepal's Terai.' *World Development*, 33(7), pp. 1101–14.

Aguirre, M. M. (2017). 'Presupeusto ni participativo ni transparente', *Nexos*, https://labrujula.nexos.com.mx/?p=1203.

Aguirre Sala, J. F. (2014). 'El potencial de los medios digitales antes la participación ciudadana tradicional y en el presupuesto participativo', *Comunicación y sociedad*, 22, pp. 211–29.

Albert, V. (2016). *The Limits to Citizen Power: Participatory Democracy and the Entanglements of the State*. London: Pluto Press.

Albó, X. (2008). *Movimientos y poder indígena en Bolivia, Ecuador y Perú*. Vol. 71. La Paz, Bolivia: CIPCA.

Alexander, J. C. (2006). *The Civil Sphere*. Oxford: Oxford University Press.

Allegretti, G. (2011). *Estudio comparativo de los presupuestos participativos en República Dominicana, España y Uruguay*. http://www.infoop.org/observ/parameters/infoop/files/File/upload/Resultados_definitivos/4o-Estudio_comparativo(V.digital).pdf.

Allegretti, G., and Copello, K. (2018). 'Winding around Money Issues: What's New in PB and Which Windows of Opportunity Are Being Opened?' in N. Dias (ed.) *Hope for Democracy: 30 Years of Participatory Budgeting Worldwide*. Faro, Portugal: Epopeia Records and Oficina, pp. 35–53.

Allegretti, G., and Falanga, R. (2016). 'Women in Budgeting: A Critical Assessment of Participatory Budgeting Experiences' in *Gender Responsive and Participatory Budgeting*. Basel, Switzerland: Springer, pp. 33–53.

Allegretti, G., and Herzberg, C. (2004). *El 'retorno de las carabelas': los presupuestos participativos de Latinoamérica en el contexto europeo*. Amsterdam/Madrid: Transnational Institute/FIM.

APSA Task Force (2012). *Democratic Imperatives: Innovations in Rights, Participation, and Economic Citizenship*. Washington, DC: American Political Science Association.

Arhip-Paterson, W., and Fouillet, C. N. (2018) 'Strife in the Construction of the Role of Citizens: Participatory Budgeting in Paris.' Unpublished Manuscript.

Arnson, C. (2001). 'El Salvador and Colombia: Lessons of the Peace Process' in M. S. Studemeister (ed.) *El Salvador: Implementation of the Peace Accords*. Washington, DC: Institute of Peace, pp. 41–6.

Avritzer, L. (2002). *Democracy and the Public Space in Latin America*. Princeton, New Jersey: Princeton University Press.

Avritzer, L. (2009). *Participatory Institutions in Democratic Brazil*. Washington, DC: Woodrow Wilson Center Press.

Avritzer, L., and Navarro, Z. (2003). *A inovação democrática no Brasil: o orçamento participativo*. São Paulo, Brazil: Cortez Editora.

Awortwi, N., and Aiyede, E. R. (eds) (2017). *Politics, Public Policy and Social Protection in Africa: Evidence from Cash Transfer Programmes*, Vol. 6. New York: Taylor & Francis.

Azarbaijani-Moghaddam, S. (2014). *Gender Inclusion Strategies in PNPM*. Jakarta, Indonesia: World Bank.

Baessa, S. (2017). *Participatory Budgeting in Mozambique*. Nairobi, Kenya: Making All Voices Count Workshop on Participatory Budgeting.

Baez, N., and Hernandez, A. (2012). 'Participatory Budgeting in the City: Challenging NYC's Development Paradigm from the Grassroots', *Interface*, 4(1), pp. 316–26.

Baierle, S. (1998). 'The Explosion of Experience: The Emergence of a New Ethical-Political Principal in Popular Movements in Porto Alegre, Brazil' in S. E. Alvarez, E. Dagnino, and A. Escobar (eds) *Cultures of Politics/Politics of Cultures: Re-Visioning Latin American Social Movements*. Boulder, Colorado: Westview Press.

Baiocchi, G. (2005). *Militants and Citizens: The Politics of Participatory Democracy in Porto Alegre*. Palo Alto, California: Stanford University Press.

Baiocchi, G., and Ganuza, E. (2014). 'Participatory Budgeting As If Emancipation Mattered', *Politics and Society*, 42(1), pp. 29–50.

Baiocchi, G., and Ganuza, E. (2017). *Popular Democracy: The Paradox of Participation*. Palo Alto, California: Stanford University Press.

Baiocchi, G., Heller, P., and Silva, S. (2011). *Bootstrapping Democracy: Transforming Local Governance and Civil Society in Brazil*. Palo Alto, California: Stanford University Press.

Barber, B. (1984). *Strong Democracy: Participatory Politics for a New Age*. Berkeley, California: University of California Press.

Bardhan, P., and Mookherjee, D. (2005). 'Decentralizing Antipoverty Program Delivery in Developing Countries'. *Journal of Public Economics*, 89(4), pp. 675–704.

Barron, P., Diprose, R., and Woolcock, M. J. (2011). *Contesting Development: Participatory Projects and Local Conflict Dynamics in Indonesia*. Yale University Press.

Baumgartner, F., and Jones, B. (1993). *Agendas and Instability in American Politics*. Chicago: University of Chicago Press.

Benton, A. L. (2016). 'How 'Participatory Governance' Strengthens Authoritarian Regimes: Evidence from Electoral Authoritarian Oaxaca, Mexico', *Journal of Politics in Latin America*, 2, pp. 37–70.

Bednarska-Olejniczak, D., and Olejniczak, J. (2018). 'Participatory Budget in Poland in 2013–2018: Six Years of Experiences and Directions of Changes' in N. Dias (ed.) *Hope for Democracy: 30 Years of Participatory Budgeting Worldwide*. Faro, Portugal: Epopeia Records and Oficina, pp. 337–54.

Berry, F. S., and Berry, W. D. (2018). 'Innovation and Diffusion Models in Policy Research' in P. Sabiatier and C. M. Weible (eds) *Theories of the Policy Process*. Abingdon: Routledge, pp. 263–308.

Best, N. J., Ribeiro, M. M., Matheus, R., and Vaz, J. C. (2010). 'Internet e a participação cidadã nas experiências de orçamento participativo digital no Brasil', *Cadernos PPG-AU/ UFBA*, 9, pp. 105–24.

Bland, G. (2011). 'Supporting Post-conflict Democratic Development? External Promotion of Participatory Budgeting in El Salvador', *World Development*, 39(5), pp. 863–73.

Bland, G. (2017). 'Sustainability as a Measure of Success: Externally Promoted Participatory Budgeting in El Salvador 10 Years Later', *Public Administration and Development*, 37(2), pp. 110–21.

Blanes, J. (2000). 'La participación popular en Bolivia: avances y retos actuales', *Síntesis: Revista documental en ciencias sociales iberoamericanas*, 33, pp. 131–50.

Boulding, C., and Wampler, B. (2010). 'Voice, Votes, and Resources: Evaluating the Effect of Participatory Democracy on Well-being', *World Development*, 38(1), pp. 125–35.

Bracamonte, J., Millán A., and Vich, V. (eds) (2005). *Sumando esfuerzos: 14 Experiencias de participación ciudadana en la gestión local 2004*. Lima, Peru: Red para el Desarrollo de las Ciencias Sociales en el Perú.

Bryan, F. (2004). *Real Democracy: The New England Town Meeting and How It Works*. Chicago: University of Chicago Press.

Cabannes, Y. (2014). *Contribution of Participatory Budgeting to Provision and Management of Basic Services Municipal Practices and Evidence from the Field*. London: International Institute for Environment and Development.

Cabannes, Y. (2018). 'Highlights on Some Asian and Russian Participatory Budgeting Pioneers' in N. Dias (ed.) *Hope for Democracy: 30 Years of Participatory Budgeting Worldwide*. Faro, Portugal: Epopeia Records and Oficina, pp. 235–54.

Cabannes, Y. (2019). *Another City Is Possible*. Chicago: University of Chicago Press.

Cabannes, Y., and Lipietz, B. (2018). 'Revisiting the Democratic Promise of Participatory Budgeting in Light of Competing Political, Good Governance and Technocratic Logics', *Environment and Urbanization*, 30(1), 67–84.

Cabannes, Y., and Ming, Z. (2014). 'Participatory Budgeting at Scale and Bridging the Rural–Urban Divide in Chengdu', *Environment and Urbanization*, 26(1), pp. 257–75.

Calabrese, T., Williams, D., and Gupta, A. (2020). 'Does Participatory Budgeting Alter Public Spending? Evidence from New York City', *Administration & Society*, 52(9), pp.1382–409.

Cameron, M., Hershberg E., and Sharpe, K. (2012). *New Institutions for Participatory Democracy in Latin America: Voice and Consequence*. Berlin: Springer.

Campbell, T. (2003). *The Quiet Revolution: Decentralization and the Rise of Political Participation in Latin American Cities*. Pittsburgh, Pennsylvania: University of Pittsburgh Press.

Carbone, M. (2005). 'Weak Civil Society in a Hard State: Lessons from Africa', *Journal of Civil Society*, 1(2), pp. 167–79.

Cárcaba, A., González, E., Ventura, J., and Arrondo, R. (2017). 'How Does Good Governance Relate to Quality of Life?', *Sustainability*, 9(4), pp. 631.

CDP and PBNYC (Community Development Project at the Urban Justice Center and the Participatory Budgeting in New York City Research Team) (2015). *A People's Budget: A Research and Evaluation Report on Participatory Budgeting in New York City*. New York: Urban Justice Center.

Ceesay, L. O. (2019). 'The Influence of Supra-institutions in Policy Making in Developing Countries: The Case of a Donor-Funded Community-Driven Development Program in The Gambia' in H. M. Grimm (ed.) *Public Policy Research in the Global South*. Cham: Springer, pp. 171–95.

Cejudo, G. M., Méza, O., Michel, C., and Velarde, G. (2019). 'Mexico' in N. Dias, S. Enríquez, and S. Júlio (eds) *Participatory Budgeting World Atlas*. Faro, Portugal: Epopeia and Oficina, pp. 96–7.

Cele, A. (2017). *Participatory Budgeting in South Africa*. Naïrobi, Kenya: Making All Voices Count Workshop on Participatory Budgeting.

Cho, B. S., No, W., and Park, Y. (2020). 'Diffusing Participatory Budgeting Knowledge: Lessons from Korean-language Research', *Asia Pacific Journal of Public Administration*, 42(3), pp. 188–206.

Choi, I. (2014). 'What Explains the Success of Participatory Budgeting? Evidence from Seoul Autonomous Districts', *Journal of Public Deliberation*, 10(2), article 9.

Cisse, A. (2019). 'Senegal' in N. Dias, S. Enríquez, and S. Júlio (eds) *Participatory Budgeting World Atlas*. Faro, Portugal: Epopeia and Oficina, pp. 78–9.

Coleman, S., and Sampaio, R. C. (2017). 'Sustaining a Democratic Innovation: A Study of Three e-Participatory Budgets in Belo Horizonte', *Information, Communication & Society*, 20(5), pp. 754–69.

Collier, D., LaPorte, J., and Seawright, J. (2012). 'Putting Typologies to Work: Concept Formation, Measurement, and Analytic Rigor', *Political Research Quarterly*, 65, p. 217.

Community Development Project with the PBNYC Research Team (2013). 'A People's Budget: A Research and Evaluation Report on Year 2 of Participatory Budgeting in New York City'. Urban Justice Center Community Development Project, https://drive.google.com/file/d/1qW3VW37gbjMSENJOMFmEhSzbOrJ-7rL_/view.

Cornwall, A., and Coelho, V. S. (eds) (2007). *Spaces for Change? The Politics of Citizen Participation in New Democratic Arenas*, Vol. 4. London: Zed Books.

Dagnino, E. (1998). 'The Cultural Politics of Citizenship, Democracy and the State' in S. E. Alvarez, E. Dagnino, and A. Escobar (eds) *Cultures of Politics/Politics of Cultures: Re-visioning Latin American Social Movements*. Boulder, Colorado: Westview Press.

Dagnino, E., and Panfichi, A. (2006). *A disputa pela construção democrática na América Latina*. Los Angeles: UniCamp.

de León, E. (2005). 'Construyendo ciudadanía: En el desarrollo local y en la reducción de la pobreza; Experiencias de presupuesto participativo septiembre-diciembre del 2004 Republica Dominicana'. http://fedomu.org.do/pp/pdfs/Construyendociudadania.pdf.

Diamond, L., and Morlino, L. (2005). *Assessing the Quality of Democracy*. Baltimore, Maryland: Johns Hopkins University Press.

Dias, N. (2014). *Hope for Democracy 25 Years of Participatory Budgeting Worldwide*. São Bras, Portugal: In-Loco Press

Dias, N. (ed.) (2018). *Hope for Democracy: 30 Years of Participatory Budgeting Worldwide*. Faro, Portugal: Epopeia Records and Oficina.

Dias, N., Júlio, S., Martins, V., Sousa, V., and Biel, F. (2018). 'Participatory Budgeting in Portugal--Standing between a Hesitant Political Will and the Impacts on Public Policies' in N. Dias (ed.) *Hope for Democracy: 30 Years of Participatory Budgeting Worldwide*. Faro, Portugal: Epopeia Records and Oficina, pp. 257–73.

Dias, N., Enríquez, S., and Júlio, S. (2019). *The Participatory Budgeting World Atlas*. Faro, Portugal: Epopeia and Oficina.

DiMaggio, P., and Powell, W. W. (1983). 'The Iron Cage Revisited: Collective Rationality and Institutional isomorphism in Organizational Fields', *American Sociological Review*, 48(2), pp. 147–60.

Dzinic, J., Svidronova, M. M., and Markowska-Bzducha, E. (2016). 'Participatory Budgeting: A Comparative Study of Croatia, Poland and Slovakia', *Journal of Public Administration & Policy*, 9(1), pp. 31–56.

ENDA-ECOPOP (2006). 'Expériences de Budget Participatif en Afrique Francophone et à Madagascar' in *Experiences de Budget Participatif en Afrique Francophone et à Madagascar*. Dakar, Senegal: ENDA-ECOPOP, p. 5.

Enríquez, S. (2019). 'France' in N. Dias, S. Enríquez, and S. Júlio (eds) *Participatory Budgeting World Atlas*. Faro, Portugal: Epopeia and Oficina, pp. 158–9.

Escamilla Cadena, A. (2019). 'El presupuesto participativo en la Ciudad de México: modalidades y resultados', *Espiral (Guadalajara)*, 26, p. 167.

Estefan, F., and Weber, B. (2012). 'Mobile-Enhanced Participatory Budgeting in the DRC' in *Information and Communications for Development*. Washington, DC: World Bank.

Falanga, R. (2018). 'The National Participatory Budgeting in Portugal: Opportunities and Challenges for Scaling up Citizen Participation in Policymaking' in N. Dias (ed.) *Hope for Democracy: 30 Years of Participatory Budgeting Worldwide*. Faro, Portugal: Epopeia Records and Oficina, pp. 447–66.

Falleti, T. G. (2005). 'A Sequential Theory of Decentralization: Latin American Cases in Comparative Perspective', *American Political Science Review*, 99(3), pp. 327–46.

Fan, Li. (2018). 'Participatory Budgeting in China: Approaches and Development' in N. Dias (ed.) *Hope for Democracy: 30 Years of Participatory Budgeting Worldwide*. Faro, Portugal: Epopeia Records and Oficina, pp. 193–210.

Fanomezantsoa, H. A. (2019). 'Madagascar' in N. Dias, S. Enríquez, and S. Júlio (eds) *Participatory Budgeting World Atlas*. Faro, Portugal: Epopeia and Oficina, pp. 70–1.

Fedozzi, L. (1998). *Orçamento Participativo: Reflexões Sobre a Experiência de Porto Alegre*. Porto Alegre, Brazil: Tomo Editorial.

Feruglio, F., and Rifai, A. (2017). *Participatory Budgeting in Indonesia: Past, Present and Future*. Making All Voices Count Practice Paper. Brighton, United Kingdom: The Institute of Development Studies.

Fishkin, J. S. (2011). *When the People Speak: Deliberative Democracy and Public Consultation*. Oxford: Oxford University Press.

Fishkin, J. S., He, B., Luskin, R. C., and Siu, A. (2010). 'Deliberative Democracy in an Unlikely Place: Deliberative Polling in China', *British Journal of Political Science*, 40(2), pp. 435–48.

Fölscher, A. (2007). *A Primer on Effective Participation: Participatory Budgeting. Public Sector Governance and Accountability Series*. Washington, DC: World Bank.

Font, J., Del Amo, S., and Smith, G. (2016). 'Tracing the Impact of Proposals from Participatory Processes: Methodological Challenges and Substantive Lessons', *Journal of Public Deliberation*, 12(1), article 3.

Font, J., Smith, G., Galais, C., and Alarcon, P. A. U. (2018). 'Cherry-picking Participation: Explaining the Fate of Proposals from Participatory Processes', *European Journal of Political Research*, 57(3), pp. 615–36.

Foroughi, B. (2017). 'Reading between the Lines of Participation: Tenant Participation and Participatory Budgeting in Toronto Community Housing', *Journal of Public Deliberation*, 13(2), article 11.

Fouillet, C. (2018). 'Through a New Spirit of Participatory Budgeting in France: Paris (2014–2020)' in N. Dias (ed.) *Hope for Democracy: 30 Years of Participatory Budgeting Worldwide*. Faro, Portugal: Epopeia Records and Oficina, pp. 385–401.

Foweraker, J. (2003). *Making Democracy in Spain: Grass-roots Struggle in the South, 1955–1975*. Cambridge: Cambridge University Press.

Fox, J. (1997). 'Transparency for Accountability: Civil-society Monitoring of Multilateral Development Bank Anti-poverty Projects', *Development in Practice*, 7(2), pp. 167–72.

Fox, J. (2015). 'Social Accountability: What Does the Evidence Really Say?', *World Development*, 72, pp. 346–71.

Francés, F., Carratalá, L., and Ganuza, E. (2018). '20 Years of Participatory Budgeting in Spain' in N. Dias (ed.) *Hope for Democracy: 30 Years of Participatory Budgeting Worldwide*. Faro, Portugal: Epopeia Records and Oficina, pp. 275–88.

Franzke, J., and Kleger, H. (2010). *Bürgerhaushalte: Chancen und Grenzen*, Vol. 36. Berlin: edition sigma.

Friedman, J. (2014). *Expanding and Diversifying Indonesia's Program for Community Empowerment, 2007–2012*. Washington, DC: World Bank.

Fung, A., and Wright, E. O. (2003). *Deepening Democracy: Institutional Innovations in Empowered Participatory Governance*. New York: Verso.

Ganuza, E., and Baiocchi, G. (2012). 'The Power of Ambiguity: How Participatory Budgeting Travels the Globe', *Journal of Public Deliberation*, 8(2), article 8.

García Bátiz, M. L., and Téllez Arana, L. (2018). 'El presupuesto participativo: un balance de su estudio y evolución en México.' *Perfiles latinoamericanos*, 2(52), pp. 1–28.

Garrido, F., and Montecinos, E. (2018). 'El Presupuesto Participativo en Chile y República Dominicana: ¿Es determinante una Ley para el fortalecimiento de la democracia participativa?', *Revista Uruguaya de Ciencia Política*, 27(2), pp. 99–120.

Gaye, B. (2008). *Le Budget Participatif en Pratique: Un guide pratique destiné aux acteurs locaux*. Dakar, Senegal: IED.

Geissel, B. (2012). 'Impacts of Democratic Innovations in Europe' in *Evaluating Democratic Innovations: Curing the Democratic Malaise*, pp. 163–83.

Genro, T. (1995). *Utopia Possível*, 2nd edition. Porto Alegre, Brazil: Artes e Ofícios, p. 27.

Genro, T. (1999). 'Um Debate Estratégico' in I. Magalhães, L. Barreto, and V. Trevas (eds) *Governo e Cidadania: Balanço e Reflexões Sobre o Modo Petista de Governar*. São Paulo, Brazil: Editora Fundação Perseu Abramo, pp. 11–17.

Genro, T., and Souza, U. D. (1997). 'A experiência de Porto Alegre' in *Orçamento Participativo: a experiência de Porto Alegre*. São Paulo, Brazil: Fundação Perseu Abramo, pp. 45–72.

Gibson, C., and Woolcock, M. (2008). 'Empowerment, Deliberative Development, and Local-level Politics in Indonesia: Participatory Projects as a Source of Countervailing Power', *Studies in Comparative International Development*, 43(2), p. 151.

Giraudy, A., Moncada, E., and Snyder, R. (2019). *Inside Countries: Subnational Research in Comparative Politics*. Cambridge: Cambridge University Press.

Goldfrank, B. (2007). 'Lessons from Latin American Experience in Participatory Budgeting' in A. Shah (ed.) *Participatory Budgeting*. Washington, DC: World Bank, pp. 91–126.

Goldfrank, B. (2011). *Deepening Local Democracy in Latin America: Participation, Decentralization and the Left*. University Park, Pennsylvania: Pennsylvania State University Press.

Goldfrank, B. (2012). 'The World Bank and the Globalization of Participatory Budgeting', *Journal of Public Deliberation*, 8(2), article 7.

Goldfrank, B. (2021). 'Inclusion without Power: Limits of Participatory Institutions' in D. Kapiszewski, S. Levitsky, and D. Yashar (eds) *The Inclusionary Turn in Latin American Democracies*. Cambridge: Cambridge University Press. pp. 133–78.

Goldfrank, B., and Landes, K. (2018). 'Participatory Budgeting in Canada and the United States' in N. Dias (ed.) *Hope for Democracy: 30 Years of Participatory Budgeting Worldwide*. Faro, Portugal: Epopeia Records and Oficina, pp. 161–76.

Goldfrank, B., and Schneider, A. (2006). 'Competitive Institution Building: The PT and Participatory Budgeting in Rio Grande do Sul', *Latin American Politics and Society*, 48(3), pp. 1–31.

Gonçalves, S. (2014). 'The Effects of Participatory Budgeting on Municipal Expenditures and Infant Mortality in Brazil', *World Development*, 53, pp. 94–110.

González, G. (2019). 'Dominican Republic' in N. Dias, S. Henriquez, and S. Júlio (eds) *Participatory Budgeting World Atlas*. Faro, Portugal: Epopeia and Oficina pp. 86–87.

Grillos, T. (2017). 'Participatory Budgeting and the Poor: Tracing Bias in a Multi-staged Process in Solo, Indonesia', *World Development*, 96, pp. 343–58.

Grupo Propuesta Ciudadana (2009). *Presupuesto participativo: Boletín de vigilancia #2*. Lima: Peru.

Gutiérrez-Barbarrusa, V. (2011). 'Análisis sobre la participación en los presupuestos participativos' in G. Alegretti (ed.) *Estudio comparativo de los presupuestos participativos en República Dominicana, España y Uruguay.* http://www.infoop.org/observ/parameters/ infoop/files/File/upload/Resultados_definitivos/4o-Estudio_comparativo(V.digital).pdf.

Hagelskamp, C., Rhinehart, C., Sillman, R., and Schleifer, D. (2016). 'Public Spending, by the People: Participatory Budgeting in the United States and Canada in 2014–15', *Public Agenda*, https://www.publicagenda.org/reports/public-spending-by-the-people-participatory-budgeting-in-the-united-states-and-canada-in-2014-15/.

Hagelskamp, C., Silliman, R., Godfrey, E., and Schleifer, D. (2020). 'Shifting Priorities: Participatory Budgeting in New York City Is Associated with Increased Investments in Schools, Street and Traffic Improvements, and Public Housing', *New Political Science*, 2(2): pp. 171–96.

Harnecker, M. (1995). *El sueño era posible.* Santiago, Chile: Lom Ediciones.

He, B. (2011). 'Civic Engagement through Participatory Budgeting in China: Three Different Logics at Work', *Public Administration and Development*, 31(2), pp. 122–33.

He, B., and Warren, M. E. (2011). 'Authoritarian Deliberation: The Deliberative Turn in Chinese Political Development', *Perspectives on Politics*, 9(2), pp. 269–89.

Heller, P. (2001). 'Moving the State: The Politics of Democratic Decentralization in Kerala, South Africa, and Porto Alegre', *Politics & Society*, 29(1), pp. 131–64.

Hernández-Medina, E. (2007). 'Globalizing Participation: "Exporting" the Participatory Budgeting Model from Brazil to the Dominican Republic', *Berkeley Journal of Sociology*, 51, pp. 69–118.

Hernández-Medina, E. (2010). 'Social Inclusion through Participation: The Case of the Participatory Budget in São Paulo', *International Journal of Urban and Regional Research*, 34(3), pp. 512–32.

Hong, S., and Cho, B. S. (2018). 'Citizen Participation and the Redistribution of Public Goods', *Public Administration*, 96(3), pp. 481–96.

Hordijk, M. (2005). 'Participatory Governance in Peru: Exercising Citizenship', *Environment and Urbanization*, 17(1), pp. 219–36.

Hunter, W., and Sugiyama, N. B. (2014). 'Transforming Subjects into Citizens: Insights from Brazil's Bolsa Família', *Perspectives on Politics*, 12(4), pp. 829–45.

Huntington, S. P. (1993). *The Third Wave: Democratization in the Late Twentieth Century*, Vol. 4. Norman, Oklahoma: University of Oklahoma Press.

Hydén, G. (2016). 'Strengthening Local Governance in Africa: Beyond Donor-Driven Approaches'. ICLD Working Paper No. 12, pp. 1–32.

Hwang, J., and Song, D. (2013). *Participatory Budgeting in Korea: A Focus on Participatory Budgeting in Yeonsu-Gu, Incheon.* Alexandria, Virginia: International Strategy Center.

Instituto Electoral del Distrito Federal (2016). *Consulta Ciudadana Presupuesto Participativo 2016.* Mexico City: Informes de la Red de Observación.

Jaramillo, M., and Alcázar, L. (2013). 'Does Participatory Budgeting Have an Effect on the Quality of Public Services?' IDB Working Paper Series No. IDB-WP-386. Washington, DC: Inter-American Development Bank.

Jaramillo, M., and Wright, G. D. (2015). 'Participatory Democracy and Effective Policy: Is There a Link? Evidence from Rural Peru', *World Development*, 66, pp. 280–92.

Johnson, C., Carlson, H. J., and Reynolds, S. (n.d.). 'Participatory Democracy and Voter Turnout: Evidence from Participatory Budgeting'. Unpublished manuscript.

Johnson, G. F. (2017). 'The Role of Public Participation and Deliberation in Policy Formulation' in M. Howlett and I. Mukherjee (eds) *Handbook of Policy Formulation*. Cheltenham, United Kingdom: Edward Elgar Publishing, pp. 198–216.

Júlio, S., Martins, V., and Dias, N. (2019). 'Portugal' in N. Dias, S. Enríquez, and S. Júlio (eds) *Participatory Budgeting World Atlas*. Faro, Portugal: Epopeia and Oficina, pp. 172–3.

Junge, B. (2012). 'NGOs as Shadow Pseudopublics: Grassroots Community Leaders' Perceptions of Change and Continuity in Porto Alegre, Brazil', *American Ethnologist*, 39(2), pp. 407–24.

Kamrowska-Zaluska, D. (2016). 'Participatory Budgeting in Poland––Missing Link in Urban Regeneration Process', *Procedia Engineering*, 161, pp. 1996–2000.

Kanouté, B., and Som-I, J. (2018). 'Participatory Budgeting in Africa: A Kaleidoscope Tool for Good Governance and Local Democracy' in N. Dias (ed.) *Hope for Democracy: 30 Years of Participatory Budgeting Worldwide*. Faro, Portugal: Epopeia Records and Oficina, pp. 77–87.

Karanja, J. (2018). Authors' interview in Makueni County. June 10, 2018.

Karpowitz, C. F., Mendelberg, T., and Shaker, L. (2012). 'Gender Inequality and Deliberative Participation', *The American Political Science Review*, 106(3), pp. 533–47.

Kasozi-Mulindwa, S. (2013). 'The Process and Outcomes of Participatory Budgeting in a Decentralised Local Government Framework: A Case in Uganda. Dissertation. Birmingham, England: The University of Birmingham.

Kingdon, J. W. (1995). 'The Policy Window, and Joining the Stream' in his *Agendas, Alternatives, and Public Policies*. NY: HarperCollins College Publisher, pp. 172–89.

Kim, S. (2016). 'Participatory Governane and Policy Diffusion in Local Governments in Korea: Implementation of Participatory Budgeting'. Research Monograph. Yeongi-gun, South Korea: Korea Development Institute

Keblowski, W., and Van Criekinger, M. (2014). 'Participatory Budgeting Polish-style: What Kind of Policy Practice Has Travelled to Sopot, Poland?' in N. Dias (ed.) *Hope for Democracy: 25 Years of Participatory Budgeting Worldwide*. São Bras, Portugal: In-Loco Press, pp. 369–77.

Kohli, A. (2004). *State-directed Development: Political Power and Industrialization in the Global Periphery*. Cambridge: Cambridge University Press.

Labonne, J., and Chase, R. S. (2009). 'Who Is at the Wheel When Communities Drive Development? Evidence from the Philippines', *World Development*, 37(1), pp. 219–31.

Lah, T. (2010). 'Public Policy Processes and Citizen Participation in South Korea' in E. M. Berman (ed.) *Public Administration in East Asia: Mainland China, Japan, South Korea, Taiwan*. London: Routledge, pp. 335–75.

Langelier, S. (2015). *Le démantèlement du budget participatif de Porto Alegre?* Paris: Harmattan Publishers.

Larangeira, S. (1996). 'Gestão e Participação: A Experiência do Orçamento Participativo em Porto Alegre', *São Paulo em Perspectiva*, 10, pp. 129–37.

Lee, W., and You, J. (2013). *Country Report: South Korea*. Washington, DC: Global Initiative for Fiscal Transparency.

Lee, Y. (2005). 'Participatory Democracy and Chaebol Regulation in Korea: State-Market Relations under the MDP Governments, 1997–2003', *Asian Survey*, 45(2), pp. 279–301.

Legard, S., and Goldfrank, B. (2020). 'The Systemic Turn and Participatory Budgeting: The Case of Rio Grande do Sul', *Journal of Latin American Studies*, 1–27, doi:10.1017/S0022216X20000954.

León, L. (2010). *Reforzando el proceso del presupuesto participativo a través de Internet: el caso de la Municipalidad de Miraflores (Lima, Perú)*. Lima, Peru: Americas Information and Communication Research Network.

Lerner, J. (2014). *Everyone Counts: Could 'Participatory Budgeting' Change Democracy?* Ithaca, New York: Cornell Selects, Cornell University Press.

Lerner, J., and Secondo, D. (2012). 'By the People, For the People: Participatory Budgeting from the Bottom Up in North America', *Journal of Public Deliberation*, 8(2), article 2.

Levitsky, S., and Way, L. (2010). *Competitive Authoritarianism: Hybrid Regimes after the Cold War*. Cambridge: Cambridge University Press.

Levitsky, S., and Ziblatt, D. (2018). *How Democracies Die*. New York: Crown Publishing Group.

Lim, S., and Y. Oh. (2016). 'Online versus Offline Participation: Has the Democratic Potential of the Internet Been Realized? Analysis of a Participatory Budgeting System in Korea', *Public Performance & Management Review*, 39(3), pp. 676–700.

Lim, P. (2017). 'Participatory Budgeting in The Philippines.' Making All Voices Count Paper. Brighton, United Kingdom: The Institute of Development Studies.

López Follega, J. L., Melgar Paz, W., and Balbín Díaz, D. (1995). *La concertación en la gestión ambiental urbana: La experiencia de Ilo*. Ilo, Peru: Asociación Civil Labor.

López Ricci, J. (2014). *Presupuesto Participativo 11 años después: ¿Cambio de rumbo o más de lo mismo?*, Lima, Peru: Cuadernos Descentralistas, p. 30.

Lorch, J. (2017). *Civil Society and Mirror Images of Weak States*. London: Palgrave Macmillan.

Lüchmann, L. H. H. (2008). 'Participação e representação nos conselhos gestores e no orçamento participativo', *Caderno crh*, 21(52), pp. 87–97.

Lund, J. F., and Saito-Jensen, M. (2013). 'Revisiting the Issue of Elite Capture of Participatory initiatives', *World Development*, 46, pp. 104–12.

Magno, F. (2013). *Country Report: Philippines*. Washington, DC: Global Initiative for Fiscal Transparency.

Mahoney, J., and Thelen, K. (2010). 'A Theory of Gradual Institutional Change' in J. Mahoney and K. Thelen (eds) *Explaining Institutional Change: Ambiguity, Agency, and Power*. Cambridge: Cambridge University Press, pp. 1–37.

Mainwaring, S. (2018). *Institutionalization, Decay, and Collapse*. Cambridge: Cambridge University Press.

Mainwaring, S., and Bizzarro, F. (2019). 'The Fates of Third-wave Democracies', *Journal of Democracy*, 30(1), p. 99.

Makaaru, J. (2017). *Participatory Budgeting in Uganda*. Nairobi, Kenya: Making All Voices Count Workshop on Participatory Budgeting.

Mansbridge, J. (1983). *Beyond Adversary Democracy*. Chicago: University of Chicago Press.

Mansuri, G., and Rao, V. (2013). *Localizing Development: Does Participation Work?* Washington, DC: World Bank.

Maratim, J. (2018). Authors' interview in Elgeyo-Marakwet County. In person interview. June 18, 2018.

Marquetti, A. (2003). 'Democracia, Equidade e Effciencia, o Caso do Orçamento Participativo em Porto Alegre' in L. Avritzer and Z. Navarro (eds) *A Inovação Democrática no Brasil: O Orçamento Participativo*. São Paulo, Brazil: Cortez Editores, pp. 129–56.

Marquetti, A., Campos, G. A., and Pires, R. (2008). *Democracia participativa e redistribuição: análise de experiências de orçamento participativo*. São Paulo, Brazil: Xamã.

Matendjua, O. (2019). 'Mozambique' in N. Dias, S. Enríquez, and S. Júlio (eds) *Participatory Budgeting World Atlas*. Faro, Portugal: Epopeia and Oficina, pp. 72–3.

Maydana, R. (2004). 'El Comité de Vigilancia, la participación y el control social', *Municipalización: diagnóstico de una década*. La Paz, Bolivia: Plural Editores.

McNulty, S. (2011). *Voice and Vote: Decentralization and Participation in Post-Fujimori Peru*. Palo Alto, California: Stanford University Press.

McNulty, S. (2012). 'An Unlikely Success: Peru's Top-down Participatory Budgeting Experience', *Journal of Public Deliberation*, 8(2), article 4.

McNulty, S. (2013). 'Participatory Democracy? Exploring Peru's Efforts to Engage Civil Society in Local Governance', *Latin American Politics and Society*, 55(3), pp. 69–92.

McNulty, S. L. (2015). 'Barriers to Participation: Exploring Gender in Peru's Participatory Budget Process', *Journal of Development Studies*, 51(11), pp. 1429–43.

McNulty, S. (2018). 'Embedded Exclusions: Exploring Gender Equality in Peru's Participatory Democratic Framework', *Global Discourse*, 8(3), pp. 532–49.

McNulty, S. (2019). *Democracy from above? The Unfulfilled Promise of Nationally Mandated Participatory Reforms*. Palo Alto, California: Stanford University Press.

Melgar, T. (2010). *Constructing Local Democracy in Post-Authoritarian Settings: A Comparison between Porto Alegre, Brazil and Naga, the Philippines*. Dissertation. Madison, Wisconsin: University of Wisconsin-Madison.

Melgar, T. R. (2014). 'A Time of Closure? Participatory Budgeting in Porto Alegre, Brazil, after the Workers' Party Era', *Journal of Latin American Studies*, 46(1), pp. 121–49.

Menser, M. (2005). 'The Global Social Forum Movement, Porto Alegre's "Participatory Budget" and the Maximization of Democracy', *Situations: Project of the Radical Imagination*, 1(1), pp. 87–108.

Meriabe, E. (2017). *Participatory Budgeting in Kenya*. Nairobi, Kenya: Making All Voices Count Workshop on Participatory Budgeting.

Miloslavich Túpac, D. (2013). *Escasa Inversión del Estado en las Mujeres: Observatorio Presupuesto Participativo 2008-2011*. Lima, Peru: Flora Tristan.

Ministerio de Economía y Finanzas (2010). 'Instructivo para el Presupuesto Participativo Basado en Resultados', *El Peruano*, March 26.

Mintrom, M. (1997). 'Policy Entrepreneurs and the Diffusion of Innovation', *American Journal of Political Science*, 41(3), pp. 738–70.

Miori, V., and Russo, D. (2011). 'Integrating Online and Traditional Involvement in Participatory Budgeting', *Electronic Journal of e-Government*, 9(1), pp. 41–57.

Montambeault, F. (2012). 'Learning to Be "Better Democrats"? The Role of Informal Practices in Brazilian Participatory Budgeting Experiences' in M. A. Cameron, E. Hershberg, and K. E. Sharpe (eds) *New Institutions for Participatory Democracy in Latin America: Voice and Consequence*. New York: Palgrave Macmillan, pp. 99–122.

Montambeault, F. (2016). 'Participatory Citizenship in the Making? The Multiple Citizenship Trajectories of Participatory Budgeting Participants in Brazil', *Journal of Civil Society*, 12(3), pp. 282–98.

Montambeault, F. (2019). '"It Was Once a Radical Democratic Proposal": Theories of Gradual Institutional Change in Brazilian Participatory Budgeting', *Latin American Politics and Society*, 61(1), pp. 29–53.

Montecinos, E. (2014). 'Diseño institucional y participación ciudadana en los presupuestos participativos: los casos de Chile, Argentina, Perú, República Dominicana y Uruguay' ('Institutional Design and Citizen Participation in Participatory Budgeting: The Cases of Chile, Argentina, Peru, Dominican Republic and Uruguay'), *Política y gobierno*, 21(2), pp. 351–78.

Navarro, Z. (2003). 'O "Orçamento Participativo" de Porto Alegre (1989-2002): um conciso comentário crítico' in L. Avritzer and Z. Navarro (eds) *A Inovação Democratica no Brasil*. São Paulo, Brazil: Cortez.

Ng, C. (ed.) (2015). *Gender Responsive and Participatory Budgeting: Imperatives for Equitable Public Expenditure*, Vol. 22. Cham: Springer.

Nebot, C. P. (2004). 'Los presupuestos participativos en España: un balance provisional. Revista de estudios locales', *Cunal* (78), pp. 64–75.

Nelson, N., and Wright, S. (1995). *Power and Participatory Development: Theory and Practice*. Bradford, United Kingdom: ITDG Publishing.

Nez, H. (2016). 'Does Participation Mean Reciprocal Learning? The Relationships between Diverse Stakeholders during Participatory Budgeting in Paris', *Journal of Civil Society*, 12(3), pp. 266–81.

No, W. (2017). *Redistribution and Deliberation in Mandated Participatory Governance: The Case of Participatory Budgeting in Seoul, South Korea*. Dissertation. Tempe, Arizona: Arizona State University.

No, W. (2018). 'History and Issues of Participatory Budgeting in South Korea' in N. Dias (ed.) *Hope for Democracy: 30 Years of Participatory Budgeting Worldwide*. Faro, Portugal: Epopeia Records and Oficina, pp. 211–21.

No, W., and Hsueh, L. (2020). 'How a Participatory Process with Inclusive Structural Design Allocates Resources toward Poor Neighborhoods: The Case of Participatory Budgeting in Seoul, South Korea', *International Review of Administrative Sciences*, doi: 0020852320943668.

Noriega, A., Aburto, F., and Montecinos, E. (2016). 'Presupuestos participativos en Chile y su contribución a la inclusión social', *Íconos Revista de Ciencias Sociales*, 56, pp. 203–18.

Nylen, W. R. (2002). 'Testing the Empowerment Thesis: The Participatory Budget in Belo Horizonte and Betim, Brazil', *Comparative Politics*, 34(2), pp. 127–45.

Nylen, W. (2003). *Participatory Democracy versus Elitist Democracy: Lessons from Brazil*. New York: Palgrave.

Nylen, W. R. (2014). *Participatory Budgeting in a Competitive-authoritarian Regime: A Case Study (Maputo, Mozambique)*. Maputo, Mozambique: Instituto de Estudos Sociais e Económicos.

O'Donnell, G. (1994). 'The State, Democratization and Some Conceptual Problems: A Latin American View with Glances at Some Post-Communist Countries' in W. C. Smith, C. H. Acuma, and E. A. Gamarra (eds) *Democracy, Markets, and Structural Reform in Latin America*. New Brunswick, Connecticut: Transaction Publishers, pp. 157–80.

Olken, B. A. (2010). 'Direct Democracy and Local Public Goods: Evidence from a Field Experiment in Indonesia', *American Political Science Review*, 104(2), pp. 243–67.

Pape, M., and Lerner, J. (2016). 'Budgeting for Equity: How Can Participatory Budgeting Advance Equity in the United States?', *Journal of Public Deliberation*, 12(2), article 9.

Park, K., Lee, H., Lee, B., and Jange, Y. (2019). 'South Korea' in N. Dias, S. Enríquez, and S. Júlio (eds) *Participatory Budgeting World Atlas*. Faro, Portugal: Epopeia and Oficina, pp. 140–3.

Paz, C. (2018). 'Youth Participatory Budgeting--Portugal' in N. Dias (ed.) *Hope for Democracy: 30 Years of Participatory Budgeting Worldwide*. Faro, Portugal: Epopeia Records and Oficina, pp. 479–90.

Peabody, L., and Lerner, J. (2019). 'Canada' in N. Dias, S. Enríquez, and S. Júlio (eds) *Participatory Budgeting World Atlas*. Faro, Portugal: Epopeia and Oficina, pp. 94–5.

Peck, J., and Theodore, N. (2015). *Fast Policy: Experimental Statecraft at the Thresholds of Neoliberalism*. Minneapolis: University of Minnesota Press.

Peixoto, T. (2009). 'Beyond Theory: e-Participatory Budgeting and its Promises for e-Participation', *European Journal of ePractice*, 7, pp. 1–9.

Peixoto, T., and Sifry, M. L. (2017). *Civic Tech in the Global South*. Washington, DC: World Bank Press.

Peixoto, T., Sjoberg, F. M., MacPhail, B., and Mellon, J. (2018). 'Policy Preferences at Different Stages of Participatory Budgeting: The Case of Paris' in N. Dias (ed.) *Hope for Democracy: 30 Years of Participatory Budgeting Worldwide*. Faro, Portugal: Epopeia Records and Oficina, pp. 553–64.

Peixoto, T., Sjoberg, F., and Mellon, J. (2019). 'A Get Out the Vote (GOTV) Experiment on the World's Largest Participatory Budgeting Vote in Brazil', *British Journal of Political Science*, 50(1), pp. 1–9.

Peixoto, T., and Steinberg, T. (2019). *Citizen Engagement: Emerging Digital Technologies Create New Risks and Value*. Washington, D.C: World Bank.

Pineda Nebot, C., Falck, A., Barros, M., Albellán López, M. Á., and Enríquez, S. (2019). 'Spain' in N. Dias, S. Enríquez, and S. Júlio (eds) *Participatory Budgeting World Atlas*. Faro, Portugal: Epopeia and Oficina, pp. 182–3.

Pinnington, E., Lerner, J., and Schugurensky, D. (2009). 'Participatory Budgeting in North America: The Case of Guelph, Canada', *Journal of Public Budgeting, Accounting & Financial Management*, 21(3), p. 454.

Portillo, M., and Jacinto, C. (2018). 'Presupuesto participativo y la calidad del gasto público en la municipalidad distrital de Inambari, Tambopata, Madre de Dios.' Masters Thesis. Universidad César Vallejo.

Porto de Oliveira, O. (2017a). *International Policy Diffusion and Participatory Budgeting: Ambassadors of Participation, International Institutions and Transnational Networks*. London: Palgrave Macmillan.

Porto de Oliveira, O. (2017b). *Participatory Budgeting in Senegal*. Nairobi, Kenya: Making All Voices Count Workshop on Participatory Budgeting.

Pradeau, G. (2018). 'A Third Wave of Participatory Budgeting in France' in N. Dias (ed.) *Hope for Democracy: 30 Years of Participatory Budgeting Worldwide*. Faro, Portugal: Epopeia Records and Oficina, pp. 373–83.

Prodescentralización (2017). *Informe anual sobre el estado del proceso de descentralización 2016*. Lima: Programa ProDescentralización.

Przeworski, A., Stokes, S. C. S., and Manin, B. (1999). *Democracy, Accountability, and Representation*, Vol. 2. Cambridge: Cambridge University Press.

Public Agenda (2016). 'Why Let the People Decide? Elected Officials on Participatory Budgeting', https://www.publicagenda.org/reports/why-let-the-people-decide-elected-officials-on-participatory-budgeting/.

Putnam, R. D., Leonardi, R., and Nanetti, R. Y. (1994). *Making Democracy Work: Civic Traditions in Modern Italy*. Princeton, New Jersey: Princeton University Press.

Randriarilala, T., and Melly, C. (2017). *Africa Regional Seminar on Participatory Budgeting. Programme SAHA-Intercooperation Madagascar*. Washington, DC: World Bank.

Ravelomanantsoa, H. (2016). *Citizen Involvement in Municipal Service Improvement (CIMSI)*. Washington, DC: Global Partnership for Social Accountability.

Remy, M. (2005). *Los múltiples campos de la participación ciudadana en el Perú*. Lima: Instituto de Estudios Peruanos.

Remy, M. I. (2011). 'Participación ciudadana y gobiernos descentralizados', *Cuadernos Descentralistas*, 28, pp. 1–82.

Rendon Corona, A. (2006). 'Distributive Justice: Participatory Budget in Porto Alegre, Brazil', *Polis*, 2(1), pp. 217–44.

Reyes, K., and González Molina, G. E. (2011). 'Presupuesto participativo República Dominicana', http://www.infoop.org/observ/parameters/infoop/files/File/upload/Seminario_Republica_Dominicana/Marcha_investigaciones_alumnos/Presentacion_de_Presupuesto_Participativo,_Karolin_Reyes.pdf.

Rifai, A. (2017). 'Participatory Budgeting in Indonesia: Past, Present and Future'. Making All Voices Count Paper. Brighton, United Kingdom: The Institute of Development Studies.

Rifai, A. (2019). 'Indonesia' in N. Dias, S. Enríquez, and S. Júlio (eds) *Participatory Budgeting World Atlas*. Faro, Portugal: Epopeia and Oficina, pp. 130–3.

Rifai, A., Asterina, N., and Hidayani, R. (2016). *Improving the transparency, inclusivity and impact of participatory budgeting in Indonesian cities*. Nairobi, Kenya: Making All Voices Count Workshop on Participatory Budgeting.

Romão, W. D. M. (2011). 'Conselheiros do Orçamento Participativo nas franjas da sociedade política', *Lua Nova: Revista de Cultura e Política*, 84, pp. 219–44.

Romero, L. C., and de Assis, W. S. (2016). 'Ciudadanía imaginada y presupuesto participativo em los pueblos indígenas de la Selva Central del Perú', *Novos Cadernos NAEA*, 19(3), pp. 71–92.

Ross, M. (2006). 'Is Democracy Good for the Poor?', *American Journal of Political Science*, 50(4), pp. 860–74.

Rose, J., Rios, J., and Lippa, B. (2010). 'Technology Support for Participatory Budgeting', *International Journal of Electronic Governance*, 3(1), pp. 3–24.

RTI International (2000). *Report of the Municipal Development and Citizen Participation Project (MDCPP)*. San Salvador: USAID/El Salvador.

Russon Gilman, H. (2016). *Democracy Reinvented: Participatory Budgeting and Civic Innovation in America*. Washington, DC: Brookings Institute Press.

Russon Gilman, H., and Wampler, B. (2019). 'The Difference in Design: Participatory Budgeting in Brazil and the United States', *Journal of Public Deliberation*, 15(1), article 7.

Saltos, T. (2008). *The Participatory Budgeting Experience Cotacachi—Ecuador*. Durban, South Africa: Africa Regional Seminar on Participatory Budgeting, March 10-13, 2008.

Sampaio, R. C., Maia, R. C. M., and Marques, F. P. J. A. (2011). 'Participation and Deliberation on the Internet: A Case Study of Digital Participatory Budgeting in Belo Horizonte', *Journal of Community Informatics*, 7, pp. 1–2.

Sanchez, M. L. M. (2013). 'Capital social y desarrollo territorial en la Ciudad de México: una reflexión a partir de los presupuestos participativos', *DRd-Desenvolvimento Regional em debate*, 3(2), pp. 100–13.

Santos, B. S. (1998). 'Participatory Budgeting in Porto Alegre: Toward a Redistributive Democracy', *Politics and Society*, 26, pp. 461–510.

Santos, B. S. (2005). *Democratizing Democracy: Beyond the Liberal Democratic Canon*. New York: Verso.

Schattschneider, E. E. (1960). *Party Government*. New Brunswick, NJ: Transaction Publishers.

Schneider, S. H., and Busse, S. (2019). 'Participatory Budgeting in Germany–A Review of Empirical Findings', *International Journal of Public Administration*, 42(3), pp. 259–73.

Schugurensky, D. (2020). Personal communication. February 2020.

Selee, A. D., and Peruzzotti, E. (eds) (2009). *Participatory Innovation and Representative Democracy in Latin America*. Washington, DC: Woodrow Wilson Center Press.

Selee, A. (2011). *Decentralization, Democratization, and Informal Power in Mexico*. University Park, Pennsylvania: The Pennsylvania State University Press.

Sellers, J. M. (2002). *Governing from Below: Urban Regions and the Global Economy*. Cambridge: Cambridge University Press.

Shah, A. (2007). *Participatory Budgeting*. Washington, DC: World Bank.

Sheely, R. (2015). 'Mobilization, Participatory Planning Institutions, and Elite Capture: Evidence from a Field Experiment in Rural Kenya', *World Development*, 67, pp. 251–66.

Shulga, I., and Sukhova, A. (2019). 'Russia' in N. Dias, S. Enríquez, and S. Júlio (eds) *Participatory Budgeting World Atlas*. Faro, Portugal: Epopeia and Oficina, pp. 138–9.

Shybalkina, I., and Bifulco, R. (2019). Does Participatory Budgeting Change the Share of Public Funding to Low Income Neighborhoods?', *Public Budgeting & Finance*, 39(1), pp. 45–66.

Simmons, B. A., and Elkins, Z. (2004). 'The Globalization of Liberalization: Policy Diffusion in the International Political Economy', *American Political Science Review*, 98(1), pp. 171–89.

Sintomer, Y., Herzberg, C., and Röcke, A. (2008). 'From Porto Alegre to Europe: Potentials and Limitations of Participatory Budgeting', *International Journal of Urban and Regional Research*, 32(1), pp. 164–78.

Sintomer, Y., Herzberg, C., Röcke, A., and Allegretti, G. (2012). 'Transnational Models of Citizen Participation: The Case of Participatory Budgeting', *Journal of Public Deliberation*, 8(2).

Sintomer, Y., Herzberg, C., Allegretti, G., Röcke, A., and Alves, M. (2013). *Participatory Budgeting Worldwide—Updated Version* (Dialog Global No. 25). Bonn: Engagement Global.

Sintomer, Y., Röcke, A., and Herzberg, C. (2016). *Participatory Budgeting in Europe: Democracy and Public Governance*. Abingdon, United Kingdom: Routledge.

Spada, P., Wampler, B., Touchton, M., and Coelho, D. (2012). 'Variety of Brazilian Participatory Budgeting Designs: 2012', http://participedia.net/en/content/brazilian-participatory-budgeting-census/.

Spada, P. (2014). 'The Diffusion of Participatory Governance Innovations: A Panel Data Analysis of the Adoption and Survival of Participatory Budgeting in Brazil', *Latin American Studies Association*, 32, pp. 1–53.

Spada, P. (2016). *The Political and Economic Effects of Participatory Budgeting*. Working Paper.

Spada, P. (2020). Dataset on Brazilian Participatory Budgeting. https://dataverse.harvard.edu/dataset.xhtml?persistentId=doi:10.7910/DVN/EDSNJS.

Spada, P., Mellon, J., Peixoto, T., and Sjoberg, F. (2016). 'Effects of the Internet on Participation: Study of a Public Policy Referendum in Brazil', *Journal of Information Technology & Politics*, 13(3), pp. 187–207.

Stolzenberg, P., and Wampler, B. (2018). 'Participatory Budgeting' in H. Heinelt (ed.) *Handbook on Participatory Governance*. Northampton, Massachusetts: Edward Elgar Publishing.

Su, C. (2012). 'Whose Budget? Our Budget? Broadening Political Stakeholdership via Participatory Budgeting', *Journal of Public Deliberation*, 8(2), article 1.

Su, C. (2016). *Re-engaging the Disenfranchised: Participatory Budgeting in the United States*. Washington, DC: Brookings Institution Press.

Su, C. (2017). 'From Porto Alegre to New York City: Participatory Budgeting and Democracy', *New Political Science*, 39(1), pp. 67–75.

Sugiyama, N. B. (2012). *Diffusion of Good Government: Social Sector Reforms in Brazil*. Notre Dame, Indiana: University of Notre Dame Press.

Sutiyo, S., and Maharjan, K. L. (2017). *Decentralization and Rural Development in Indonesia*. Singapore: Springer Nature.

Sześciło, D., and Wilk, B. (2018). 'Can Top Down Participatory Budgeting Work? The Case of Polish Community Fund', *Central European Public Administration Review*, 16(2), pp. 179–92.

Torrens, A. (2005). *Economic Impact Analysis of Kecamatan Development Program Infrastructure Projects*. Report prepared for the Government of Indonesia and the World Bank.

Touchton, M., and Wampler, B. (2014). 'Improving Social Well-being through New Democratic Institutions', *Comparative Political Studies*, 47(10), pp. 1442–69.

Touchton, M. and Wampler, B. (2020). 'Participatory Budgeting in Kenya: Piloting New Techniques for Project Monitoring' (No. 149808, pp. 1–29). World Bank.

Touchton, M., Borges, N., and Wampler, B. (2017). 'Democracy at Work: Moving beyond Elections to Improve Well-being', *American Political Science Review*, 111(1), pp. 68–82.

Touchton, M., Wampler, B., and Peixoto, T. (2019). *Of Governance and Revenue: Participatory Institutions and Tax Compliance in Brazil*. Washington, DC: World Bank.

Tranjan, R. (2015). *Participatory Democracy in Brazil: Socioeconomic and Political Origins*. Notre Dame, Indiana: University of Notre Dame Press.

UN-Habitat; ENDA-ECOPOP (2008). 'Le Budget Participatif en Afrique: Guide pour la formation en pays francophones' in *Vol. II: Méthodes et Approches*. Nairobi, Dakar: UN-Habitat, p. 92.

Valverde Viesca, K. (2017). 'Cinco años de presupuesto participativo en el Distrito Federal: Un balance de la participación ciudadana' in K. Valverde Viesca, E. Gutiérrez Márquez, and J. A. Flores López (eds) *Ciudadanía y Calidad de Vida: Debates, retos, y experiencias al desarrollo social en México y América Latina*. Mexico City: Universidad Nacional Autónoma de Mexico, pp. 177–208.

Van Cott, D. L. (2008). *Radical Democracy in the Andes*. New York: Cambridge University Press.

Villas Boas, R., and Telles, V. (1995). *Poder local, participação popular, constução de Cidadania*. São Paulo, Brazil: Fórum Nacional de Participação Popular nas Administrações Municipais and Instituto Pólis.

Vincent, S. (2012). *Dimensions of Development: History, Community, and Change in Allpachico, Peru*. Toronto: University of Toronto Press.

Walker, J. (1969). 'The Diffusion of Innovations among the American States', *The American Political Science Review*, 63, pp. 880–99.

Wampler, B. (2007). *Participatory Budgeting in Brazil: Contestation, Cooperation, and Accountability*. University Park, Pennsylvania: Pennsylvania State University Press.

Wampler, B. (2008). 'When Does Participatory Democracy Deepen the Quality of Democracy? Lessons from Brazil', *Comparative Politics*, 41(1), pp. 61–81.

Wampler, B. (2015). *Activating Democracy in Brazil: Popular Participation, Social Justice, and Interlocking Institutions*. Notre Dame, Indiana: University of Notre Dame Press.

Wampler, B., and Avritzer, L. (2004). 'Participatory Publics: Civil Society and New Institutions in Democratic Brazil', *Comparative Politics*, 36(3), pp. 291–312.

Wampler, B., and Avritzer, L. (2004). 'Participatory Publics: Civil Society and New Institutions in Democratic Brazil', *Comparative Politics*, 36(3), pp. 291–312.

Wampler, B., and Avritzer, L. (2005). 'The Spread of Participatory Democracy in Brazil: From Radical Democracy to Participatory Good Government', *Journal of Latin American Urban Studies*, 7(1), pp. 1–32.

Wampler, B. (2012). 'Participatory Budgeting: Core Principles and Key Impacts.' *Journal of Public Deliberation*, 8(2), pp. 1–13.

Wampler, B., McNulty, S., and Touchton. M. (2018). *Participatory Budgeting: Spreading Across the Globe*. Washington, DC: Transparency and Accountability Initiative.

Wampler, B., and Touchton, M. (2019). 'Designing Institutions to Improve Social Well-being: Evidence from across Brazil's Participatory Budgeting Programs', *European Journal of Political Research*, 58(3), pp. 915–37.

Wampler, B., Touchton, M., and Spada, P. (2019). 'The Digital Revolution and Governance in Brazil: Evidence from Participatory Budgeting', *Journal of Information Technology & Politics*, 16(2), pp.154–68.

Warren, M. E. (2007). 'Institutionalizing Deliberative Democracy' in S. W. Rosenberg (ed.) *Deliberation, Participation and Democracy*. London: Palgrave Macmillan, pp. 272–88.

Weyland, K. G. (ed.) (2004). *Learning from Foreign Models in Latin American Policy Reform*. Washington, DC: Woodrow Wilson Center Press, p. 203.

Wong, S. (2012). 'What Have Been the Impacts of World Bank Community-driven Development Programs? CDD Impact Evaluation Review and Operational and Research Implications'. Washington, DC: World Bank.

World Bank (2003a). *World Development Report 2004: Making Services Work for Poor People*. Washington, DC: World Bank.

World Bank (2003b). *Better Governance for Development in the Middle East and North Africa: Enhancing Inclusiveness and Accountability (MENA Development Report)*. Washington, DC: World Bank.

World Bank (2008). 'Brazil: Toward a More Inclusive and Effective Participatory Budget in Porto Alegre'. Report No. 40144-BR. Washington, DC: World Bank.

World Bank (2010a). *Governance and Development Effectiveness Review: A Political Economy Analysis of Governance in Madagascar*. Washington, DC: World Bank.

World Bank (2010b). *Peru: Evaluación del Presupuesto Participativo y su relación con el presupuesto por resultados*. Washington, DC: World Bank.

World Bank (2013). *Participatory Budgeting and Operations: Case Examples from Africa: Madagascar and Mozambique*. Washington, DC: World Bank.

World Bank (2015). *Republic of Madagascar Second Governance and Institutional Development Project*. Washington, DC: World Bank.

World Bank (2017). *The Kenya Participatory Budgeting Initiative*. Washington, DC: World Bank.

World Bank (2020). *Citizen Engagement Brief*. World Bank. Retrieved July 20, 2020 from https://www.worldbank.org/en/about/what-we-do/brief/citizen-engagement.

Wu, Y. (2014). 'Participatory Budgeting: A Way to Reinforce the Power of the People's Congress' in B. Wai Yip and Y. Kao (eds) *The Changing Policy-making Process in Greater China: Case Research from Mainland China, Taiwan, and Hong Kong*. New York: Routledge, pp. 59–77.

Wu, Y., and Wang, W. (2011). 'The Rationalization of Public Budgeting in China: A Reflection on Participatory Budgeting in Wuxi', *Public Finance & Management*, 11(3), pp. 262–83.

Wu, Y., and Wang, W. (2012). 'Does Participatory Budgeting Improve the Legitimacy of the Local Government? A Comparative Case Study of Two Cities in China', *Australian Journal of Public Administration*, 71, pp. 122–35.

Index

Note: Figures are indicated by an italic "*f*", Tables are indicated by an italic "*t*", respectively, following the page number.

For the benefit of digital users, indexed terms that span two pages (e.g., 52–53) may, on occasion, appear on only one of those pages.

Abers, R. 17–18
accountability 16, 51
  Asia 129–30
  Brazil 86, 89
  China 127, 197
  external accountability 161, 177–8, 185
  horizontal accountability 89, 183–4
  Indonesia 125
  Kenya 165–6
  Latin America 101, 183–4
  Mozambique 169–70
  North Atlantic countries 156, 186
  oversight and 101
  PB: Deepening Democracy through
    Community Mobilization 76
  PB: Digital Participation 77–9, 189–90
  PB: Efficient Governance 78–9, 189–90
  PB: Social Development and
    Accountability 48, 188–9
  PB: theory of change 51–2, 58, 60–2, 76–9, 181
  PB as technical tool and 182
  Peru 81, 93–4
  Philippines 110, 130
  Senegal 173
  social accountability 21, 38, 60–1, 78, 199
  South Korea 130, 189
  sub-Saharan Africa 159–60, 162, 177–9, 185
  vertical accountability 89, 161, 183–4
Aceron, J. 129–30
Africa 35–7
  see also sub-Saharan Africa
Aguirre, M. M. 98
Alarcon, P. A. U. 144
Albert, Victor 87
Alcázar, L. 94
Allegretti, G. 134–5
Aquino, B. III 65–6, 107–8
Aquino, C. 106
Argentina 81–2, 90–1
Asia 18, 20, 35–6, 105*t*, 129–32, 155
  accountability 129–30
  Asian Development Bank 129

case studies 80, 105
citizen participation 104, 129
civil society 129–30
comparative analysis 127–9
democratization 102–4, 129
donors 199
PB: adoption 129
PB: Deepening Democracy through
  Community Mobilization 105
PB: diffusion 104
PB: impact 129–31, 184–5
"PB-like" programs 102–5
PB: Mandated by National Government
  102–3, 105, 127–9
PB: mimetic adaptation 102–3
PB: political and social change 184–5
resource allocation 184–5
social justice 102–3, 193
well-being 129–31
World Bank 37, 129
see also China; Indonesia; Philippines;
  South Korea
Asterina, N. 117, 120
Australia 35–6
authoritarian regime 9–11, 38–9, 64–5,
  125–6, 195–8
  malleability of PB's rules 104–5
  PB principles 38–9
  PB as radical bodies of change 131
  PB as technical tool 127, 131
  PB as tool for legitimation of 127, 131,
    175, 196–8
  semi-authoritarian regime 4, 64–5,
    197–8
  see also China; Mozambique; Russia
Avritzer, L. 17–18

Baessa, S. 169–70
Baierle, Sergio 137
Baiocchi, G. 15–18, 34, 36–9, 59, 88–9,
  181, 193
Bednarska-Olejniczak, D. 152–3

Belo Horizonte (Brazil) 1, 30–1
　citizen participation 87–8
　community leaders 1, 55, 60
　PB: Digital Participation 85
　PB: Empowered Democracy and
　　Redistribution 45
　PB: success 2–3, 85, 87
　PB Housing 30–1, 85
　Quality of Life Index 30, 85
Biel, F. 145
Bifulco, R. 142
Bland, G. 96–7
Bolivia 22, 41–2
Brazil 81–2, 83t, 182–3
　1988 Constitution 84
　accountability 86, 89
　"best practice" award 31–2, 90–1
　Blumenau 9–10, 30
　civil society 86, 88–9
　community-level outcomes 86, 88–90
　creation of PB 4, 27–8, 39, 81
　decentralization 27, 84
　democratization 83–4
　favela 1, 60
　individual-level outcomes 86–8
　Londrina 27–8
　PB: adaptation 85
　PB: decline and end 9, 86
　PB: Digital Participation 85
　PB: Empowered Democracy and
　　Redistribution 81–90, 187–8
　PB: impact 86–90, 182–4, 187–8
　PB: political and social change 7, 17, 182–4
　PB: success 8–9, 17
　PB: underperformance and
　　challenges 9–10, 71
　Recife 27–8, 30, 45
　Rio Claro 9–10, 30
　Rio Grande do Sul 85
　Santo André 30–2, 87
　social inclusion 88
　social justice 84, 90, 187–8
　well-being 61–2, 86, 89–90
　women's participation 87–8
　World Bank 61–2
　see also Belo Horizonte; Porto Alegre
　　PB Model
Busse, S. 151–2

Cabannes, Y. 28–9, 33, 43, 127
Calabrese, T. 141–2
Canada 37, 133
　see also North Atlantic countries; Toronto
Carratalá, L. 144, 150

CDD programs (community-driven
　　development) 12, 41, 115–16, 158–9
Cejudo, G. M. 98
change see PB: political and social change; theory
　of change
Chicago (United States) 21, 39, 133–4, 190–1
　PB: Deepening Democracy through
　　Community Mobilization 47, 138–43
　PB: impact 140, 142–3
　social inclusion 133–4, 140, 142–3, 194
　social justice 140
China 38–9, 64–5, 125–7, 195–7
　accountability 127, 197
　"administration, political reform, citizen
　　empowerment" logics 126–7
　CCP (Chinese Communist Party) 126–7, 197
　Chengdu 127, 197
　citizen empowerment 126–7
　Deliberative Polling 125–6
　PB: consultative nature 131
　PB: Efficient Governance 126, 131
　PB: principles 38
　PB as tool for reinforcing CCP's authority 126
　PB as top-down process 126–7
　resource allocation 126
Cho, B. S. 115
citizen apathy 50, 131–3, 155–6
citizen empowerment 3–4, 86, 126–7, 129, 159,
　　182–3, 203–4
　China 126–7
　marginalized/minority groups 14, 16,
　　193–4
　North Atlantic countries 136, 157, 185–6
　PB and 6, 8, 14–16, 36–7, 39, 158–9
　PB: Empowered Democracy and
　　Redistribution 45–7
　PB: theory of change 53–6, 74–5
　PB as radical democratic project and 182
　sub-Saharan Africa 158–9
citizen participation 4–6, 8–9, 16, 53–5
　Asia 104, 129
　budget decisions 2, 12–13
　deepening democracy 3–4
　Indonesia 121
　Kenya 165–6
　marginalized groups 64
　Porto Alegre PB Model 30–1, 87–8
　public decision-making 3–5, 13
　South Korea 111–12, 114–15
　sub-Saharan Africa 162, 185
civil society 26–7
　Asia 129–30
　Brazil 86, 88–9
　Canada 37

Indonesia 116–17, 125, 129–30
key lessons for civil society activists
    201–3
Latin America 101–2
PB: creation of 27–8
PB: Deepening Democracy through
    Community Mobilization 76, 188
PB: Digital Participation 189–90
PB: Efficient Governance 189–90
PB: Social Development and
    Accountability 78, 188–9
PB: theory of change 51–2, 58–60, 62,
    76, 78, 181
PB theory of change: civil society
    configuration 69, 71–2, 184
Peru 93–4
Philippines 108–10, 129–30
South Korea 114–15, 129–30, 189
sub-Saharan Africa 159, 162, 177–9, 185
United States 37
    see also CSO; NGO
class-related issues 55–6
clientelism 17, 80, 93–4, 98, 141–2, 170, 201
    see also PB: challenges and shortcomings
Colombia 81–2, 90–1
community leaders 1, 55
    Belo Horizonte 1, 55, 60
    Indonesia 10, 116–17, 119, 128
consensus-based model 49, 74
    from majoritarian secret ballot to consensus-
        based model 11–12, 192
    Indonesia 119
    Social Development and Accountability 48
    sub-Saharan Africa 159, 163–5, 169–70,
        177–9, 185, 192
    see also vote
corruption 3, 6, 17, 31–2, 62, 201
    Madagascar 167–8
    Mozambique 169
    Peru 93–4
CSO (civil society organization) 12, 16,
    26–8, 35–6
    Córdoba 143–4
    Indonesia 59
    Kenya 166
    Madagascar 168
    Mexico 97–8
    Peru 59, 93–4
    Senegal 173
    Spain 143–4
    Uganda 174
    see also civil society; NGO
Cuba 64–5
cynicism 9–11, 51, 62

decentralization 3, 21, 26–7, 33, 41, 201
    Brazil 27, 84
    Kenya 162–3
    Latin America 81
    Madagascar 167
    Mozambique 168–9
    PB: theory of change 65–7
    Peru 92
    PT 27–8, 84
    Senegal 171–2
    South Africa 173
    sub-Saharan Africa 161
    Uganda 174–5
Deepening Democracy through Community
    Mobilization (PB type) 22–3, 47,
    49–50, 202
    accountability 76
    Asia 105
    Chicago 47, 138–43
    civil society 76, 188
    Europe 47, 143–7, 154
    Indonesia 105, 115–16
    Latin America 82, 97–100
    Mexico 82, 97–100
    New York City 47, 138–43
    North Atlantic countries 47, 135–6, 146–7
    paradox in 188
    Philippines 105
    Portugal 145–6
    resource allocation 188
    social inclusion 99–100
    South Korea 105, 111
    Spain 47, 143–5
    theory of change and 74–6, 188
    Toronto 47, 137–8
    well-being 188
Deliberative Polling 12, 125–6
democracy 3–4, 19–20, 195
    deepening democracy 3–4, 19–20, 31–2,
        51, 88–9
    democratic socialism 28
    "illiberal" democracy 3
    North Atlantic democracies 133–4
    PB and 2, 4, 8–9, 16, 200
    PB "as hope for democracy" 5–6, 145, 181
    PB as radical democratic project 8, 15, 17–18,
        21, 28, 34–5, 51, 81, 136, 181–2, 203
    PB as "school of democracy" 34, 54–5, 64, 149
    PB theory of change and 63–4
    Third Wave of 26–7, 40
    see also democratization; participatory
        democracy; representative democracy
Democratic Republic of the Congo 159, 161,
    171, 175–6

democratization 3, 22, 26–7, 63–4, 195
　Asia 102–4, 129
　Brazil 83–4
　El Salvador 81, 95–6
　Indonesia 104, 116, 124–5, 129
　Latin America 81
　Peru 81, 92
　Philippines 104, 129
　Porto Alegre PB Model 81
　South Korea 104, 111, 129
DFID (Department for International
　　Development, UK) 26, 48, 77–8, 158, 168–9
Dias, N. 145, 181, 187
Digital PB (PB type) 22–3, 38, 47–50,
　　194–5, 203
　accountability 77–9, 189–90
　Brazil 85
　civil society 189–90
　Democratic Republic of the Congo 175–6
　Europe 149–51, 154
　from ballots in meetings to online PB 194–5
　Global North 74–5
　Kenya 176
　North Atlantic countries 135–6, 149–51,
　　156, 186
　Paris 38, 47–8, 133–4, 147–9, 154, 194–5
　resource allocation 189–90
　South Korea 111
　Spain 47–8, 133–4, 144, 147–51, 154, 194–5
　sub-Saharan Africa 175–6
　theory of change and 74–5, 77, 189–90
　see also technology
DiMaggio, P. 25–6, 187
Dominican Republic 34–5, 82
　PB: Mandated by National Government 47,
　　74–5, 102, 127–8
　PB: underperformance and challenges 102, 184
donors 20, 33–4, 40, 197–9, 203
　El Salvador 96–7, 100, 128–9
　external accountability 161, 178
　Mozambique 168–9
　PB: Mandated by National Government 198
　PB: Social Development and Accountability
　　188–9
　Senegal 171, 173
　sub-Saharan Africa 158–9, 161, 177–8, 180,
　　185, 199
　see also DFID; USAID; World Bank
Dutra, O. 85

Ecuador 32–3, 82, 90–1
Efficient Governance (PB type) 22–3, 48–50
　accountability 78–9, 189–90
　China 126, 131
　civil society 189–90

Europe 136, 151–2
　France 48, 133–4, 146
　Germany 48, 133–4, 136, 151–2, 154
　Poland 48–9, 153
　resource allocation 126
　South Korea 48–9
　state capacity 151
　theory of change and 74–5, 78–9, 189–90
　well-being 78–9, 189–90
elite capture 17, 109, 139–40, 149, 159, 164,
　　177, 192–3
　see also PB: challenges and shortcomings
El Salvador 33–4, 82, 83t
　democratization 81, 95–6
　DLGA (Democratic Local Governance
　　Activity) 95–6
　PB: Social Development and
　　Accountability 48, 82, 95–7, 100
　potential sustainability of donor-led
　　process 96–7, 100, 128–9
　RTI International 95–7
　USAID 33–4, 95–7, 100, 128–9
Empatía 36, 39–40
Empowered Democracy and Redistribution
　　(PB type) 22–3, 45–7, 49
　Belo Horizonte 45
　Brazil 81–90, 187–8
　disappearance of 187–8
　France 146
　Latin America 81–90, 99–100
　social justice 84, 90, 99–100
　theory of change 74–6, 79, 187–8
　see also Porto Alegre PB Model
ENDA-ECOPOP (Espaces Co production
　　et d'Œ res Populaires pour l'Environnement
　　et le Développement en Afrique) 172
Escamilla Cadena, A. 98
Ethiopia 37, 159
Europe 17–18, 32–3, 35–6, 133, 183
　case studies 80
　PB: Deepening Democracy through
　　Community Mobilization 47, 143–7, 154
　PB: Digital Participation 149–51, 154
　PB: Efficient Governance 136, 151–2
　PB: impact 146–7, 154
　PB: Mandated by National Government 152–4
　PB normative adoption 37
　see also France; Germany; North Atlantic
　　countries; Poland. Portugal; Spain
European Union 33, 36, 134–5, 168–9

Fedozzi, L. 17–18
Fölscher, A. 106–7
Font, J. 144
Ford Foundation 40, 116, 129, 161–2

France 146, 154
  PB: Efficient Governance 48, 133–4, 146
  PB: Empowering Democracy through
    Community Mobilization 146
  see also Paris
Francés, F. 144, 150
Fujimori, A. 33, 92

Galais, C. 144
Ganuza, E. 15–16, 34, 36–9, 59, 144, 150, 181, 193
García Bátiz, M. L. 98
gender issues *see* women/women's participation
Genro, T. 28
Germany
  PB: Efficient Governance 48, 133–4, 136,
    151–2, 154
  PB: impact 151–2, 154
Global North 32–3
  PB: Digital Participation 74–5
  see also North Atlantic countries
Global South 31–2, 51, 191
  PB: Social Development and
    Accountability 74–5, 77–8, 188
  PB transformation 10
  reform agenda and PB 35–6
Godfrey, E. 142
Goldfrank, B. 86
Gonçalves, S. 89–90
government 5–6, 8–9, 20, 26–7
  executive/legislative officials 13, 68–9, 165–6
  government officials and PB 56–7
  Indonesia 10, 12
  PB: challenges 9–10, 34–5
  PB: theory of change and civil servants 57–8
  PB: theory of change and government
    officials 56–7
  see also Mandated by National Government;
    policy; state capacity
government support 35, 67, 71–2, 181, 184,
  188–9, 202
  Madagascar 168
  Peru 128
  South Korea 115
  stronger government support 67–8
  see also state capacity
Grillos, T. 121, 201
GTZ (Gesellscha für Technische
  Zusammenarbeit, Germany) 158
Gupta, A. 141–2

Hagelskamp, C. 140, 142
He, B. 126–7, 197
Heller, P. 88–9
Herzberg, C. 43, 134–5, 145–7, 151
Hidayani, R. 117, 120

Hong, S. 115
Hope for Democracy 145, 187
Hordijk, M. 59
Hsueh, L. 115

IEED (Institut International pour
  l'Environnement et le Développement) 172
India 42, 68
Indonesia 10, 39–40, 105*t*, 115–25, 191
  accountability 125
  citizen participation 121
  civil society 116–17, 125, 129–30
  Community-Driven Development 41, 115–16
  community leaders 10, 116–17, 119, 128
  consensus-based model 119
  CSOs 59
  democratization 104, 116, 124–5, 129
  government 10, 12
  Ministry of Finance 128, 191
  Musrenbang process 117, 122–3
  NGOs 120–1
  PB: adaptation 117–19, 122–3
  PB: Deepening Democracy through
    Community Mobilization 105, 115–16
  PB: impact 118, 120, 124–5
  PB: Mandated by National Government 47,
    74–5, 102–3, 105, 115–17, 128
  PB: Social Development and
    Accountability 105, 115–16
  PB: success 124–5, 128–9
  PB: underperformance and
    challenges 10, 128
  resource allocation 120, 123–5, 191
  social inclusion 121, 123–4
  social justice 119–21
  technology 120–1, 124
  well-being 120, 124–5, 130–1
  women's participation 119, 123–5
  World Bank 37, 41, 123–4, 128–9, 191
Indonesian cities 41, 115–16, 120*t*, 129–30
  City-Wide PB, PB 117–18
  Neighborhood PB 117–18
  Surakarta 59, 116–17, 120–1
  see also Indonesia
Indonesian villages 105, 115–16, 121,
  128–9, 171–2
  KDP (Kecamatan Development Project)
    121–5, 128–31
  PNPM (Program Nasional Pemberdayaan
    Masyarakat Mandiri) 122–4, 129–30
  see also Indonesia
IN LOCO (NGO) 168–9
isomorphism (institutional isomorphism) 22, 25
  coercive, mimetic, normative
    isomorphism 22

Jaramillo, M. 94
Júlio, S. 145, 187

Kasozi-Mulindwa, S. 175
Keblowski, W. 153
Kenya 21, 56, 158, 160–1, 197–8
   accountability 165–6
   Accountable Devolution Program 33–4
   citizen participation 165–6
   consensus-based model 163–5
   CSOs 166
   decentralization 162–3
   NGOs 176
   PB: Digital Participation 176
   PB: impact: 165–6, 179, 197–8
   PB: Social Development and
      Accountability 48, 162–6
   PB: underperformance and
      challenges 164, 166
   social justice 163–5
   women's participation 164
   World Bank 37, 162–3
Kota Kita (NGO) 120–1

Langelier, S. 86
Latin America 4, 18, 20, 28–9, 32, 83t, 100–3, 183
   accountability 101, 183–4
   as birthplace of PB 81, 100
   case studies 80–2
   civil society 101–2, 183–4
   community-level outcomes 100–1
   comparative analysis 99–100, 102
   decentralization 81
   democratization 81
   from Empowered Democracy to Mandated by
      National Government 90–5
   individual-level outcomes 100–1
   mimetic and normative adoption 82–3
   national laws and PB 82–3
   PB: Deepening Democracy through
      Community Mobilization 82, 97–100
   PB: Empowered Democracy and
      Redistribution 81–90, 99–100
   PB: impact 82–3, 99–103, 183–4
   PB: Mandated by National Government
      74–5, 81–2, 91–5, 100, 102
   PB: political and social change 17, 183–4
   PB: Social Development and
      Accountability 82, 95–7, 100
   social justice, weakening of 82–4
   well-being 101, 183–4
   see also Brazil; El Salvador; Mexico; Peru
left-wing politics 3, 31–3, 35–6, 68, 90–1
   North Atlantic countries 136, 154–5
   participatory democracy 40

Portugal 145, 154
South Korea 111
Spain 143, 154
   see also PT
Lim, P. 108
Lipietz, B. 43

Madagascar 160–1
   corruption 167–8
   CSOs 168
   decentralization 167
   PB: impact 167–8
   PB: Social Development and
      Accountability 166–8
   PB: underperformance and challenges 167–8
   World Bank 166–7
Making All Voices Count project (Institute for
   Development Studies, University of
   Sussex) 19
Mandated by National Government (PB
   type) 22–3, 34, 37, 47, 49–50, 198
   Asia 102–3, 105, 127–9
   Dominican Republic 47, 74–5, 102, 127–8
   donors 198
   Indonesia 47, 74–5, 102–3, 105, 115–17, 128
   Latin America 74–5, 81–2, 91–5, 100, 102
   North Atlantic countries 136, 152–4
   PB: theory of change and 74–7, 79, 189, 198
   PB: underperformance and challenges 76,
      100, 102
   Peru 47, 74–5, 91–5, 102, 127–8, 198
   Philippines 102–3, 105
   Poland 47–9, 74–5, 127–8, 136, 152–5
   Portugal 136, 152
   resource allocation 189
   South Korea 47–9, 74–5, 102–3, 105, 111–15,
      128, 189
   sub-Saharan Africa 174–6
   Uganda 127–8, 160, 174–5
   "unfunded mandates" 67–8, 76, 128, 175, 189
Marcos, F. 40–1, 106
Marquetti, A. 89
Martins, V. 145
McNulty, S. 55, 59, 82, 93–4101, 198
Melgar, T. 106–7
Mexico 59, 82, 83t, 90–1
   CSOs 97–8
   Mexico City 47, 63, 97–8
   PB: Deepening Democracy through
      Community Mobilization 82, 97–100
   PB: impact 98–9
   PRD (Party of the Democratic
      Revolution) 97–8
   PRI (Institutional Revolutionary Party) 97–9
   World Bank 99

Miloslavich Túpac, D. 94
Ming, Z. 127
Montambeault, F. 59, 86–7, 98, 101
Moore, A. J. 21, 138–9
Mozambique 1–3, 158, 160–1
    accountability 169–70
    authoritarian regime 168–9
    corruption 169
    decentralization 168–9
    DFID/UKAID 168–9
    international donors 168–9
    NGOs 168–9
    PB: impact 170–1
    PB: politicization 169–70
    PB: Social Development and Accountability
        48, 168–71
    World Bank 37, 168–9

neoliberalism 33, 92
New York City (United States) 39, 64,
        133–4, 190–1
    PB: Deepening Democracy through
        Community Mobilization 47, 138–43
    PB: impact 140–3
    PB: success 140–1
    resource allocation 141–2, 186, 194
    social inclusion 73, 114, 133–4, 140–3, 194
    social justice 140, 142
NGO (non-government organization) 12, 40
    Indonesia 120–1
    Kenya 176
    Mozambique 168–9
    PB: diffusion 29–30, 137
    Porto Alegre PB Model 84–5
    Senegal 172
    sub-Saharan Africa 158, 161–2
    see also civil society
No, W. 112, 114–15
North Atlantic countries 134, 135t, 155–7
    accountability 156, 186
    case studies 80
    citizen empowerment 136, 157, 185–6
    comparative analysis 154–5
    left-wing politics 136, 154–5
    North Atlantic democracies 133–4
    PB: adaptation 133–4, 136–7, 155
    PB: adoption 134–5, 155, 185–6
    PB: Deepening Democracy through
        Community Mobilization 47,
        135–6, 146–7
    PB: Digital Participation 135–6, 149–51,
        156, 186
    PB: impact 155–7
    PB: Mandated by National Government
        136, 152–4

PB: political and social change 184–6
PB: South-to-North diffusion 131–2,
        134–6
resource allocation 141, 186
social inclusion 136–7, 155–6, 185–6
social justice 136–7
technology 155
well-being 156–7, 186
see also Canada; Europe; Global North;
        United States

OIPD (International Observatory of
        Participatory Democracy) 4, 35–6, 134–5
Olejniczak, J. 152–3
Open Government Partnership 4, 36, 107
Open Society Foundation 161–2
oversight 5, 14–15, 177, 181
    accountability and 101
    PB: theory of change and 60, 72, 74
    Philippines 108–9
    see also PB: principles
Oxfam International 40

parallel evolutionary development 26–7
    parallel development of similar PB
        programs 26–7, 40–3
    PB: distinction from other participatory
        institutions 6, 12, 22, 181–2
Paris (France) 133–4, 146
    allocation of resources 38
    PB: adaptation 133–4, 148–9
    PB: Digital Participation 38, 47–8, 133–4,
        147–9, 154, 194–5
    PB: underperformance and challenges 149
Park, Y. 115
Participatory Budgeting World Atlas 81, 187
participatory democracy 4, 40, 67, 88
    South Korea 111–12
    see also democracy
participatory development 3–4, 26–7,
        41–2, 90–1
PB (Participatory Budgeting)
    actors 21, 31, 79–80
    binding nature of programs 5, 13, 201
    consultative nature of programs 35
    creation of 4, 27–8
    definition 4–6, 8, 15, 21, 181
    distinction from other participatory
        institutions 6, 12, 22, 181–2
    enhancing PB's effectiveness 201–3
    "as hope for democracy" 5–6, 145, 181
    key lessons for policymakers and civil society
        activists 201–3
    operational process 5–7, 201–2
    popular appeal of 51

PB (Participatory Budgeting) (*cont.*)
  as radical democratic project 8, 15, 17–18, 21,
    28, 34–5, 51, 81, 136, 181–2, 203
  as "school of democracy" 34, 54–5, 64, 149
  as technical tool 8, 15–16, 21, 33–9, 95, 100,
    127, 131, 161, 181–2, 193
PB: adaptation and transformation 8–12, 20–2,
  49, 72, 181, 187, 203
  1st wave of PB diffusion (1989–mid-1990s):
    key adaptations 30
  2nd wave of PB diffusion (mid-1990s–
    mid-2000s): key adaptations 34
  3rd wave of PB diffusion (mid-2000s–2020):
    key adaptations 39
  Brazil 85
  coercive adaptation 25
  context and PB adaptation 25
  groupings of PB adaptation 50
  Indonesia 117–19, 122–3
  key design adaptations 12, 194–5
  mimetic adaptation 25–6, 42, 102–3
  normative adaptation 25, 39
  North Atlantic countries 133–4, 136–7, 155
  Paris 133–4, 148–9
  PB diffusion: isomorphic adoption and
    adaptation 28–40
  Peru 92–3
  political/social change and 15–16
  Spain 133–4, 143–4
  sub-Saharan Africa 158–9
  timing of PB adoption and adaptation of basic
    PB design 15–16, 22, 42
  see also PB: design
PB: adoption of 22, 136
  1st wave 22
  2nd wave 22, 133–4
  3rd wave 22, 133–4, 199
  coercive adoption 25, 30–1, 35–7, 48–9, 177
  location/region 22
  mimetic adoption 25–6, 30–1, 33, 35–8, 47–9,
    82–3, 95, 111, 129, 139, 146, 155,
    187, 196–7
  motivations for 11–12, 25–6, 31, 36–7,
    44–5, 49, 181
  normative adoption 25, 30–2, 35–7, 45, 47–9,
    82–3, 111, 129, 136, 139, 143, 155,
    181, 185–6
  North Atlantic countries 134–5, 155, 185–6
  PB diffusion: isomorphic adoption and
    adaptation 28–40
  timing of PB adoption and adaptation of PB
    design 15–16, 22, 42
PB: benefits 8–9, 16, 51, 200, 203
  accountability 16, 51
  democracy 2, 4–6, 8–9, 16, 200

  development 2, 5–6
  human development 8–9, 16
  policy change 5–6
  redistributive outcomes 13–14
  resource allocation 8–9, 16
  transparency 8–9, 14, 16, 36–7, 48
  see also accountability; citizen empowerment;
    citizen participation; civil society;
    democratization; well-being
PB: challenges and shortcomings 9–11, 17, 51,
  62, 199–200, 203
  authoritarian regimes 9, 195–8
  Brazil 9–10, 71
  costs of implementation 9–10
  Dominican Republic 102, 184
  governments 9–10, 34–5
  Indonesia 10, 128
  "invited participation" 9–10, 34–5, 116,
    119, 166
  Kenya 164, 166
  lack of goals achievement 9, 19–20, 86
  Madagascar 167–8
  Paris 149
  participation fatigue 9, 62, 86
  "partici-washing" 9, 195–8
  PB: Mandated by National Government 76,
    100, 102
  PB as "good"/"bad" way to give decision-
    making power to citizens 199–200
  PB as partisan project 86, 169–70, 197–8
  PB as technical tool 15–16, 33, 36–7, 100,
    127, 181
  Peru 10, 60, 71, 91–5, 100, 102, 128, 184
  Philippines 71, 110
  Poland 154
  Senegal 172
  sub-Saharan Africa 179–80
  Uganda 175
  underperformance 9–10
  unresolved issues 195–201
  see also clientelism; corruption; cynicism;
    elite capture
PB: design 181
  enhancing PB's effectiveness 201–2
  key design adaptations 12, 194–5
  oversight 60, 72, 74
  PB impact and 11, 184
  scale 72–3, 190–2, 199
  social inclusion 53–4, 72–4, 192–4
  social justice requirement 72–3, 192–4, 201
  theory of change: variation in program
    design 72–4, 184
  voting rules 74, 192
  see also PB: adaptation and transformation;
    theory of change

PB: diffusion
  1st wave (1989–mid-1990s): spreading
    throughout Brazil 29
  2nd wave (mid-1990s–mid-2000s): moving
    beyond Brazil 31, 100
  3rd wave (mid-2000s–2020): rapid spread
    around the globe 35, 104
  Asia 104
  isomorphic adoption and adaptation 28–40
  NGOs 29–30, 137
  Philippines 107
  PT and 29–30, 32, 84–5
  South-to-North diffusion 131–2, 134–6
  sub-Saharan Africa 158–9
  see also PB: global adoption
PB: global adoption 2, 4, 11, 15–18, 20–1,
    49–50, 181, 203
  experimentation 31
  PB as international "best practice" 31–2,
    35–7, 47, 95, 181
  tracing the spread of PB 27–43
  see also PB diffusion
PB: impact 8–11, 20, 50, 181–2, 203
  Asia 129–31, 184–5
  Brazil 86–90, 182–4, 187–8
  Chicago 140, 142–3
  Europe 146–7, 154
  Germany 151–2, 154
  Indonesia 118, 120, 124–5
  Kenya 165–6, 179, 197–8
  Latin America 82–3, 99–103, 183–4
  Madagascar 167–8
  Mexico 98–9
  Mozambique 170–1
  New York City 140–3
  North Atlantic countries 155–7
  PB mimetic adoption 38
  Peru 93–5
  Philippines 108–9
  Portugal 145
  Senegal 173
  South Korea 128
  Spain 154
  sub-Saharan Africa 159, 177–9, 185
  Uganda 175
  see also accountability; civil society; PB:
    benefits; PB: challenges and shortcomings;
    theory of change; well-being
PB: levels of adoption 11–12, 72–3
  district level 39
  from municipal governments to villages,
    city sub-districts, and nations 11–12,
    190–2, 199
  municipal/sub-municipal 39, 49, 65
  national level 2

  state/provincial level 2
  subnational level 2, 8, 34, 36–8, 47, 65, 76
PB: political and social change 10–11, 23–4,
    51–2, 182
  Asia 184–5
  Brazil 7, 17, 182–4
  institutional adaptations and 11, 15–16
  Latin America 17, 183–4
  North Atlantic countries 184–6
  PB: motivations for adoption 49
  sub-Saharan Africa 184–5
  see also PB: impact; theory of change; theory
    of change and PB typology
PB: principles 5–6, 11, 21–2, 181–2, 195
  different emphasis on principles and
    institutional variation 11–12, 15, 21–2
  oversight 5, 14–15
  participatory democracy and 40
  PB adaptation and 11–12
  PB institutional design and 72
  PB mimetic adoption 38
  PB's distinction from other participatory
    institutions 12
  social inclusion 5, 14
  social justice 5, 13–15, 30, 34
  voice 5, 12–15
  vote 5, 13, 15
  see also oversight; PB: typology and PB
    principles; social inclusion; social justice;
    voice; vote
PB: research on 15–19, 51–2, 200–1, 203–4
  case-study research 17–19, 33–4, 55,
    100–1
  medium and large-N studies 17–19, 78, 86,
    89–90, 94, 100–1, 187, 200–1
  "state of the art" analysis 19
  statistical analyses 18
PB: success 7–8, 10–11, 17
  Belo Horizonte 2–3, 85, 87
  Brazil 8–9, 17
  Indonesia 124–5, 128–9
  New York City 140–1
  Porto Alegre PB Model 4, 31–2, 84, 87–9
  South Korea 115, 189
  Toronto 138
PB: typology 11–12, 22–3, 43–9, 46t, 182
  PB adaptation and 50
  see also Deepening Democracy through
    Community Mobilization; Digital
    Participation; Efficient Governance;
    Empowered Democracy and
    Redistribution; Mandated by National
    Government; Social Development and
    Accountability; theory of change and PB
    typology

PB: typology and PB principles 43–5, 46*t*, 49, 181–2
  actors driving adoption 43–5
  degree of local control over resources 43–4
  internal decision-making process 43–4
  participant engagement 43–4
  resource allocation 43–4
PB ambassadors 15, 134, 137, 200–1
PBP (Participatory Budgeting Project) 4, 35–6, 138–41
Peck, J. 15, 28–9
Peixoto, T. 89, 176
Peru 2, 32, 34, 59, 81–2, 83*t*, 90–1, 202–3
  accountability 81, 93–4
  civil society 94
  corruption 94
  CSOs 59, 93–4
  decentralization 92
  democratization 81, 92
  government support 67
  Lambayeque 59, 67
  PB: adaptation 92–3
  PB: impact 93–5
  PB: Mandated by National Government 47, 74–5, 91–5, 102, 127–8, 198
  PB: underperformance and challenges 10, 60, 71, 91–5, 100, 102, 128, 184
  PB Law 81, 91–3
  transparency 93
  universal PB adoption 33
  well-being 94
  women's participation 94–5
Philippines 21, 40–1, 105*t*, 106–11
  accountability 110, 130
  BuB (Bottom-up Budgeting) 107–10, 129–30
  civil society 108–10, 129–30
  democratization 104, 129
  Naga City 40–1, 106–7
  oversight 108–9
  PB: Deepening Democracy through Community Mobilization 105
  PB: diffusion 107
  PB: impact: 108–9
  "PB-like" programs 106
  PB: Mandated by National Government 102–3, 105
  PB: underperformance and challenges 71, 110
  state capacity 109–10
  well-being 108–10, 130–1
Poland
  PB: Efficient Governance 48–9, 153
  PB: Mandated by National Government 47–9, 74–5, 127–8, 136, 152–5
  PB: underperformance and challenges 154

Solecki Fund 152–3
Sopot 153–4
policy
  adaptation 25–6
  creation of 23–4
  diffusion 24–5
  "fast policy" 15
  PB: key lessons for policymakers 201–3
  policy change 5–6, 109, 140–1
  policy entrepreneurs 23–4, 27–9, 68, 81, 84–5, 92, 197
  policy innovation, key driver mechanisms of 23–7
  policy translation 15
  reform agenda and PB 35–7
  windows of opportunity 23, 27, 39, 42, 129
Porto Alegre PB Model (Brazil) 6–8, 50, 84, 86, 202
  citizen participation 30–1, 87–8
  democratization 81
  internationalization and alignment with 111–13, 133–4, 143, 145–6, 177
  NGOs 84–5
  PB: Empowered Democracy and Redistribution 45, 84
  PB: origins 4, 21, 27–8, 83–4, 190–1
  PB: success 4, 31–2, 84, 87–9
  resource allocation 8, 89
  social justice 13, 84, 89
  technology 84
  voting system 74, 177
Porto de Oliveira, O. 15, 28–9, 31–2, 134, 200–1
Portugal 1–2, 64–5, 133–4, 145
  left-wing politics 145, 154
  Palmela 145
  PB: Deepening Democracy through Community Mobilization 145–6
  PB: impact 145
  PB: Mandated by National Government 136, 152
Powell, W. W. 25–6, 187
"pro-poor" projects/impact 55–6, 79, 114–15, 184–5, 193
  prioritization of 71, 94, 202
PT (*Partido dos Trabalhadores*/Worker' Party—Brazil) 3–4, 28, 83–5, 89–90, 187–8
  decentralization 27–8, 84
  democratization 84
  end of office 86
  PB creation 27–8, 81, 83–4
  PB diffusion and adoption 29–30, 32, 84–5
  social justice 13–14, 30, 84
public sphere 12–13, 28, 63–4

Quality of Life Index 30, 73, 85, 192–3

race-related issues 55–6
Rendon Corona, A. 89
representative democracy 3–4, 64, 69, 144,
    192–3, 203
    North Atlantic democracies 133–4
    PB and 4, 35, 37
    South Korea 111–12
    see also democracy
resources/resource allocation 8–9, 16, 202–3
    Asia 184–5
    Belo Horizonte 30–1
    China 126
    decrease in resource allocation for PB
        programs 187–8, 194
    Indonesia 120, 123–5, 191
    New York City 141–2, 186, 194
    North Atlantic countries 141, 186
    Paris 38
    PB: Deepening Democracy through
        Community Mobilization 188
    PB: Digital Participation 189–90
    PB: Efficient Governance 126
    PB: Mandated by National Government 189
    PB: Social Development and
        Accountability 188
    PB typology and PB principles: local control
        over resources 43–4
    PB typology and PB principles: resource
        allocation 43–4
    Porto Alegre PB Model 8, 89
    South Korea 194
Rifai, A. 117, 120
right-wing politics: PB's decline and end 86
Robredo, J. 107
Röcke, A. 43, 145–7, 151
Roh Moo-hyun 112
Rousseau, J. 40
Russia 37–9, 64–5, 188, 195–7
    mimetic adoption 196–7
    PB: Social Development and Social
        Accountability 131

Sanchez, M. L. M. 98
Santos, B. S. 17–18, 63
Schleifer, D. 142
Schneider, S. H. 151–2
Schugurensky, Daniel 137
Scotland 152
secret ballot (decision-making mechanism) 7,
    44–5, 74, 139–40
    from majoritarian secret ballot to consensus-
        based model 11–12, 192
    see also vote

Senegal 40–1, 158, 160–1
    accountability 173
    CSOs 173
    decentralization 171–2
    international donors 171, 173
    NGOs 172
    PB: impact: 173
    PB: Social Development and
        Accountability 171–3
    PB: underperformance and challenges 172
    women's participation 172
Shybalkina, I. 142
Silliman, R. 142
Silva, S. 88–9
Sintomer, Y. 43, 145–7, 151
Smith, G. 144
Social Development and Accountability (PB
        type) 22–3, 48, 50
    accountability 48, 78, 188–9
    civil society 78, 188–9
    consensus-based model 48
    DFID 48, 77–8
    donors 188–9
    El Salvador 48, 82, 95–7, 100
    Global South 74–5, 77–8, 188
    Indonesia 105, 115–16
    Kenya 48, 162–6
    Latin America 82, 95–7, 100
    Madagascar 166–8
    Mozambique 48, 168–71
    resource allocation 188
    Senegal 171–3
    South Africa 173–4
    state capacity 77–8, 160
    sub-Saharan Africa 160, 173–4, 176–8
    theory of change and 74–5, 77–8, 188–9
    USAID 48, 50, 77–8
    well-being 78, 188
    World Bank 48, 50, 77–8
social inclusion 5, 14, 100, 182, 202
    Brazil 88
    Chicago 133–4, 140, 142–3, 194
    Indonesia 121, 123–4
    marginalized/minority groups 88, 187–8, 193
    New York City 73, 114, 133–4, 140–3, 194
    North Atlantic countries 136–7, 155–6, 185–6
    PB: Deepening Democracy through
        Community Mobilization 99–100
    PB: theory of change and 53–4, 72–4,
        187–8, 192–4
    shift from social justice to social
        inclusion 11–12, 100, 187–8, 192–4, 201
    South Korea 114–15, 194
    Toronto 133–4, 138
    see also PB: principles

social justice 5, 13–15, 30, 34, 182, 203
    Asia 102–3, 193
    Brazil 84, 90, 187–8
    Chicago 140
    Indonesia 119–21
    Kenya 163–5
    New York City 140, 142
    North Atlantic countries 136–7
    PB: Empowered Democracy and
        Redistribution 84, 90, 99–100
    PB: theory of change and 72–3, 187–8,
        192–4, 201
    Porto Alegre PB Model 13, 84, 89
    PT 13–14, 30, 84
    shift from social justice to social
        inclusion 11–12, 100, 187–8, 192–4, 201
    South Korea 114–15, 194
    Spain 144
    sub-Saharan Africa 159, 193
    weakening of 34–5, 82–4, 97
    see also PB: principles
Sousa, V. 145
South Africa 3, 64, 68, 158–61
    ANC (African National Congress Party) 173–4
    decentralization 173
    PB: decline and end 173
    PB: Social Development and
        Accountability 173–4
South Korea 32–3, 47, 74–5, 100, 104, 105t,
    111–15, 183
    accountability 130, 189
    citizen participation 111–12, 114–15
    civil society 114–15, 129–30, 189
    democratization 104, 111, 129
    Gwangu 111–12
    left-wing politics 111
    participatory democracy 111–12
    PB: Deepening Democracy through
        Community Mobilization 105, 111
    PB: Digital Participation 111
    PB: Efficient Governance 48–9
    PB: impact 128
    PB: Mandated by National Government 47–9,
        74–5, 102–3, 105, 111–15, 128, 189
    PB: success 115, 189
    representative democracy 111–12
    resource allocation 194
    Seoul 113–15, 128
    social inclusion 114–15, 194
    social justice 114–15, 194
    technology 113
    well-being 130–1, 184–5, 189
Spada, P. 86
Spain 32–3, 134–5, 143

Barcelona 21, 47–8, 147–51, 154, 194–5
Córdoba 32–5, 47, 133–6, 143–5
CSOs 143–4
left-wing politics 143, 154
Madrid 21, 47–8, 133–4, 144, 147–51,
    154, 194–5
PB: adaptation 133–4, 143–4
PB: Deepening Democracy through
    Community Mobilization 47, 143–5
PB: Digital Participation 47–8, 133–4, 144,
    147–51, 154, 194–5
PB: impact 154
Sevilla 32–5, 47, 133–6
social justice 144
state capacity 44, 66–7, 70, 196–7, 199, 202
    high state capacity 151
    low state capacity 77–8, 104–5, 109–10,
        157–60, 177, 179, 196–7, 199
    PB: Efficient Governance 151
    PB: Social Development and Accountability
        77–8, 160
    Philippines 109–10
    sub-Saharan Africa 157–60, 177, 179
Su, C. 140
sub-Saharan Africa 20, 159, 160t, 177–80
    accountability 159–60, 162, 177–9, 185
    case studies 80, 159–61
    citizen empowerment 158–9
    citizen participation 162, 185
    civil society 159, 162, 177–9, 185
    comparative analysis 176–7
    consensus-based model 159, 163–5, 169–70,
        177–9, 185, 192
    decentralization 161
    DFID 158
    international donors 158–9, 161, 177–8, 180,
        185, 199
    NGOs 158, 161–2
    PB: adaptation 158–9
    PB: diffusion 158–9
    PB: Digital Participation 175–6
    PB: impact 159, 177–9, 185
    PB: Mandated by National Government 174–6
    PB: political and social change 184–5
    PB: Social Development and
        Accountability 160, 173–4, 176–8
    PB: underperformance and
        challenges 179–80
    social justice 159, 193
    state capacity 157–60, 177, 179
    transparency 162
    USAID 158, 178–9
    well-being 159, 177–9, 185
    World Bank 36–7, 158–9, 161–2, 176, 178–9

see also Democratic Republic of the Congo;
    Kenya; Madagascar; Mozambique; Senegal;
    South Africa; Uganda
Suharto 41, 59, 115–16, 175
Sześciło, D. 152–3

technology 39–40
    from ballots in meetings to online
        PB 194–5
    Indonesia 120–1, 124
    North Atlantic countries 155
    Porto Alegre PB Model 84
    South Korea 113
    see also Digital Participation
Téllez Arana, L. 98
Theodore, N. 15, 28–9
theory of change 12, 52–3, 79–80, 182–7
    accountability 51–2, 58, 60–2, 76–9, 181
    causal mechanisms promoting social and
        political change 12, 51–2, 79–80, 182
    caveats 52, 186–7
    citizens: engaging, deliberating, empowering
        53–6, 74–5
    civil servants 57–8
    civil society 51–2, 58–60, 62, 76, 78, 181
    community-level outcomes 51–2, 61–2, 75,
        79–80, 182
    conceptual model of change 52, 53f
    government officials 56–7
    individual-level outcomes 51–2, 57–8, 182
    variation in program design 72–4
    well-being 51–2, 58, 61–2, 78–80, 181
    see also PB: design
theory of change: macro-level factors 51–2,
        62–7, 74–5, 79–80, 182–3
    decentralization 65–7
    economic conditions 65
    political context 63
    see also theory of change
theory of change: meso-level factors 51–2, 62–3,
        67–72, 74–5, 79–80, 182–3
    civil society configuration 69, 71–2, 184
    government support 67, 71–2, 181, 184
    state capacity 70
    see also theory of change
theory of change and PB typology 51–2,
        78–9, 187–90
    Deepening Democracy through Community
        Mobilization 74–6, 188
    Digital Participation 74–5, 77, 189–90
    Efficient Governance 74–5, 78–9, 189–90
    Empowered Democracy and
        Redistribution 74–6, 79, 187–8
    macro-level factors 74–5, 77–8

Mandated by National Government 74–7, 79,
        189, 198
    meso-level factors 74–5, 77–8
    Social Development and Accountability 74–5,
        77–8, 188–9
    see also theory of change
"Think Globally, Act Locally" 190–1
Toledo, A. 33, 92
Toronto 47, 133–6
    PB: Deepening Democracy through
        Community Mobilization 47, 137–8
    PB: success 138
    social inclusion 133–4, 138
    Toronto Housing Corporation 32–3, 39, 137–8
Touchton, M. 19, 59, 82, 89–90
transparency 8–9, 14, 16, 36–7, 48, 60–1
    Peru 93
    sub-Saharan Africa 162

UCLG (United Cities and Local Governments)
        134–5
Uganda 64–5, 158, 160–2
    CSOs 174
    decentralization 174–5
    NPM (New Public Management) 174–5
    PB: impact 175
    PB: Mandated by National Government 127–8,
        160, 174–5
    PB: underperformance and challenges 175
    UN agencies and 174
    World Bank 37, 174
UN (United Nations) 24–5, 31–2, 174
    UN-Habitat 23–4, 31–2, 90–1
United States 17–18, 64, 133, 138–9, 155,
        183, 190–1
    Boston 39, 133–4, 138–9, 155
    civil society 37
    PB: adoption 134–5
    PB and government officials 56–7
    PB normative adoption 37, 39
    Seattle 133–4, 138–9, 155
    Vallejo 39, 55
    see also Chicago; New York City; North
        Atlantic countries
URB-AL (European Union-sponsored Urban
        Program) 33, 134–5
Uruguay 32, 82, 90–1
USAID (United States Agency for International
        Development) 26
    El Salvador 33–4, 95–7, 100, 128–9
    PB: Social Development and
        Accountability 48, 50, 77–8
    PB as technical tool 34
    sub-Saharan Africa 158, 178–9

Van Criekinger, M. 153
Venezuela 32, 81-2
Villarán, S. 94-5
voice 5, 12-15
    see also PB: principles
vote 5, 13, 15
    PB: theory of change and 74, 192
    see also consensus-based model;
      PB: principles; secret ballot

Wampler, B. 9-10, 19, 55, 82, 87-90
Washington Consensus 33
well-being, impact on
    Asia 129-31
    Brazil 61-2, 86, 89-90
    Indonesia 120, 124-5, 130-1
    Latin America 101, 183-4
    North Atlantic countries 156-7, 186
    PB: Deepening Democracy through
      Community Mobilization 188
    PB: Efficient Governance 78-9, 189-90
    PB: Social Development and Accountability
      78, 188
    PB: theory of change 51-2, 58, 61-2,
      78-80, 181
    Peru 94
    Philippines 108-10, 130-1
    South Korea 130-1, 184-5, 189
    sub-Saharan Africa 159, 177-9, 185

Wilk, B. 152-3
William and Flora Hewlett Foundation 19
Williams, D. 141-2
women/women's participation 55, 94-5
    Brazil 87-8
    empowerment 94-5
    Indonesia 119, 123-5
    Kenya 164
    Peru 94-5
    Senegal 172
World Bank 1-2, 21, 31-4, 36-7, 61-2, 90-1
    Africa 37
    Asia 37, 129
    Brazil 61-2
    decentralization and 3
    Digital Engagement Evaluation Team 176
    Indonesia 37, 41, 123-4, 128-9, 191
    Kenya 37, 162-3
    Madagascar 166-7
    Mexico 99
    Mozambique 37, 168-9
    PB: Social Development and
      Accountability 48, 50, 77-8
    PB as technical tool 34, 36-7
    sub-Saharan Africa 36-7, 158-9, 161-2,
      176, 178-9
    Uganda 37, 174
World Social Forum 32
Wright, G. D. 94